Social Reinsurance

A New Approach to Sustainable Community
Health Financing

Editors
David M. Dror and **Alexander S. Preker**

THE WORLD BANK
Washington, D.C.

INTERNATIONAL LABOUR OFFICE
Geneva

World Bank
1818 H Street, NW
Washington, DC 20433
Telephone: 202-473-1000
Internet: www.worldbank.org
E-mail: feedback@worldbank.org

International Labour Office
4, route des Morillons
CH-1211 Geneva 22
Switzerland
Fax: (+41 22) 799 6938
Internet: www.ilo.org/publns
E-mail: pubvente@ilo.org

The findings, interpretations, and conclusions expressed here are those of the author(s) and do not necessarily reflect the views of the Board of Executive Directors of the World Bank or the governments they represent, or the views of the International Labour Office.

The World Bank and the International Labour Office cannot guarantee the accuracy of the data included in this work. The boundaries, colors, denominations, and other information shown on any map in this work do not imply on the part of the World Bank or the International Labour Office any judgment of the legal status of any territory or the endorsement or acceptance of such boundaries.

ISBN 0-8213-5041-2
ISBN 92-2-112711-7

Library of Congress Cataloging-in-Publication Data

Social reinsurance : a new approach to sustainable community health financing / David M. Dror and Alexander S. Preker, editors.
     p.cm.
   ISBN 0-8213-5041-2
   1. Community health services--Developing countries--Finance. 2. Medical economics--Developing countries. 3. Reinsurance--Developing countries. I. Dror, David M. II. Preker, Alexander S., 1951-

RA410.5.S63 2002
362.1'2'091724--dc21

2002025883

Contents

APPENDIXES

BOXES

FIGURES

TABLES

Foreword

A
ction to improve health and facilitate access to health care is important
for individual well-being and national economic performance. But paying for health care is problematic. Equally vital elements of well-being,
such as food, are paid through out-of-pocket payments. But that approach does
not work well for health care. Unlike food, it is needed unpredictably and can be
very expensive. On the face of it, the solution is private insurance. But this approach, too, does not work well because major information problems make individually risk-rated private insurance inefficient, expensive, and unable to cover
all medical risks. The U.S. system, substantially reliant on private medical insurance, faces problems that are entirely predicted by economic theory.

All other advanced industrial countries finance health care out of a mixture of
(limited) out-of-pocket payments, together with funding through social insurance, and taxation, or from a mixture of the two. Neither approach is perfect.
Systems with taxpayer funding of publicly produced health care can be slow to
innovate and to respond to consumer preferences; systems based on social insurance combined with private production face continual upward pressures on medical spending. Yet either is capable of delivering a reasonable combination of quality, access, and cost containment.

What, however, of poorer countries with limited (or minimal) fiscal and institutional capacity? Public budgets in such countries cannot afford more than minimal health care systems; and individually risk-rated insurance is likely to face
even more problems than in the West because of the limited regulatory ability of
government. As a result, when illness strikes, the poor—and especially the rural
poor and people working in the informal economy—have to rely on private resources to pay for health care. For poorer people in low-income countries, out-of-
pocket expenditure on health care can reach 80 percent of total medical spending, and a recent study of hospital visits in India showed that between one-third
and one-half of patients needing inpatient care became impoverished because of
inadequate risk management techniques.

Enter Dror, Preker, and their coauthors! This volume discusses community-
based approaches to insuring people against medical risk—not based on individual risk rating like private insurance, but along the lines of decentralized social
insurance based on the average risk. Recent studies of community savings, loans,

and financing schemes show how even the poor can insure themselves against unexpected events. Community-level health insurance programs improve access to essential drugs, primary care, and basic hospital care for rural populations and informal sector workers, offering at least some protection against the impoverishing effects of illness.

Tapping into experience from other sectors, the authors argue that subsidies can be used more effectively to expand insurance coverage, and that reinsurance can improve the financial viability of community-financed health schemes in settings where larger or more formal health financing mechanisms fail to reach large parts of the population. Reinsurance makes it possible to spread and transfer medical risks previously regarded as common shocks (and hence, uninsurable), such as environmental hazards (risks of pollution), earthquakes, meteorological and electrical storms, and retroactive coverage of asbestos damage.

The authors suggest that reinsurance techniques could also be used to improve the viability of small risk pools typical of community health financing schemes. This is an innovative application to the health sector and to poor populations of lessons learned from other sectors.

This book shows how the underlying idea of social insurance can be made operational in countries without the capacity to finance or organize large-scale systems, thus making it possible to improve access to health care for poor people in poor countries. There is no need to belabor the importance of the topic.

Nicholas Barr
Professor of Public Economics
London School of Economics
June 2002

Acknowledgments

P roduction of this book was supported by a World Bank Development Marketplace 2000 Award (www.DevelopmentMarketplace.org/html/report118.html). The International Labour Office (ILO) provided additional funding.

The editors and authors are grateful to Eduardo Doryan (currently Special Representative of the World Bank to the United Nations in New York), who acted as sponsor for the Social Re Development Marketplace 2000 Project, and to Charlie Griffin (currently Director Human Development South Asia), who acted as adviser for the project. Valuable support was also provided by Assane Diop (Executive Director, Social Protection Sector, ILO), Christopher Lovelace (Director for Health, Nutrition and Population at the World Bank) and Michael Cichon (Chief, Financial, Actuarial and Statistical Branch, Social Protection Sector, ILO).

The following individuals contributed directly to the book: *Erwin Alampay* (Institute of Public Health Management Manila, and professor at the University of the Philippines National College of Public Administration and Governance); *Jean-Paul Auray* (director of the Laboratoire d'Analyse des Systèmes de Santé, UMR-5823 of CNRS, University of Lyon 1 Claude-Bernard, France); *Bernd Balkenhol* (Director of Social Finance Programme, ILO); *Yolanda Bayugo* (Institute of Public Health Management Manila , and consultant on provincial health systems in Cambodia); *Sara Bennett* (senior research adviser, Partners for Health Reform, and lecturer on Health Economics and Financing, London School of Hygiene and Tropical Medicine); *Stéphane Bonnevay* (research fellow, MA2D Group, Laboratoire d'Analyse des Systèmes de Santé University of Lyon 1 Claude-Bernard, France); *Logan Brenzel* (senior program associate/health economist, Management Science for Health); *Reinhard Busse* (professor and department head for health care management at Technische Universität Berlin, and until April 2002, head of the Madrid hub of the European Observatory on Health Care Systems); *Craig Churchill* (Social Finance Programme, ILO, Geneva, and formerly director of research and policy at Calmeadow); *Gérard Duru* (professor of mathematics and econometrics at University of Lyon 1 Claude-Bernard, France); *Frank G. Feeley* (clinical associate professor, Boston University School of Pubic Health); *Jonathan Flavier,* (a community-based health specialist, Philippine Rural Reconstruction Movement); *Robert Fonteneau* (senior specialist, Caisse Nationale d'Assurance Maladie, Paris, detailed to the Social Protection Sector, ILO); *Donato J.*

Gasparro (president of NiiS/APEX Consulting Group, N.J.); *George Gotsadze* (director, Curatio International Foundation, Tbilisi, Georgia); *Jeannie Haggerty* (professor in the Départements de Médecine familiale and Médecine sociale et préventive at the Université de Montréal); *Melitta Jakab* (was a researcher, Human Development Network, the World Bank, Washington, D.C., currently completing a Ph.D. in health economics at Harvard University); *Avi Kupferma* (country director, then regional director, of ORT-Asia, a branch of the World ORT Union, an international nongovernmental organization); *Michel Lamure* (professor of computer sciences [informatics] and applied mathematics, University of Lyon 1 Claude-Bernard, France); *Jack Langenbrunner* (senior economist, the World Bank, Washington, D.C.); *William Newbrander* (director, MSH's Center for Health Reform and Financing); *Anne Nicolay* (adviser of the "Social Health Insurance" component [formerly the SHINE Project] of the German Support to the Philippine Health Sector); *J. François Outreville* (Executive Secretary, United Nations Staff Mutual Insurance Society, Geneva, and previously with the United Nations Conference on Trade and Development (UNCTAD) and Associate Professor of Finance and Insurance at Laval University, Quebec); *M. Kent Ranson* (research consultant at SEWA Social Security in Ahmedabad, Gujarat); *Rakesh Rathi* (IT Systems Manager, World Health Organization [WHO], Geneva); *Tracey Reid* (epidemiological research specialist, University of Montreal); *Aviva Ron* (until July 2002, director, Health Sector Development, World Health Organization, Western Pacific Regional Office, Manila, and previously with the WHO International Cooperation Office, Geneva, and the ILO's South-East Asia and Pacific Multidisciplinary Advisory Team [SEAPAT], based in Manila); *Elmer S. Soriano* (Institute of Public Health Management, Manila); *Katherine Snowden* (senior consultant, Third Sector New England, Boston); *Michel Vaté* (professor of economics, IEP Lyon, Université Lumière Lyon 2, France); *Axel Weber* (social protection specialist, the Asian Development Bank, and previously an independent consultant in health insurance and social protection); *Hiroshi Yamabana* (actuary in the Financial, Actuarial, and Statistical Services Branch, ILO, Geneva). Our thanks go to all.

Valuable guidance on methodological issues was provided by Dyna Arhin, Cris Atim, Cristian Baeza, Clive Bailey, Alejandro Bonilla, Krzysztof Hagemejer, Guido (Guy) Carrin, Michael Cichon, Lucy Firth, Robert Fonteneau, Wouter van Ginneken, Charles Griffin, Patrick Goergen, Soledad A. Hernando, Jürgen Hohmann, Christian Jacquier, Ruth Koren, Joe Kutzin, Ivan Lavallée, Volker Leienbach, Marilyn E. Lorenzo, Wendy K. Mariner, Michael McCord, Anne Mills, Christian Mumenthaler, Phillip A Musgrove, Nicolas Nicoloyannis, Manuel L. Ortega, Jean François Outreville, John W. Peabody, Dominique Peccoud, Joyce Pickering, Benito Reverente, Emmanuel Reynaud, George Schieber, Paul Siegel, Nicole Tapay, Nancy Turnbull, Daniel Tounissoux, Madeleine R. Valera and David Wilson

The authors of the book are grateful for the access provided to parallel and ongoing research on community financing by the World Bank, World Health Organization, and International Labour Office, with important inputs from Harvard University, London School of Hygiene and Tropical Medicine, London School of Economics and Political Science, Laboratoire d'Analyse des Systèmes de

Santé, University of Lyon 1 Claude-Bernard, France, Abt Associates Inc. (Partnerships for Health Reform USA), MSH, Institute for Public Health Management, Manila Philippines, University of Philippines-Manila, College of Public Health and National Institute of Health Policy (Manila), GTZ-SHINE project (Manila, Philippines), ORT Health Plus Scheme (La Union, Philippines), Tarlac HMO (Tarlac Philippines) and Kisiizi Mission Hospital (Kisiizi, Uganda).

Several participants in two meetings, one held in Geneva and the other in Washington, D.C., to review earlier drafts of this book have also provided insights and many pertinent questions. The editors are indebted to these anonymous contributors as well.

Kathleen A. Lynch provided valuable assistance in editing the manuscript. Mariko Ouchi provided research and administrative assistance. Catherine Atnony, Margaret Antosik, Dominique Blanvillain, Mary Hall, and Naz Mowlana provided essential and much appreciated secretarial and administrative support. Last but not least, Noam and Emma Braslavsky designed the book cover, the logo, and our website (http://www.ilo.org/socialre). Thanks to all.

David M. Dror and Alexander S. Preker,
Editors

Abbreviations and Acronyms

ACDECO	Angono Credit and Development Cooperative, the Philippines
ART	Alternative risk transfer
ASA	Association for Social Advancement
ATP	Ability to pay
BAHAO	Barangay Health Workers Aid Organization, the Philippines
BRAC	Bangladesh Rural Advancement Committee
BRI	Bank Rakyat Indonesia
BSMPC	Bagong Silang Multi-Purpose Cooperative, the Philippines
CBHCO	Community-based health care organization
CBO	Community-based organization
CGE	Cost-generating event
DALE	Disability-adjusted life expectancy
DfID	Department for International Development (United Kingdom)
DHS	Demographic health surveys
DOH	Department of health
FR	Finite-risk reinsurance
GDN	Global Development Network
GDP	Gross domestic product
GNP	Gross national product
GRDP	Gross regional domestic product
GTZ	German Technical Corporation
HDI	Human Development Index
HMO	Health maintenance organization
IEC	Information, education, and communication
ILC	International Labour Conference
ILO	International Labour Organization
IMR	Infant mortality rate
ITRMC	Illocos Training and Regional Medical Centre, the Philippines
LGU	Local government unit (the Philippines)
M&E	Monitoring and evaluation
MIU	Microinsurance unit
MFI	Microfinance institution
MGA	Mutual guarantee association

MLE	Maximum likelihood estimator
MMG	Medical Mission Group Hospital and Health Services Cooperative, the Philippines
MMR	Maternal mortality rate
MOH	Ministry of health
NATCCO	National Confederation of Cooperatives, the Philippines
NBFI	Nonbank financial institution
NCR	National capital region, the Philippines
NDHS	National Demographic and Health Survey
NESSS	National Epidemic Sentinel Surveillance System
NGO	Nongovernmental organization
NGT	Nominal group techniques
NHIP	National Health Insurance Program
NHS	National Health Services
OECD	Organisation for Economic Co-operation and Development
OHPS	ORT Health Plus Scheme, Philippines
ORT	Organization for Educational Resources and Training, the Philippines
PHIC	Philippines Health Insurance Corporation (PhilHealth)
PO	People's organization
PPC	Physicians per capita
ROSCA	Rotating savings and credit associations
RC	Risk characteristics
SEWA	Self-Employed Women's Association, India
SHINE	Social Health Insurance Networking and Empowerment, the Philippines
SSS	Social Security System, the Philippines
STEP	Strategies and Tools against Social Exclusion and Poverty, ILO
SU	Social utility
U.N.	United Nations
UNDP	United Nations Development Programme
USAID	U.S. Agency for International Development
U5MR	Under-five mortality rate
WHO	World Health Organization
WTP	Willingness to pay

Introduction

W hy look to the community for health care financing? Traditional sources of funding are often inadequate, leaving many of the 1.3 billion poor people in low- and middle-income countries without access to even the most basic health services. Most of these excluded people are poor, many living on less than US$1 a day. Many are children and other dependents of rural agricultural workers in the informal economy. Those who work, including children, are often exposed to high health risks—walking barefoot in fields and quarries, climbing makeshift scaffolding, inhaling toxic fumes in poorly ventilated cottage industries. Many young women are unprotected against and during pregnancy, and only the lucky few have professionally trained birth attendants.

This story is not new. Governments in low- and middle-income countries have tried to reach these excluded populations through public clinics and hospitals. To pay for these services governments usually use a combination of broad-based general revenues, contributions from the formal labor force, and user fees, similar to the time-tried financing mechanisms used by Western industrial countries. But the same formal financing instruments do not work as well in many developing countries, leaving many of the poor without needed health care or financial protection against the cost of illness.

Community-financing schemes have evolved in the context of two sets of failures:

- *Government failure* to collect taxes and organize public finance, to provide social protection for vulnerable populations, and to exercise oversight of the health sector

- *Market failure* to offer an effective exchange between supply and demand, partly because of the gap between needs, demand, and ability to pay, and partly because of the prevalence of nonmonetary transactions in the informal sector

Under these circumstances many rural populations and informal-sector workers have turned to local community organizations to help meet their health care needs.

The strengths of community financing in mobilizing and managing health care resources—where more formal financing mechanisms have failed—are based on three factors. The first factor is *social capital*. When hard times strike, family, friends, and community are often the ultimate safety net for low-income groups. The second factor is the preexistence of some community institutions that organize successful reciprocal arrangements, including *microinsurance,* among members of the community. Low-income households often feel more confident about contributing to community-financing programs that operate credit, savings, and insurance organizations and already have a positive track record locally, rather than to broad-based national health insurance. The third factor is the *interconnectivity* between local communities and external institutions committed to advance the general welfare of society. Schemes that build such connections early on have a better chance of expanding their membership, resources, risk pool, and benefit package as the community they serve grows and evolves.

But to serve the poor well, community-financing programs must overcome important limitations. Such schemes usually cover only small groups of people. They lack insurance and reinsurance mechanisms to spread risks across large populations and are isolated from formal financing and provider networks. Often, they have difficulty mobilizing enough resources to cover the cost of priority health services for the poor, fail to encourage prevention or to use therapies effectively, and rely on management staff with limited professional training. The survival and mainstreaming of community-financing schemes depend in large measure on remedying these problems from inception.

DEFINITION OF COMMUNITY-BASED HEALTH FINANCING

Community-based financing has evolved into a generic expression used to cover a large variety of health-financing arrangements. Different authors use the term in different ways. Microinsurance, community health funds, mutual health organizations, rural health insurance, revolving drug funds, and community involvement in user-fee management have all been referred to as community-based financing. A common feature of all these programs is the predominant role of collective action in raising, pooling, allocating, purchasing, and supervising the management of health-financing arrangements. A second common feature is that the people covered often have no other financial protection or collective financing arrangement to pay for their health care, and government-provided services do not reach them. A third common feature is the voluntary nature of these schemes and the tradition of self-help and social mobilization that are embraced by the poor in many low-income countries.

The volume revolves around micro-level health insurance units, including community-financing schemes designed to spread costs and risks among their members. These organizations could benefit from the application of insurance principles to improve risk-management and reinsurance mechanisms.

OBJECTIVE AND SCOPE OF THIS VOLUME

This volume discusses strategies and public policies that countries and donors can use to mitigate the shortcomings of community-financing schemes designed along the lines of microinsurance. Reinsurance is emphasized as a mechanism for enlarging the risk pool and spreading risks across larger population groups, which no single microinsurance scheme could do on its own.

The volume also discusses other measures to strengthen microinsurance-based community-financing schemes, including improving the actuarial basis for determining the insurance premium needed to protect against expenditure fluctuations; introducing subsidies to pay for the premiums of low-income populations; using effective prevention and case-management techniques to limit expenditure fluctuations, notably through enhancements of benefits with high externalities; enlisting technical support to strengthen local schemes' management capacity; and establishing and strengthening links with formal financing and provider networks. Through such action, the volume demonstrates, community financing can be the important first stepping stone toward improved financial protection and access to health services for the poor.

The volume does not address some of the specific problems associated with other forms of community-financing schemes such as community involvement in user-fee management, facility-based mutual health organizations, revolving drugs funds, or subregional or district-level social health insurance programs. Nor does the volume address the intersectoral determinants of health outcomes, although policies that influence activities in these areas may have a profound impact on health and demand for health services. These include policies on education, water, sanitation, transport, national security, agriculture and food, and the multiple social and economic dimensions of development policy.

TARGET AUDIENCE

This volume provides a useful review of health-financing policy for rural and informal-sector workers in low- and middle-income countries. Its target audiences are both general and specialized readers. General readers such as policymakers, health care workers, and staff from the international development community who may have few quantitative skills can skim the detailed technical chapters on theoretical issues in part 2 without losing the book's flow or core messages. Specialized readers such as health-financing experts, health economists, and academics will find most of the volume useful. For these readers, the volume provides a useful review of social health care financing at low-income levels, complementing other work on this topic. Specialists who want to skim the general context presented in part 1 can go straight to the detailed technical issues in parts 2 and 3. Although the story and the material unfold progressively throughout the book, each chapter is written to be self-contained, allowing readers to dip into individual chapters of particular interest.

BACKGROUND TO RESEARCH

The conceptual and technical underpinnings for this volume were developed over 18 months by a team of experts from the International Labour Office (ILO), the World Bank, the University of Lyon-1, and other collaborating organizations. It included field studies in Uganda and the Philippines. The research benefited from financial support provided by a World Bank Development Marketplace Award 2000 and core budget funding from the ILO.

ROADMAP FOR VOLUME

The following sections provide a roadmap for the volume.

Part 1—Development Challenges in Health Care Financing

This part gives an overview of the problems that low- and middle-income countries face in securing sustainable financial protection and access to health care for rural and informal-sector workers. The focus is on the roles played by local communities.

In *chapter 1*, Preker, Langenbrunner, and Jakab remind readers of the great progress made during the twentieth century in improving health outcomes and financial protection against illness. Yet many of the causal links leading to im- proved financial protection and sustainable health care have bypassed the world's 1.3 billion poor, living on less than US$1 per day, who have been largely excluded from the advances and improvements in health services delivery, organization, and financing. The authors trace financing to three factors: demand for and utili- zation of health services by households and communities; collective health care financing arrangements, inputs, and services that influence health; and govern- ment policies that affect the previous two. The authors identify three obstacles to extending financial protection against the cost of illness at low-income levels: low revenue-raising capacity, lack of risk sharing, and inefficient and inequitable resource allocation patterns.

In *chapter 2*, Dror, Preker, and Jakab review the role communities have played in addressing the problems identified in chapter 1 and in combating social exclu- sion. The authors review the history of financial protection against the cost of illness and the origins of social exclusion of rural and informal-sector workers. They conclude that governments, often unwittingly, contribute to social exclu- sion through different economic and social policies. In response to such exclu- sion, communities have begun to bridge the gap in social protection between people covered against the cost of illness through formal schemes and those with no protection at all. It is shown that the problem of exclusion is not only explainable by lack of resources, but also by a lack of overlap between needs, demand, and supply of health services. The authors suggest that success of community-based financing arrangements rests on three interrelated factors. Success is strongly correlated with the level of reciprocal risk-sharing arrangements among the members of the community. Such risk-sharing arrangements have often developed around microfinance instruments for the poor. These, in turn, depend on trust and other aspects of the social capital created through community networks. And public policies that emphasize the need for more inclusive and empowering social policies have also played an important role. The authors conclude by summarizing policy measures that governments can take to strengthen community-based financing schemes. These measures include improving insurance and reinsurance mechanisms; subsidizing the health insurance premiums of the poorest; promoting more effective prevention and case-management techniques, notably through (subsidized) enhancements of benefits with high externalities; providing technical support to strengthen local schemes' management capacity; and strengthening links with formal financing and provider networks.

Part 2—Insurance, Microinsurance, and Reinsurance

Part 2 reviews the basic principles of dealing with financial risk of illness through insurance, microinsurance, and reinsurance. It looks at how to determine whether or not a risk is insurable, presents statistical approaches to calculating risks, and develops a model for estimating risk profiles and calculating reinsurance premiums under different scenarios. The section concludes by reviewing known insurance-market failures and ways of dealing with them at the community level.

In *chapter 3*, Outreville reminds readers that insurance was created in response to a pervasive need for protection against the risk of losses. Yet no single insurance company has the financial capacity to provide unlimited coverage in any line of business because of restrictions in size and variations in risk. Experience has shown that reinsurance is a more efficient and less costly mechanism for sharing the assumed risk with others than having individual insurers underwrite separate portions of a potential loss. The author reviews the traditional reinsurance methods and a variety of contract methods. Nontraditional reinsurance methods that blend elements of insurance, reinsurance, and capital markets are thought to be particularly relevant to community-based microinsurance programs by insulating the primary insurer from the peaks and troughs of volatile underwriting results during the contract period and by establishing mechanisms to set aggregate stop-loss provisions for potential catastrophic events. The chapter also looks at some of the principles that should govern a reinsurance program. The primary decisions to be made by the insurer and reinsurer are how much risk the insurer should cede to the reinsurer for coverage and how much risk the insurer should retain. The author concludes that four functions are required to protect a reinsurance company's development: financing, program-management capacity, stabilization against fluctuations, and protection against catastrophe risk.

In *chapter 4*, Balkenhol and Churchill trace the evolution of microfinance back to the original microcredit movement in Bangladesh in the mid-1970s. Although the authors recognize that the idea of applying microinsurance to health care is still being tested in many countries, they suggest that the learning curve could be shortened if lessons learned from the delivery of other microfinance services are made more accessible to the health field. The authors describe several market imperfections the microcredit movement had to overcome to enable the poor to access such financial services. Remedies included using social capital and peer pressure as collateral, requiring a business plan to overcome information asymmetries, instituting frequent repayment periods with zero tolerance for delinquency, streamlining the application process, introducing high processing fees, and staffing with local people who know the clients. The authors define *microfinance* as a range of financial services, available to the poor and sustainable in the medium term. The authors introduce a topology of such microfinance institutions, where microinsurance is one arrangement (others are microcredit and microsavings). They summarize lessons learned from the microinsurance movement, including specific recommendations regarding institutional arrangements, management style, staffing issues, portfolio quality, human capacity, information management, transparency, client retention, affordability, and regulatory environment. Reinsurance is seen as one of the critical success factors to the microinsurance business, suggesting that the same may be true of microinsurance applied to health. The authors conclude that experience from microfinance indicates that local culture, the economic context, and external assistance all matter. Given the great variety of such arrangements, they suggest that any development of micro health insurance should start with market research and that "one size may not fit all."

In *chapter 5*, Dror looks at the application of insurance and reinsurance to the financing of health care at the community level. First he traces the history of the microinsurance movement, highlighting microinsurers' ability to attract excluded groups and the poor as members. Recognizing that management weaknesses may be a deterrent factor, he suggests that introducing coherent risk-management principles into the scene of community-based health schemes would increase their efficiency and their attractiveness to prospective members at the community level. The author looks at some of the factors communities must consider when establishing and running such programs. The author concludes that simplicity, affordability, and proximity to members are critical to their success.

In the second section, Dror reviews some of the vulnerabilities of microinsurance and possible remedies. He identifies weaknesses on both the income and expenditure side. The author points out that the small group size of many microinsurance schemes is the root cause for fluctuations in risk and that reinsurance mechanisms can effectively address these two related vulnerabilities. Reinsurance requires reliable data on the sources of instability: variance of unit costs and probability of occurrences. To establish these, knowledge has to be transferred to strengthen management. Adding benefits with high externalities and high cost-benefit ratios to the benefit package can reduce some risk. Backup linkages to formal health-financing mechanisms are also necessary to allow communities to enjoy financial support that would otherwise probably not reach them.

In *chapter 6,* Vaté and Dror raise the basic but difficult question of which risks and associated costs are insurable and which are not. The question is particularly pertinent in the context of applying risk-management principles, as they can only be applied to insurable events. The benefit package of health schemes is not normally limited to insurable events. In the context of small health schemes, the distinction must be made since different financing mechanisms must be applied to insurable and uninsurable benefits. The authors present three types of limit to insurability: actuarial, economic, and sociopolitical. To be insurable from an actuarial point of view, a risk must be random, observable, and diversifiable. The risk of a nonrandom event that occurs frequently and with great certainty cannot be spread across a homogeneous group of people because each individual will have an equally high chance of being affected. Hence, the premium collected from each individual would have to be equal to each individual's cost of the event. In the health sector, a number of events do not meet the actuarial insurability criteria. Although some insurance companies still cover them, these events have to be fully charged back or subsidized to meet the cost and profit margin. Examples are death benefits (everyone dies) and dental care for children (most children end up with cavities). And the event must be observable so that the risk can be calculated and the event can be validated. The authors then describe the economic and sociopolitical limits to insurability. First, to be insurable, the premium has to be high enough to cover the cost. If it is not high enough *(economic limit),* the insurer will be exposed to a high risk of insolvency even without unexpected variance. Second, to be insurable there must not be any unreasonable policy or political impediments. For example, a policy requiring microinsurance units to cover the poor without receiving a subsidy for doing so may leave the scheme vulnerable if those clients default on payments. The authors conclude that there is a large gray area in the insurable/uninsurable debate that depends as much on economic, legal, ethical, and cultural factors as on actuarial circumstances.

In *chapter 7,* Bonnevay, Dror, Duru, and Lamure present a mathematical model to demonstrate the ability of reinsurance to stabilize the variance in risk experienced by multiple microinsurance units. The reinsurance model uses two assumptions: that the reinsurance will deal only with random insurable events and their related costs; and that the reinsurance covers a share of the microinsurance costs above a certain level in exchange for a premium. The mathematical model deals with the sources of financial instability that are specific to small health schemes, and shows the mechanism through which reinsurance can compensate such schemes for these specific vulnerabilities. The model does not deal with predictable nonrandom events, which are a standard part of any microinsurance scheme's benefits outlay. In other words, the model assumes that the reinsurer will pay the cost of insured benefits that exceed a defined amount and that the microinsurance scheme will pay for the cost of the benefits up to that amount *(reinsurance threshold)*. Using various assumptions and simulating various scenarios the authors demonstrate the insurer's tradeoff between low contributions (to attract members) without reinsurance, and higher contribution levels to cover the additional cost of reinsurance. The authors conclude that microinsurance units will benefit from reinsurance in two ways. First, reinsurance buffers the microinsurer from unexpected expenditure fluctuations. Second, it reduces the microinsurer's need to accumulate contingency reserves and provides a mechanism to predict the level of surpluses that can be used to enhance the benefit package.

In *chapter 8,* Auray and Fonteneau deal with the following problem: application of risk-management principles requires estimation of the risk related to cost-generating events. Because of poor or no recordkeeping by microinsurers, risk estimates are prone to error. The authors deal with the problem of estimating risk without sufficient data and with the confidence intervals associated with using relatively inaccurate estimates. Auray and Fonteneau review some of the standard techniques such as the normal distribution, the Monte Carlo simulation method, construction of confidence intervals, and consensus methods such as Delphi and Bayesian Maximum Likelihood Estimation. They conclude by reminding the reader that, regardless of the technique used, "probability" is only a guide and the results must be validated against empirical evidence from the field.

In *chapter 9,* Weber examines the insurance market failure well known to the health insurance industry and shows that microinsurance schemes are not immune from such problems. Weber reviews key causes of insurance market failure, including information asymmetry, adverse selection, moral hazard, free-rider phenomenon, distrust, cost escalation, limited competition, high transaction cost, lack of financing and financial intermediaries, high dropout rates, failure of risk coverage, disclaimers, corruption, and fraud. Insurmountable as these problems may seem, innovative approaches at the community level may provide some useful lessons for mainstream private and social health insurance. Weber points out that microinsurance schemes often stimulate the local health provider market, thereby overcoming supply shortages. Information campaigns have been successful in explaining the need for insurance to local communities. Posting official price lists has been one way of countering the abuses of local monopoly providers. Since many microinsurance schemes offering health benefits are attached to other community-based financial services, they are able to share some of their fixed overhead expenses, thereby cutting the high transaction costs often associated with freestanding health insurance schemes. Discounts and local information campaigns have been used successfully to counter dropout. Many microinsurance schemes have found innovative ways to deal with adverse selection. These methods include compulsory waiting periods, compulsory membership (for example, in the case of marriage, or affiliation with a local cooperative), and group coverage (for example, family membership and minimum percentage of a community). To reduce moral hazard from members, some schemes set limits for claims on minor expenses (moral hazard is less problematic for catastrophic care since few people elect to have unnecessary serious surgery just to collect benefits). Other schemes have successfully reduced moral hazard by providers *(supplier-induced demand)* through appropriate reimbursement mechanisms (for example, case coverage payments) and referral systems.

Part 3—Implementation Issues

Part three presents a set of critical implementation issues related to community-based microinsurance schemes. It explores such issues as the role of governments in regulating and subsidizing such schemes, ability and willingness to pay, and market competition. The section concludes with a summary of operational data requirements needed to operate a successful microinsurance and reinsurance system.

In *chapter 10,* Bennett and Gotsadze look at the growing empirical evidence in implementing microinsurance schemes for health care, focusing closely on financial stabilization and risk management. The authors distinguish between two types of capacity often missing during design and early implementation. The first capacity requirement is the need for specific human skills to perform certain tasks: organizational management, knowledge of the regulatory environment, actuarial skills to compute premiums, and data-processing skills to run information systems. The second requirement is organizational capacity: infrastructure, human resources, technology, management structure, and incentive regime. Despite the paucity of well-documented evidence on design experiences, effective management and stabilization of financial risk appear to be recurrent themes. In particular, proper actuarial analysis of potential revenue and expenditure flows is often omitted during the design phase. Information on scheme implementation is better documented than scheme design. Three factors appear salient to success during the implementation period: aggressive marketing and community mobilization to maintain and increase enrollment; strong financial management to ensure that revenues and expenditures continue to balance, and to prevent fraud and abuse; and strategic purchasing from providers to achieve the best value for scarce money mobilized by the community schemes. The authors suggest that there is an inherent tension between sound financial management and the need for external assistance in strengthening capacity, and the need to preserve social capital and the sense of community ownership, a major strength of microinsurance schemes. They conclude with an appeal for better learning from experience in the future through improved monitoring and evaluation during the situational analysis, design, and implementation phases.

In *chapter 11,* Ranson and Bennett examine action that governments can take to facilitate the development, sustainability, and impact of community-financing schemes. The authors suggest that a first responsibility of governments should be to determine if microinsurance is serving the broad goals of the society. Assuming that it does, the authors then describe three types of government action: well intentioned and well executed, well intentioned but poorly executed, and poorly intentioned and poorly executed. Community-financing schemes often develop precisely in the context of weak government ability to secure national or regional financing for health care. Expectations about what such governments can do to help microinsurance schemes should be approached with caution. Examples of positive government action would include development of a broad policy framework and mandates for community involvement in reaching excluded groups (legal recognition and control of corruption), parallel to other public policies in this area. Such positive action would include information, monitoring, and regulation of existing schemes and the providers that serve their members. Governments can support microinsurance schemes through indirect subsidies to pay for the premiums of the poor, direct financial support to schemes themselves and the providers that serve their members, and nonfinancial support in the form of drugs, equipment, staff, other inputs, and discounted access to publicly financed facilities. Government support may also include access to public services for catastrophic care, supplemental insurance, and reinsurance. But the authors conclude that good intentions are not enough. Even well-executed government support can change the nature of community-based action, thereby undermining its very essence. Transparency, voice, community ownership, and innovation may suffer from even minor external intervention. Worse, schemes that become dependent on government subsides may be hard hit after a change in mandate or administration. Finally, many government bureaucrats prefer government-provided health insurance because it gives them greater control over resources or may preserve self-interested corruption.

In *chapter 12,* Feeley emphasizes that the reinsurance scheme's regulatory environment usually has a major impact on its optimal design and operation. The regulatory environment can determine the amount of capital *(policyholder surplus)* and can influence the corporate structure, management, and cost of information and accounting systems. The author emphasizes that insurance regulation in developed countries is often designed to protect consumers. Rules are written to keep the companies solvent, force them to meet insurance obligations, and protect consumers in the event of a carrier's bankruptcy. The lack of consumer protection in many developing countries often leaves both insurer and insured vulnerable. Since there are no models to review, the author proposes a set of standard regulatory provisions and a set of additional regulatory considerations. The minimal provisions would include rules governing licensing, ownership, and mandatory reporting (financial and other). In addition, regulations should cover benefit requirements and a range of restrictions (benefit exclusion, underwriting and risk selection, provider selection, and marketing). In concluding, Feeley raises a question about the ability of the reinsurance scheme to also act as a primary insurer and indicates some advantages and disadvantages of such arrangements.

In *chapter 13,* Busse emphasizes that no matter how well a reinsurance mechanism is designed to deal with insolvency related to random fluctuations of risk, it cannot deal with a systematic recovery gap. This gap occurs when a scheme's expenditure always exceeds its income, even without expenditure fluctuation resulting from variance. Many microinsurance schemes are established with too little history of cost experience, leading to poor prediction whether the contributions will cover the outlay on claims. But even when an attempt at projection has been made, several things can still go wrong. First, on the expenditure side, some of the newly insured may use health services more frequently than they did without insurance *(moral hazard)*. Providers, knowing that their patients are covered by insurance, may also encourage unnecessary utilization. Second, on the income side, rural and informal-sector workers with irregular employment may not be able to keep up with regularly scheduled contributions. Other patients may simply be too poor to contribute. And financial resources may be lost through poor financial management, high administrative costs, and even fraud and abuse by scheme managers. Busse reviews three of the most common methods of closing the recovery gap through subsidies, based on Europe's experience during the past century: subsidizing the premiums of poor individuals by paying the poor directly; subsidizing the microinsurance scheme for "taking on" poor patients who cannot pay; and paying providers who serve the poor for their services. The author reviews the key advantages and disadvantages of each of these methods. He concludes by highlighting three lessons learned from the European experience. First, even with a perfectly designed insurance scheme, some subsidy will be needed to cover rural areas and the poor, offer selective incentives to providers, and encourage standardization of the scheme's benefit package. Second, the way the subsidy is administered will have a powerful impact on the behavior of the microinsurance scheme and providers. And third, the way the resources for the subsidies are raised and spent directly affect equity, efficiency, and the poor.

In *chapter 14,* Brenzel and Newbrander look at the ability and willingness of rural and informal-sector workers to pay contributions to microinsurance schemes covering health care benefits. The authors review surveys that indicate that the contribution rate, design, and contents of the benefit package, quality of health services provided, and choice among providers are often critical factors influencing willingness to pay. Willingness is also directly related to household income (ability to pay). The authors suggest that ability to pay may be a better predictor of enrollment, continuity, and sustainability than willingness, where intent expressed through surveys may not materialize as a payment. The authors highlight the often narrow margin between revenues collected and expenditure obligations experienced by many microinsurers, which leaves them extremely vulnerable to both economic and health shocks. The authors conclude that, although reinsurance could be designed to protect most schemes against catastrophe losses, the premium could be unaffordable for most members. Instead of recovering the full cost of the reinsurance premium from the membership, the authors suggest leveraging public funds or using government subsidies targeted to the poor for this purpose.

In *chapter 15,* Newbrander and Brenzel identify some of the market forces that affect the development of microinsurance and factors that will improve their environment. The authors explain recent growth in microinsurance schemes as a

response partly to government's failure to provide coverage for excluded population segments and partly to increased grass-roots involvement by communities in
their own social development. The authors examine the potential market for reinsurance, highlighting both enabling factors and constraints. They review three
supply-side factors that have affected the proliferation of microinsurance schemes.
These factors include a greater willingness of providers and facilities to participate
in such schemes, a greater willingness of community management committees to
support the schemes' development and implementation, and an increase in the
local capacity to manage such schemes. On the demand side, the ability and willingness to pay is closely related to the microinsurance unit's sustainability. The
authors warn that an uncontrolled proliferation of poorly designed microinsurance
schemes is likely to feed people's skepticism about joining such schemes.
Newbrander and Brenzel identify several activities as creating a favorable environment for future growth of microinsurance schemes: introducing an appropriate
regulatory environment to address the issues raised by Feeley in chapter 12; helping local communities develop a capacity to design and run such schemes; enact-
ing measures to mitigate against insurance market failure (preventing cream skimming, moral hazard, adverse selection, unfair benefit restrictions, cost escalation,
and fraud); and improving existing schemes' financial viability. The authors stress
that subsidies and reinsurance have two reinforcing effects. Such mechanisms,
therefore, improve the schemes' financial viability by encouraging expanded membership and enlargement of the risk pool through greater numbers. Subsidies also
allow poorer households to participate, thereby strengthening the social capital
and the sense of solidarity at the community level. The authors conclude that
microinsurers can reinsure themselves by pooling insurance funds, accepting reciprocal arrangements with other funds, obtaining state subsidies to cover risks
above a certain level, and joining in a subregional, regional, national, or international reinsurance pool.

In *chapter 16,* Dror focuses on the data needed in the relationship between
reinsurer and microinsurer. He points out that the main purpose of a statistical
and accounting framework is to provide the data needed to operate the reinsurance and defines this cluster of data. Essential data elements include information on the scheme's income, expenditure, risk *(utilization patterns),* provider
behavior, and management. The author emphasizes that the amount, type, and
quality of data can have a significant impact on a reinsurance scheme's success
or failure. As a first-line insurer, the typical microinsurance scheme needs a
reliable database on its financial flows—income and expenditure patterns, for
which the demographic parameters of its members and their utilization pattern
of health benefits are necessary. A historical record of the income and expenditure of the different microinsurance schemes participating in a reinsurance pool
is also essential for designing the reinsurance program and its cost. The author
emphasizes that, although many microinsurance schemes exist in technology-
deficient environments, in today's world even the smallest and poorest scheme

can operate a minimal accounting and statistical framework that can provide automatic audit trails, validation, data security, and user support. A standard software program, developed through the proposed ILO/Bank–supported *Social Re* project (described in part 4), simplifies the tasks of recording, analyzing, and transmitting such information. The main advantages of the data framework are a user-friendly basis for determining the contribution schedule needed to cover the benefit package offered, and a database to maintain good business relations with the reinsurer.

Part 4—Toward a Reinsurance Pilot in the Philippines

Part 4 reviews the preparations toward piloting the reinsurance concept, through a framework called *Social Re*. This section provides much of the background material that was elaborated in the process of selecting the Philippines as a location for the pilot. The selection criteria included such considerations as government interest, level of literacy (female literacy in particular), electrification, access to telecommunications and computers, and the existence of microinsurance schemes and a significant informal sector. This part looks at the experience with microinsurance schemes, cultural aspects determining attitudes to risk and its aversion, epidemiological risk profiles of several communities, experience in setting up a scheme, its actuarial assessment, and a business plan for launching a pilot of *Social Re* in the Philippines.

In *chapter 17*, Flavier, Soriano, and Nicolay present a case study of social health insurance in the Philippines. The authors review the Philippines health care delivery system, health care financing, and expenditure trends. They also review issues relating to household income and ability to pay in the Philippines. The National Health Insurance Program that was set up in 1995 has been successful in reaching part of the urban population, which is able to pay the premiums set by this scheme. But many rural and informal-sector workers are both too poor and too mistrusting of programs sponsored by the central government to contribute the premiums for a national insurance plan that gives them, potentially, less than residents in the capital and in large cities. Based on this background, the chapter sets out the reasons for the growth of community-based financing and provider organizations. It reviews a recent survey of 66 community-based health insurance schemes conducted in the Philippines, looking at their benefit packages, contributions system, user fees, subsidies and other income, membership, management, and resource base (financial and staff). The authors conclude that one strategy toward implementing universal coverage under the National Health Insurance Program could be to have community groups play a predominant role in health insurance coverage of the informal sector.

In *chapter 18*, using the Philippines as a case example, Haggerty and Reid describe how epidemiological data—data on demographic patterns, mortality, morbidity, and risk factors—can furnish important clues about people's health needs and demands for health care. The authors emphasize that, although official data are usually based on national aggregates, important clues about the risk profile for microinsurance schemes can often be obtained from surveys and data on local service utilization. Using this approach, the authors conclude that since the Philippines (used as a case study for their analysis) remains a country with a high fertility rate and young population age structure, members of microinsurance units will want coverage for maternal and child services, much of which can be provided in ambulatory settings. But the country is also entering the demographic and epidemiological transition toward lower fertility rates and a shift from infectious to chronic diseases. The authors suggest that this will lead to increased use of more expensive hospital services for such conditions. Microinsurance schemes that are aggressive in the early detection and management of conditions such as diabetes, hypertension, breast cancer, cervical cancer, and colon cancer are likely to avoid later expensive treatment for these conditions. The authors also stress the importance to microinsurance schemes of managing lifestyle-related risk factors such as smoking, drinking, obesity, depression, and domestic violence. The authors conclude that observed differences in utilization patterns in the Philippines are probably related more to differences in access to affordable health services, the nature of payment systems, and the range of available benefits, than to the underlying epidemiological patterns. Active management of the benefit package is therefore likely to be critical to microinsurance schemes' sustainability.

In *chapter 19*, Soriano, Dror, Alampay, and Bayugo provide a brief overview of the social history of the Philippines, tracing its roots to the Malay people and others who came from China, India, the Arabian peninsula, Spain, and the United States. Based on the assumption that social capital is a determining factor in the success of microinsurance, optimal mobilization of this force requires adherence to local cultural, sociological, and ethical values. Four periods were formative. During the pre-colonial period prior to the sixteenth century, society was fragmented at village level into three classes—nobility, commoners, and helpers. There was no national culture or state. The Spanish colonial experience from the mid-sixteenth to late nineteenth centuries introduced a military administration and the religious doctrines associated with the Roman Catholic Church. The Americans who arrived in the late nineteenth century combined their political and economic strength into a semifeudal society, with power based on land ownership. In the post-American period, the old power elite has continued to dominate national and regional politics. But at the local level, the traditional cultural reliance on the community has prevailed as the basic social unit, offering people mutual support and reciprocity. In recent years, well-educated professionals have been acquiring power through their personal authority and entrepreneurial activities to challenge the established order of things. The authors believe that this background is critical to understanding the social capital and the local people's firm attachment to grassroots organizations such as microinsurance schemes. Still prevalent within the community is a deep distrust of central-government schemes and the formal top-down power structure, based on exclusion of most rural and informal-sector workers. Likewise, the central government, with periodic challenges to its authority from local movements, is reluctant to hand over too much power to local communities. In this context, the authors conclude that a microinsurance scheme's acceptance depends less on its objectives and technical design than on the degree to which local dignitaries support and promote it; the reciprocity it offers all players; and its ability to address locally recognized and frequently occurring problems (instead of offering protection against unknown and unappreciated risk that may or may not happen sometime in the distant future). As long as the Philippines' current national health insurance scheme fails in these areas, community involvement in health care financing remains pertinent.

In *chapter 20,* Kupferman and Ron review some of the conditions that led to the establishment of community-financing mechanisms during the past two decades. They identify key factors including changes in the perceived role of the state, reductions in government spending, transfer of financial autonomy to health care providers, decentralization, erosion of traditional social support systems, and emergence of gaps in social protection. The authors assert that it is in this context that community-based social protection has flourished. The authors claim that, to secure the financial and operational viability of the microinsurance schemes as part of the social safety net, supply and demand cannot be left only to market forces. Instead, they advocate a type of managed competition they call "structuring demand and supply." The authors identify the key target population for microinsurance schemes as a combination of individual informal-sector workers (economically active and inactive) and members of civil society organizations with strong grass-roots connections (agricultural cooperatives, local lending and savings schemes, and organizations with religious or international affiliations). These population groups have three common characteristics: their community solidarity, their unfamiliarity with insurance concepts (let alone reinsurance), and their traditional approach to illness. Once the target population has been identified, the authors claim that the key to success in community financing is to link the scheme's design to factors relevant to the target population, its health status, behavior patterns, and available health care resources. Simplicity, responsiveness to the local people's expectations, and ability to meet health needs are seen as paramount. The authors' personal experience leads them to favor schemes that favor a family subscription unit (rather than individuals); offer a range of benefits, including ambulatory care, inpatient care, and prescription drugs; are subject to community oversight of management; and pay both ambulatory and inpatient providers according to capitation-based contracts. Related supply-side factors include the availability of insurance, health care resources, and an appropriately skilled health workforce. The authors conclude by saying that "microinsurance is what the term implies. It is insurance on a small scale." The underlying objective should be to use such microinsurance to spread the understanding of the need for insurance among rural and informal-sector workers to broaden access to health care and eventually achieve universal coverage.

In *chapter 21,* Yamabana provides an actuarial assessment of the ORT Health Plus Scheme in the Philippines. The author describes the scheme's benefits and analyzes its contribution income, benefit expenditure, and other expenditure. He points out its high membership turnover but states that the compliance rate is satisfactory. Nevertheless, the author concludes that the scheme is running a deficit that will likely increase as result of the systemically increasing gap between expenditure and income, which is unrelated to random fluctuations in expenditure. The author suggests that this gap has to be closed before the scheme can set out to protect itself, through reinsurance, against random fluctuations in expenditure or other income shortfalls. The simple tool for mid-term financial projections developed during this assessment can be used to determine which risks should be considered for a possible reinsurance contract.

In *chapter 22,* Feeley, Gasparro, and Snowden propose a three-phased approach to setting up a reinsurance program for the Philippines *Social Re*: a start-up phase, an infrastructure development phase, and an operational phase. The authors emphasize that during the start-up phase the planners have to decide where to locate, find start-up capital, determine personnel requirements, and find out the legal requirements for setting up a reinsurance scheme. During development of the organization's infrastructure, the focus will be on establishing networks and systems for technical support, claims administration, auditing, and operational administration. Once up and running, the social insurance scheme will focus on operational issues such as premium collection, marketing, actuarial analysis, regulatory reporting, and claims management. The authors elaborate a detailed business plan, including break-even estimates under best-case and worst-case scenarios. The authors conclude that many of the necessary elements for running a reinsurance scheme are similar to the institution building needed to strengthen the microinsurance schemes. Success will depend on careful planning, technical assistance to client microinsurers, social marketing, and strong linkages with the government. Additionally, monitoring and evaluation at the initial implementation phases will also be instrumental for feedback into planning.

In *appendix A,* Dror and Rathi present a shortened version of the user manual for the *Social Re Data Template* software. In *appendix B,* Bonnevay, Duru, and Lamure describe the *Social Re Toolkit* software for calculating the reinsurance premium from the input data coming from the *Social Re Data Template.* The toolkit is the simulation module, whose theoretical and mathematical underpinnings are described in chapter 7. (Both software packages can be ordered separately from the book.)

CONCLUSIONS

This volume treats community-based microinsurance as an incremental first step to improved financial protection and access to health services for poor, rural, and informal-sector workers. It challenges the ability of low- and middle-income countries to leapfrog the long developmental process needed to build among excluded population segments the trust in central government–run schemes that could extend coverage to the whole population as a "big-bang" top-down endeavor.

In the meantime, governments could introduce more pro-poor policies that would build on existing social capital to strengthen community action in securing financial protection against the cost of illness. Enhanced access to needed health care would occur by:

- Encouraging and supporting the development of insurance and reinsurance mechanisms at the community level that can protect against expenditure variance and enlarge the effective size of the risk pool;

- Increasing targeted subsidies to pay for the insurance and reinsurance premiums of low-income populations (in part or in full);

- Including the use of prevention and case-management techniques to avoid unnecessary expenditure variance, notably through provision of benefits with high externalities;

- Providing technical assistance to strengthen the schemes' management capacity; and

- Forgoing stronger links between microinsurance units and the benefits of existing formal financing and provider networks.

David M. Dror
Senior Health Insurance Specialist
Social Re Team Leader
International Labour Office, Geneva

Alexander S. Preker
Chief Economist
Health, Nutrition, and Population
Human Development Network
World Bank, Washington, D.C.

PART 1

Development Challenges in Health Care Financing

CHAPTER 1

Rich-Poor Differences in Health Care Financing

Alexander S. Preker, Jack Langenbrunner, and Melitta Jakab

T he twentieth century witnessed greater gains in health outcomes than any other time in history. These gains resulted partly from improvements in income with accompanying improvements in health-enhancing social policies (housing, clean water, sanitation systems, and nutrition) and greater gender equality in education. The gains also resulted from new knowledge about the causes, prevention, and treatment of disease and from the introduction of policies, financing, and health services that made such interventions accessible more equitably (Preker and others 2001b).

ACHIEVING FINANCIAL PROTECTION AGAINST THE COST OF ILLNESS

Improving ways to finance health care and protect populations against the cost of illness has been central to this success story. Prior to the nineteenth century, most health-related transactions took place directly between patients and their healers. Patients could express their preference directly as consumers. Subsidies for the poor and collective risk-sharing arrangements did not exist.

With industrialization and the scientific revolution, there was a rapid expansion in knowledge about good health and illness and in the range and cost of available diagnostic methods and interventions. As expensive treatments became available for rare and complex conditions, health systems became differentiated into several subfunctions—financing, input generation, and provision of services (WHO 2000). The *financing function* includes the collection and pooling of revenues and their use by allocating resources or purchasing services from providers. The *input generation function* includes the production, import, export, distribution, and retail of human resources, knowledge, pharmaceuticals, medical equipment, other consumables, and capital. The *service delivery function* includes both population-based public health services and clinical services provided through

For their helpful comments on a draft of this chapter, the authors thank George Schieber, Sector Leader, World Bank Health, Nutrition, and Population Team and Sector Manager of its Middle East and North Africa Region, and Philip A. Musgrove, Lead Economist, World Bank, Human Development Network, Health, Nutrition, and Population Team.

public and private diagnostic, ambulatory, and inpatient facilities for individuals and households. These core functions of health systems are influenced by governments through their stewardship function and by the population through political processes, demand, and markets.

One of the great achievements in financing health care during the twentieth century was the move away from direct out-of-pocket payment and spot market transactions between patients and providers to broad-based insurance and subsidy-based financing (Preker 1998, pp. 103–24). In 1938, New Zealand became the first country with a market economy to introduce compulsory participation and universal entitlement to a comprehensive range of health services, financed largely through the public sector. The United Kingdom followed a similar path 10 years later when it established the National Health Services (NHS) in 1948. Universal access to health care in many East European countries—Albania, Bulgaria, the Czech Republic, Hungary, Poland, Romania, the Slovak Republic, and the former Soviet Union—was achieved through similar legislative reforms. Today, the population in most industrial countries (with the exception of Mexico, Turkey, and the United States) enjoys universal access to a comprehensive range of health services, financed through a combination of general revenues, social insurance, private insurance, and user charges.

As a result of these developments, the share of the world's population protected against the catastrophic cost of illness increased significantly during the twentieth century. Global spending on health rose from 3 percent to 8 percent of global gross domestic product (GDP) (US$2.8 trillion). At the current 3.5 percent global growth rate for GDP, spending on health-enhancing activities will grow by about US$98 billion a year worldwide. The matching figures for low- and middle-income countries are 4 percent of the GDP (US$250 billion), and an expected growth of some US$8 billion a year.

EXCLUSION OF LOW-INCOME RURAL POPULATIONS AND INFORMAL WORKERS

Costa Rica, Malaysia, Sri Lanka, Zambia, and a number of other countries have tried to follow a similar path, but the quest for financial protection against the cost of illness in middle- and low-income countries has been a bumpy ride.

As described by various reports, many of the world's 1.3 billion poor still do not have access to effective and affordable drugs, surgeries, and other interventions because of weaknesses in the financing of health care (World Bank 1993, 1997; World Health Organization [WHO] 2000; International Labour Organisation [ILO] 2000). Low-income populations still rely heavily on out-of-pocket expenditure instead of risk-sharing arrangements to pay for care, thereby exposing themselves to added risk of impoverishment from the double effect of income loss during illness, the high cost of health care, and variations in the prices charged by providers (Diop, Yazbeck, and Bitran 1995).

When ill, low-income households in rural areas continue to use home remedies, traditional healers, and local providers who are often outside the formal health system. Often, only the rich and urban middle classes have access to the health care advances of the twentieth century. In many low-income countries—where public revenues are scarce (often less than 10 percent of GDP) and institutional capacity in the public sector is weak—a large share of financial resources is still not channeled through formal risk-sharing arrangements.

As a result, although 84 percent of the world's poor shoulder 93 percent of the global burden of disease, only 11 percent of the US$2.8 trillion spent on health care reaches the low- and middle-income countries (WHO 2000). Two observations stand out. Poor countries spend less in both relative (spending per GDP) and absolute (U.S. dollars per capita) terms (figure 1.1A). Poor countries rely much more on out-of-pocket expenditure than on financial resources channeled through risk-sharing arrangements (figure 1.1B).

UNDERSTANDING THE ORIGINS OF RICH-POOR DIFFERENCES IN HEALTH CARE FINANCING

Health care financing through collective arrangements has two independent objectives: it provides the financial resources to diagnose, prevent, and treat known illness and to promote better health; and it provides an opportunity to protect individuals and households against the direct financial cost of illness

FIGURE 1.1   Spending and Risk-Sharing Arrangements

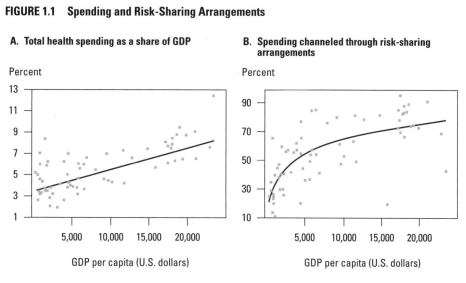

A. Total health spending as a share of GDP

B. Spending channeled through risk-sharing arrangements

Source: World Bank data.

when channeled through risk-sharing mechanisms (Hsiao 1994; Mossalios, Figueras, and Dixon 2002; Schieber and Maeda 1997).[1] Different issues arise in the case of the public and private engagement in health care financing and service delivery. The need for collective arrangements and strong government action in health care financing is often confused with public production of services. The poor and other excluded populations often seek care from private providers because public services in rural and low-income urban areas are often scarce or plagued by understaffing, supply shortages, and low-quality care. Poor households and community-financing schemes therefore often turn to private providers for the care they need. Such engagement by private providers can still be pro-poor if there are mechanisms to exempt the poor or subsidize user fees (Preker, Harding, and Girishankar 2001, pp. 209–52) and if purchasing arrangements include coverage for the poor (Preker and others 2001a, pp. 80–108).

The causal links leading to financial protection and sustainable health care financing are complex (figure 1.2). The following four-part framework summarizes the key outcomes of improved health and better financial protection; demand and utilization patterns; supply in the health system and related sectors; and policy actions by governments, civil society, the private sector, and donors (adapted from Claeson and others 2001).

Outcome indicators. First, although financial protection is highlighted as the key outcome indicator in this report, the WHO (2000) has highlighted three broad goals of most health systems: financial fairness (an indicator that combines progressivity and financial protection into one indictor); disability-adjusted life expectancy (DALE, an indicator that combines life-expectancy and disability measures); and responsiveness (a consumer satisfaction indicator that combines ethical and consumer quality dimensions).

Demand and utilization in influencing financial protection. Second, there is a complex interplay among household assets (human, physical, financial, and social), household behavior (risk factors, needs, and expectation for services), ability and willingness to pay, and availability of insurance or subsidies (Soucat and others 1997). This part of the analysis emphasizes the importance of household and community behavior in improving health and in reducing the financial risks.

Supply in health system and related sectors. Third, there is a hierarchy of interest from non-health-sector factors in improving financial protection (such as GDP, prices, inflation, availability of insurance markets, effective tax systems, credit, and savings programs) to more traditional parts of the health system (preventive and curative health services, health financing, input markets, and access to effective and quality health services—preventive, ambulatory, and inpatient). In respect to the latter, organizational and institutional factors contribute to the incentive environment of health financing and service delivery systems in addition to the more commonly examined determinants such as management, input, throughput, and output factors (Harding and Preker 2001).

FIGURE 1.2   Determinants of Outcome: Health and Financial Protection

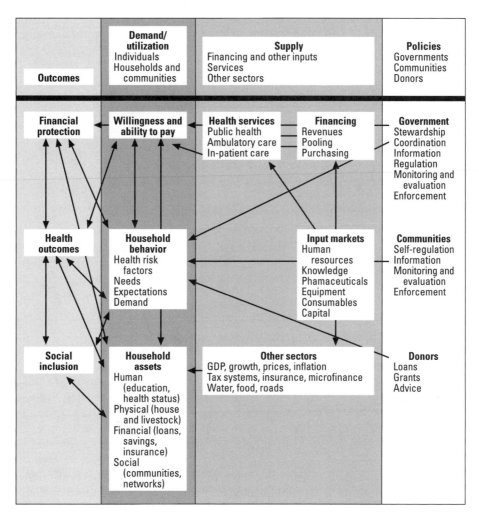

Source: Based on World Bank Poverty Reduction Framework; Claeson and others 2001.

Policy actions by governments, civil society, and the private sector. Finally, through their stewardship function, governments can deploy a variety of policy instruments to strengthen the health system, the financing of services, and the regulatory environment within which the system functions (Saltman and Ferroussier-Davis 2000). These policy instruments include access to information, creation of an appropriate regulatory framework, use of contracts, subsidies for the poor, and direct public production of services. In countries with weak government capacity, civil society and donors can be encouraged to play a similar role.

KEY OBSTACLES IN EXTENDING FINANCIAL PROTECTION THROUGH FORMAL ARRANGEMENTS

In many low-income countries, the poor are often excluded from formal arrangements, lacking both a sustainable source of financing to pay for health care and financial protection against the cost of illness. The following section summarizes some of the key obstacles to extending social protection against the cost of illness through formal health care financing arrangements (see box 1.1 for a summary of the complex flow of funds through the health system).

Problems in Mobilizing Financial Resources at Low-Income Levels

Several factors make the policy options for financing health care at low-income levels different from those at higher income levels. In resource mobilization, these factors include:

- A lower absolute level of financial resources can be mobilized at low-income levels and in poor communities.

BOX 1.1   FLOW OF FUNDS THROUGH THE HEALTH SYSTEM

The flow of funds through the health care system and public/private mix is complex, as shown in the figure below. This flow can be differentiated into three discrete activities: collecting revenues (source of funds), pooling funds and spreading risks across larger population groups, and purchasing services from public and private providers of health services (allocation or use of funds).

In very few countries do organizational and institutional structures correspond, one-to-one, with the three core subcomponents of the health financing function. In most countries, these three subfunctions of health care financing coexist under different organizational configurations. In all countries, the ministry of finance collects and pools public resources through general taxation. Through the budgetary process, some of these funds are allocated to the ministry of health or directly to providers. Parallel to these arrangements, many countries also integrate the collection of premiums and pooling of financial resources through social insurance funds, voluntary private insurers, community-financing schemes, or employers.

Finally, in all countries, providers collect some revenues directly as out-of-pocket payments at the time of treatment. As seen earlier, the poorer the country, the more likely is significant "leakage" of financing through such direct patient/provider channels, thereby exposing individuals and households to the financial risk of illness and exposing providers to an inability by poor populations to pay (heavy black arrow in the figure).

(Box continues on the following page.)

BOX 1.1 (continued)

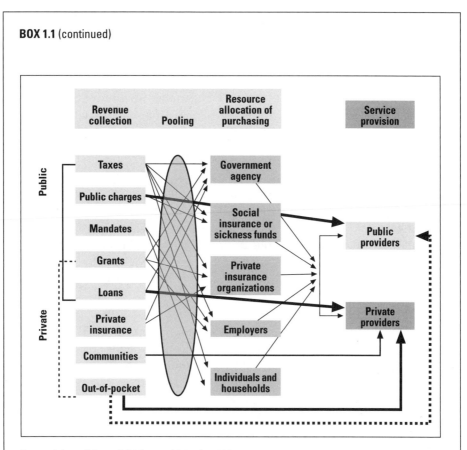

Source: Adapted from Schieber and Maeda 1997.

A combination of general taxation, social insurance, private health insurance, and limited out-of-pocket user charges has become the preferred health financing instruments for middle- and higher-income countries where income is readily identifiable and taxes or premiums can be collected at the source. By contrast, in low-income countries where income is not readily identifiable and collecting taxes or premiums at the source is difficult, other instruments such as community financing, personal savings, and direct out-of-pocket fees play a larger role in health care financing—by design or default.

- A larger proportion of the population lives in rural areas, relies on barter transactions, has irregular seasonal employment, and works in the informal sector. This makes it difficult to link the collection of premiums with employment, to enforce compulsory membership (membership in community schemes is usually voluntary), and hence to secure a steady income stream for health care.

- Willingness and ability to pay are difficult to assess—hence, the high reliance on consumption taxes at low-income levels and the regressive nature of the general revenues tax structure.

- The transaction costs are high and governments' or social insurance agencies' capacity is weak to collect taxes and social insurance premiums in low-income countries from rural and low-income workers. This problem reduces the resources that can be made available to subsidize care for the poor.

The macroeconomic instability that often exists at low-income levels (fiscal deficits, inflation, and fluctuating exchange) contributes to the instability of the income stream through formal taxation mechanisms (figure 1.3). This problem is seen even in countries that once had public financing and universal entitlement to health care such as some of the countries that underwent severe economic shock following the transition from central planning to more market-oriented economies. In those countries with large rural and informal employment sectors, collective health care financing arrangements have all but collapsed (Preker, Jakab, and Schneider 2002).

When a country's taxation capacity is low, 10 percent of GDP or lower, it would take 30 percent of government revenues to meet a 3 percent of GDP health expenditure target through formal collective health care financing channels. In most countries, public expenditure on health care is much lower than this, often not surpassing 10 percent of public expenditure. Hence, less than 1 percent of GDP of public resources is available for the health sector. At an income level of US$300 per capita or less, the resulting US$3 per capita often cannot cover even minimal basic care for the poor (World Bank 1997).

FIGURE 1.3   Low-Income Countries Have Weak Capacity to Raise Revenues

Total government revenues as a percentage of GDP

- Governments in many countries often raise less than 20 percent of GDP in public revenues; and

- The tax structure in many low-income countries is often regressive.

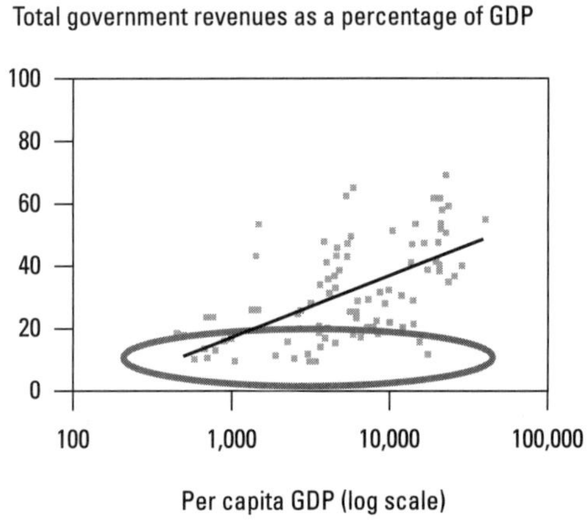

Per capita GDP (log scale)

Source: World Bank data.

Individuals and households in low-income countries often have a greater capacity and willingness to pay through direct out-of-pocket payments to providers and community-financing schemes than through the scarce resources that can be mobilized through formal channels (Sari and Langenbrunner 2001). Coupled with the low quality and strict rationing of services, even the poor often bypass public providers to seek the care they need directly from the informal sector and private providers. This exposes the poor to a significant risk of impoverishment from the cost of illness (Wagstaff, Watanabe, and van Doorslaer 2001), especially when their illness requires hospitalization (Peters and others 2001). In many countries, community-financing schemes have developed to offer less formal prepayment schemes that offer limited services (Arhin-Tenkorang 1995; Atim 1999). However, many of these schemes operating among low-income groups encounter both a recovery gap (chapter 13, this volume) and a compliance gap (chapter 17, this volume, presents data from the Philippines).

Problems in Revenue Pooling at Low-Income Levels

A different set of problems is faced during the pooling of financial resources at low-income levels. Although the rich are better able to contribute than the poor, the poor bear a much larger share of the disease burden. Sharing costs across income groups is, therefore, a fundamental aspect of financial protection in the health sector. Furthermore, people use health care most during childhood, the childbearing years, and old age—when they are the least productive economically. Smoothing out income across the life cycle can, therefore, also contribute to financial protection in the health sector. Based on these observations, three types of revenue transfers occur in the health sector during the revenue-pooling process: from rich to poor (subsidies); from healthy to sick (insurance); and from the economically active part of the life cycle to the inactive early and later years (savings), as shown in figure 1.4.

Such revenue pooling often falls apart at low-income levels for several reasons:

- Tax evasion is widespread among the rich and middle class in the informal sector, allowing higher income groups to avoid contributing their share to the revenue pool.

- Any pooling that does exist is usually fragmented along income levels, preventing effective cross-subsidies between higher- and lower-income groups. For example, many countries have separate financing systems for formal-sector and government workers (social insurance), the poor (general revenue subsidies), the rich (private insurance and personal savings), populations in rural areas and the informal sector, and other excluded segments of the population (self-help and community financing schemes).

- Personal and household savings are often the main source of intertemporal transfers.

FIGURE 1.4   Revenue Pooling Equalizes Inequities

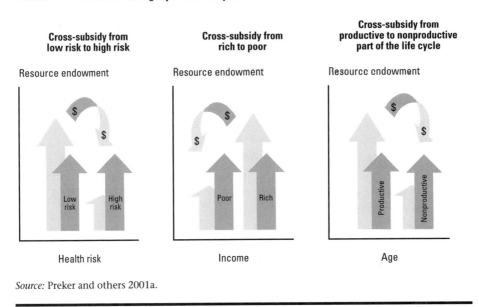

Source: Preker and others 2001a.

- Dissatisfaction with the quality and scope of services provided through ministries of health and other public providers leads many low-income groups to bypass formal financing systems to obtain the services they think they need directly from the informal sector and private providers through direct out-of-pocket payments. This undermines all three pooling systems described above.

In many countries, local community-financing schemes have emerged partially as an informal-sector response to these shortcomings in revenue pooling at low-income levels. (See box 1.2 for conceptualization of various risk sharing arrangements.)

Problems in Allocating Resources and Rationing Care at Low-Income Levels

In most countries, the potential range and scope of services that can be provided through resource allocation or purchasing services in the formal public sector is unsustainable without some form of care rationing.

How to ration such care is a critical policy decision that all countries face. Yet there is surprisingly little consensus among either professionals or practitioners on this topic (Musgrove 1999, 2000; Jack 2000). Rationing may occur through: *low-end truncation* by introducing copayments or excluding from the publicly financed package high-frequency, low-cost interventions such as dental care, drugs, eyeglasses, hearing aids, and allied health services; *high-end truncation* by excluding low-frequency,

BOX 1.2   DIFFERENT APPROACHES TO SHARING RISKS

The financial burden of health risks can be shared in many ways. Different health care systems approach this issue differently. Three common approaches are:

- Primitive (no insurance)—All risk shouldered by the patient

- National (full insurance)—All risk shouldered by the insurer at the broadest possible level (national)

- Community (partial insurance)—Risk shared among insurers, patients, and providers

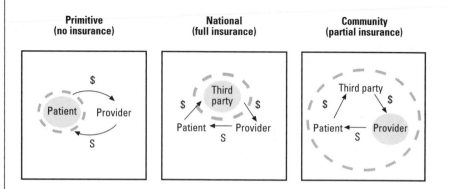

$ Money

S Services

Note: The dashed circle indicates the flow of risk.

Many low-income countries still expect patients to shoulder most health risks, as they offer no insurance. Examples include India and every country in sub-Saharan Africa. In most other countries, the state assumes some patient risks through their ministries of health or national health insurance programs. For reasons described in this chapter, few low-income countries have the capacity or resources to implement this type of risk-sharing arrangement for the whole population. Most therefore restrict their national health service coverage to a subsegment of the population.

Community-financing schemes have stepped in to fill this gap by assuming some but not all the risks of health care financing. These schemes share risks across the insurer, patients, and providers. Patients share some risk since most community schemes put ceilings on benefits or exclude certain services or conditions. Costs not covered by the plan remain with the patient. And providers that work with these schemes also shoulder some risk, since they cannot turn away patients who have partial coverage but cannot pay the difference. In these circumstances the providers become insurer of last resort.

very expensive interventions such as high-technology diagnostic services and he-roic aggressive surgery or chemotherapy that can extend life only by a few weeks or days; *elimination of ineffective care* such as alternate therapies and unproven inter-ventions; and *random quality deterioration* by not making any explicit decision but allowing the quality to erode slowly over time (figure 1.5).

Many low-income countries opt to ration services by not making any explicit decisions regarding the scope and range of services. Instead, they use nonspecific broad expenditure caps that push rationing decisions to lower levels of the pro-vider system. Faced with enormous expectations and demand from the popula-tion, providers often find it easier to allow service quality to deteriorate—through drug shortages, equipment breakdowns, capital stock depreciation, and lowering of hygiene standards—than to make politically and ethically difficult rationing decisions. Politically and ethically difficult rationing decisions about the target-ing of public expenditure to the poor are also difficult in such an environment. As a result of such difficulties, the rich often benefit more from public subsidies and public expenditure than do the poor (Gwatkin 2001, pp. 217–46).

As in the case of problems in resource mobilization and pooling at low-income levels, even the poor often prefer to bypass such quality rationing by publicly financed providers when they think they can find services in the informal sector and from private providers that will respond more directly to their needs and expectations for care. (See box 1.3 for a more detailed discussion on selected is-sues relating to resource allocation and purchasing.)

FIGURE 1.5   Cost-Risk Concentration Curve

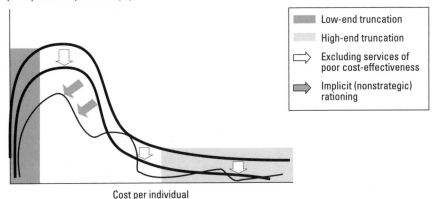

BOX 1.3   WHAT TO BUY USING PUBLIC FUNDS, IN WHICH FORM, HOW MUCH TO BUY, AND HOW TO PAY FOR IT?

Musgrove (1999) provides a decision tree on the rational use of public financing in the health sector.

What to buy using public funds. It starts with the overarching issue of allocative efficiency by asking if the proposed expenditure is for public goods, generally population-based services. If the answer is "yes," the next step is to rank such expenditures in terms of cost-effectiveness—or even better, cost-benefit analysis—to decide which will be funded. If proposed expenditures do not meet public goods criteria, the tree asks whether significant externalities or risks of catastrophic costs are involved and whether the proposed beneficiaries are poor. Thus, allocative efficiency, risk, equity, and cost-effectiveness interact to determine public-financing decisions in health. Economic principles govern each decision point but, because many other factors are often weighed, the outcomes will vary considerably across countries. The overriding principle is to maximize the potential impact on populations and the poor. In most countries there are important tradeoffs between achieving overall population health impact and targeting maximum benefits of public expenditure on the poor.

In which form? Risk-sharing arrangements may buy or allocate resources across a continuum, ranging from simple to complex units obtained. At the lower end of complexity, resources may be spent on suppliers of inputs such as pharmaceuticals, equipment, supplies, or labor. Moving up the ladder, resources may be spent on suppliers of specific interventions such as vaccinations or diagnostic services. At a higher level of complexity, resources may be spent on suppliers of complex services such as integrated ambulatory and inpatient care. Finally, at the highest level of complexity, resources may be spent on suppliers that may try to maximize outcomes such as a reduction in morbidity or mortality. Risk-sharing arrangements that choose suppliers that provide the desired units of care are more likely to get good value for money than those that blindly follow historical resource allocation.

If the unit desired is periodic blood pressure checks, a low-complexity intervention, coordination among providers is not necessary. Individual doctors, nurses, medical aids, and others are all able providers. But if the desired unit of care is a reduction in morbidity from cardiovascular disease, the range of providers able to deliver that service would change dramatically. Integrated provision of such care often requires a much greater range of services and complex coordination of networks of doctors, ambulatory care centers, lab and imaging facilities, and hospitals, as well as public health services that can do outreach and health promotion. The risk-sharing arrangement would no longer want to identify individual doctors or nurses as eligible providers, but complex networks of provider organizations already coordinating their operations. Although integrated population interventions would be the most effective way to provide

(Box continues on the following page.)

BOX 1.3 (continued)

health services, it is extremely demanding organizationally and institutionally for both insurers and providers. Improving overall health status would be the most desirable unit to focus on, but risk-sharing arrangements do not usually have direct control over the non-health-sector determinants such as education, income, and housing that affect health outcomes. Therefore, output proxies are usually used instead.

How much to buy? How much to buy should be determined by a balance between the supply of services, their prices, and the demand for such services, based on willingness and ability to pay. Most individuals and households will defy this logic when faced with the prospect of long-term disability and death. In those circumstances, patients are often willing to go deeply into debt and pay a much higher price than the market would otherwise bear. This imbalance is further distorted by subsidies and third-party insurance that reduce the cost of care to the individual consumer. Supply, instead of the usual market signals, is therefore often the limiting factor that determines how much to buy.

How to pay for it? Patients can pay directly out-of-pocket, but the high and unexpected costs of care encourage that costs be mediated through third-party insurers or organizations that pool resources. When providers are reimbursed indirectly through intermediaries, it is the payment mechanism used rather than prices and demand that creates the incentive environment for suppliers of services. The payment mechanism can be analyzed and is developed along two different axes: (a) unit of payment and (b) level of payment. Each aspect is technically difficult. The larger the unit of payment, the more difficult it is to develop an appropriate price for it. The level of payment, if too high, could encourage overutilization. If the level is too low, access could be hurt or informal payments extracted from patients. An optimal payment system for providers should induce providers to perform high-quality, effective treatments, while at the same time promoting a rational allocation of resources to and within the health sector. In reality, international experience and the literature reflects tensions across these multiple objectives. No payment system addresses all objectives equally well (Langenbrunner and Wiley 2002, pp. 150–76).

NOTE

1. We will not deal with the indirect impact of illness on loss of income from interruption in employment, although this is clearly another important dimension of financial protection against the cost of illness.

REFERENCES

Arhin-Tenkorang, D.C. 1995. *Rural Health Insurance: A Viable Alternative to User Fees*. Discussion Paper. London: School of Hygiene and Tropical Medicine.

Atim, C. 1999. "Social Movements and Health Insurance: A Critical Evaluation of Voluntary, Non-profit Insurance Schemes with Case Studies from Ghana and Cameroon." *Social Science and Medicine* 48(7):881–96.

Claeson, M., and others. 2001. *Health, Nutrition, and Population Sourcebook for the Poverty Reduction Strategy Paper.* Discussion Paper. Washington, D.C.: World Bank.

Diop, F., A.Yazbeck, and R. Bitran. 1995. "The Impact of Alternative Cost Recovery Schemes on Access and Equity in Niger." *Health Policy Planning* 10(3):223–40.

Gwatkin, D. 2001. "Poverty and Inequalities in Health within Developing Countries: Filling the Information Gap." In D. Leon and G. Walt, eds., *Poverty, Inequality, and Health: An International Perspective.* Oxford: Oxford University Press.

Harding, A., and A.S. Preker. 2001. *A Framework for Understanding Organizational Reforms in the Hospital Sector.* HNP Discussion Papers. Washington, D.C.: World Bank.

Hsiao, W.C. 1994. "Marketization—The Illusory Magic Pill." *Health Economics* 3(6):351–57.

ILO (International Labour Organisation). 2000. *World Labour Report: Income Security and Social Protection in a Changing World.* Geneva: ILO.

Jack, W. 2000. "Public Spending on Health Care: How Are Different Criteria Related? A Second Opinion." *Health Policy* 53(1):61–7.

Langenbrunner, J.C., and M.M. Wiley. 2002. "Hospital Payment Mechanisms: Theory and Practice in Transition Economies." In M. McKee and J. Healy, eds., *Hospitals in a Changing Europe.* Buckingham: Open University Press.

Mossalios, E., J. Figueras, and A. Dixon, eds. 2002. *Funding Health Care: Options for Europe.* Buckingham: Open University Press.

Musgrove, P. 1999. "Public Spending on Health Care: How Are Different Criteria Related?" *Health Policy* 47(3):207–23.

_____. 2000. "Cost-Effectiveness as a Criterion for Public Spending on Health: A Reply to William Jack's 'Second Opinion'." *Health Policy* 54(3):229–33.

Peters, D., A. Yazbeck, G.N.V. Ramana, and R. Sharma. 2001. *India—Raising the Sights: Better Health Systems for India's Poor.* Washington, D.C.: World Bank.

Preker, A.S. 1998. "The Introduction of Universal Access to Health Care in the OECD: Lessons for Development Countries." In S. Nitayarumphong and A. Mills, eds., *Achieving Universal Coverage of Health Care.* Bangkok: Ministry of Public Health.

Preker, A.S., and others. 2001a. *Resource Allocation and Purchasing (RAP) Arrangements that Benefit the Poor and Excluded Groups.* HNP Discussion Papers. Washington, D.C.: World Bank.

_____. 2001b. "Role of Communities in Resource Mobilization and Risk Sharing: A Synthesis Report." Report Submitted to Working Group 3 of the Commission on Macroeconomics and Health, Jeffrey D. Sachs (chairman). Geneva: World Health Organization.

Preker, A.S., A Harding, and N. Girishankar. 2001. "Private Participation in Supporting the Social Contract in Health: New Insights from Institutional Economics." In A. Ron and X. Scheil-Adlung, eds., *Recent Health Policy Innovations in Social Security*, International Social Security Series, Vol. 5. London: Transaction Publishers.

Preker, A.S., M. Jakab, and M. Schneider. 2002. " Health Financing Reform in Central and Eastern Europe and the Former Soviet." In E. Mossalios, J. Figueras, and A. Dixon, eds., *Funding Health Care: Options for Europe.* Copenhagen: WHO Observatory.

Saltman, R.B., and O. Ferroussier-Davis. 2000. "The Concept of Stewardship in Health Policy." *Bulletin of the World Health Organization* 78(6):732–39.

Schieber, G., and A. Maeda. 1997. "A Curmudgeon's Guide to Health Care Financing in Developing Countries." In G. Schieber and A. Maeda, eds., *Innovations in Health Care Financing.* Proceedings of a World Bank Conference, March 10–11, 1997. Washington, D.C.: World Bank.

Sari, N., and J.C. Langenbrunner. 2001. "Consumer Out-of-Pocket Spending for Pharmaceuticals in Kazakhstan: Implications for Sectoral Reform." *Health Policy Planning* 16(4):428–34.

Soucat, A., T. Gandaho, D. Levy-Bruhl, X. de Bethune, E. Alihonou, C. Ortiz, P. Gbedonou, P. Adovohekpe, O. Camara, J.M. Ndiaye, B. Dieng, and R. Knippenberg. 1997. "Health Seeking Behavior and Household Expenditures in Benin and Guinea: The Equity Implications of the Bamako Initiative." *International Journal of Health Planning and Management* 12(S1):137–63.

Wagstaff, A.N., N. Watanabe, and E. van Doorslaer. 2001. *Impoverishment, Insurance, and Health Care Payments.* HNP Discussion Paper. Washington, D.C.: World Bank.

WHO (World Health Organization). 2000. *World Health Report 2000—Health Systems: Measuring Performance.* Geneva: WHO.

World Bank. 1993. *World Development Report—1993: Investing in Health.* Washington, D.C.: World Bank.

_____. 1997. *Sector Strategy: Health, Nutrition, & Population.* Washington, D.C.: World Bank, Human Development Network.

CHAPTER 2

The Role of Communities in Combating Social Exclusion

David M. Dror, Alexander S. Preker, and Melitta Jakab

The link between employment and health insurance has been central to the extension of coverage to entire populations in most industrial countries where urbanization and formal labor-market participation are high. This link is more difficult—if not impossible—to forge in the case of rural, agricultural, or self-employed workers or the urban poor who have neither formal employers nor steady work. These groups make up most of the population in most low- and middle-income countries. For these *excluded populations,* access to health services is still inadequate (WHO 2000; ILO 2000a; and Sen 2000).

ORIGINS OF SOCIAL EXCLUSION FROM FORMAL HEALTH CARE FINANCING

The following section summarizes the origin of social exclusion from formal health care financing.

Where Does Social Exclusion in the Health Sector Originate?

Excluded populations share some similar characteristics: little cash income, limited education, poor health, and difficult access to services because of residential remoteness, minority status, ethnic or tribal affiliation, or gender inequality. Thus, the root causes of exclusion from health services are multifactorial but not always or only related to poverty. This exclusion often translates into a low ability on the part of the excluded to identify their health needs, set priorities, and pay for their care. In addition to their inability to pay and to express demand, several other underlying reasons account for their exclusion from health care.

First, the economic interactions of excluded populations are often nonmonetary (for example, barter, share-cropping work, or intertemporal lending of goods). In rural areas, even the poorer segments of the population can and do engage in

The authors acknowledge, with thanks, the insightful comments on this work from Wouter van Ginneken, Senior Social Security Specialist, Planning, Standards, and Development Branch, Social Protection Sector, International Labour Office; and of Charles C. Griffin, Sector Manager, World Bank, Latin America and the Caribbean Region, Health Sector.

economic activity, but it is often based on full or partial exchanges of goods or services rather than on cash. Cash has a premium because of its commutability outside a local barter economy. Hence, requiring cash payments for access to health services (or health insurance) may create an additional difficulty for certain population segments.

Second, health insurance schemes frequently require a fixed monthly payment. This periodicity, modeled on wage earners' circumstances, is too rigid for people with irregular income patterns. Excluded populations may be reluctant or unable to assume an obligation to pay a fixed amount each month when their income is irregular.

Third, living, working, and societal circumstances in the informal economy are less amenable to risk-averse choices, quite apart from the relatively high— often unavoidable—exposure to risks (including, but not limited to, health). An environment that is both less health conscious and less risk averse, and which simultaneously also needs to ration spending, may be inhospitable to insurance in general and health insurance in particular (Soriano, Dror, Alampay, and Bayugo, chapter 19, this volume).

This state of affairs explains why excluded populations' health needs are often not expressed in terms of *demand* (priority requirements that the needy can satisfy by paying money). It also explains why the link between health services and health insurance is not self-explanatory, since solvent demand is materialized in spot transactions between patient and healer, whereas health insurance occurs through prepayment to a financial intermediary.

Demand for health services (as distinct from demand for health insurance) does not in itself reflect coherent priorities. The informal sector shares with the formal sector the characteristic that needs and demand are not identical in health. Thus, a more accurate description of the situation underlying the lack of a market would require an examination of the interactions of three parameters: needs, demand, and supply (figure 2.1). Seven different zones can be distinguished, each

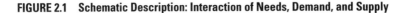

FIGURE 2.1   Schematic Description: Interaction of Needs, Demand, and Supply

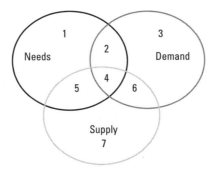

representing a different equilibrium in market interactions. These zones are particularly valid where health services are partial and severely rationed:

- *Zone 1—Undetected and unmet needs.* This may include public goods with large externalities for which the population will rarely demand services.

- *Zone 2—Needs in demand but inadequate market to offer services.* This could occur, for example, in low-density and low-income areas where the transaction cost of services may be much higher than potential revenues, shifting some of the operating costs to providers.

- *Zone 3—Demand for unavailable services corresponding to consumer preferences, not urgent medical needs.* Such services might include, for example, cosmetic surgery and medically unnecessary, excessive diagnostic services.

- *Zone 4—Adequate supply and priority needs for which the population is willing to pay (solvent demand).* This zone represents the area of activity of community-funded health schemes, and the ideal balance would be to maximize this zone.

- *Zone 5—Needs but no real demand.* This situation often occurs in the case of communicable diseases, which have large externalities but often little demand for prevention even when public financing and production of services are adequate.

- *Zone 6—Supplier-induced demand unrelated to real medical needs and perhaps medically unnecessary or medically damaging.* Aggressive marketing of diagnostic services, C-sections, or prostatectomies could result in this situation.

- *Zone 7—Excess supply but neither need nor demand.* This often happens in the case of low- quality, poorly equipped and staffed public clinics in rural areas.

This graphic presentation illustrates the impact of certain forms of subsidization or service targeting. For example, when subsidies are directed toward suppliers (as often done by missionary and disaster-relief organizations that operate field hospitals or sell medical material below cost), an increase will occur in Zone 4 but also in Zones 5, 6, and 7. In other words, an increase in supply could enhance the overlap of supply and need, but at the same time an undesirable increase could occur in excess supply and in supply-induced demand (figure 2.2).

Subsidizing the poor instead of the supply would produce an increase in Zones 2, 3, and 6, in addition to Zone 4, the province of community-funded health schemes. Since there is no theoretical or practical assurance the subsidy would be used only to enlarge Zone 4, such a subsidy could provoke feelings of unfairness and dissatisfaction among donors, providers, and the target population (figure 2.3).

These pitfalls could be avoided by expanding Zone 4 by enhancing overlap of all the zones (figure 2.4). An allocative system operating only (or predominantly) in Zone 4 would do this. In later chapters, we will see how the community can fill this role in the informal sector, both by mobilizing societal structures that encourage the poor to contribute to a prepayment scheme and by serving as the

FIGURE 2.2   Subsidizing Supply

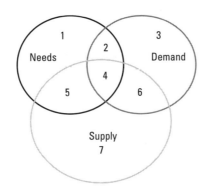

FIGURE 2.3   Subsidizing Demand

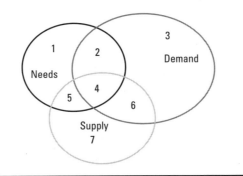

FIGURE 2.4   Enhancing Overlap

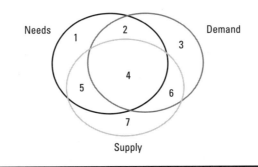

beneficiary of subsidies to improve the cost-benefit ratio of voluntary contributions (through external financing of some components of the benefit package), particularly services that—if unsubsidized—would fall into Zones 1 and 5.

Measuring the gap between needs and demand (Zones 1 and 3) to identify Zones 2 and 4 is complex, and not just because of methodological difficulties. It would also require a comparison of modern medical care with alternative, traditional, or ethnic forms of healing. This raises qualitative issues such as: Should microinsurance schemes cover the cost of traditional medicine? If people trust traditional healers and are willing to pay for their care, can microinsurance units completely ignore that trust? As the target population of microinsurance schemes is normally less educated, the influence of traditional beliefs may be more pervasive there than in other population groups. Willingness to affiliate with microinsurance units may be dampened by traditional beliefs about metaphysical causes of illness rather than cause-effect links to exogenous elements (microbial infection, viruses, unhealthy lifestyle, malnutrition) and endogenous elements (heredity, predisposition, psychosomatic responses). On this topic, there is very little knowledge, yet it is essential in the assessment of financial impact.

Exclusion also occurs when some segments of the population cannot access certain services. The reality in low- and middle-income countries is that a disproportionately low share of public spending reaches the lower-income deciles of the population, even when governments try to target public expenditure (figure 2.5). Global strategies to extend coverage are often too far removed from the grass-roots level where the problem is situated. Without finely calibrated

FIGURE 2.5   Pro-Rich Bias of Public Subsidies

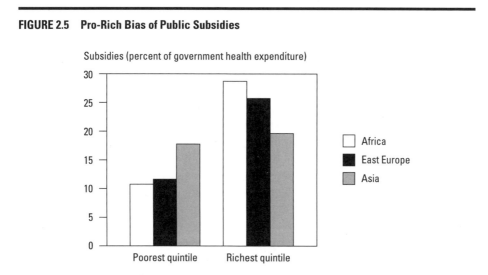

Source: Adapted from Gwatkin 2000.

targeting, such communities may never gain access to adequate services or financial protection against the cost of illness.

In summary, exclusion from health services can manifest itself as—and originate directly from—unstructured demand for health services, or an inadequate supply, or both.

Mentioning sparse supply as one cause of exclusion does not mean that the market for health services is supply based or that health service providers also create the market and facilitate the transfer. Precisely because insufficient private supply of health services to the poor and rural dwellers is a reaction to insufficient demand, spot transactions have to be shifted to some form of prepayment, from risk segregation to risk pooling, and from fee-for-service to averaging out unit costs.

Historical Roots

The realization that communities can play a role in addressing exclusion is neither new nor can it be construed to excuse the government from assuming some responsibility in health care financing. The international community has, since World War II, recognized the need to provide universal access to health care, but the consensus on how to achieve this goal has evolved slowly. As early as 1944, the Declaration of Philadelphia, adopted by the International Labour Conference (ILC), recognized "the solemn obligation of the International Labour Organisation to further among the nations of the world programmes which will achieve... the extension of... comprehensive medical care...." [1] In 1952, the ILC adopted the Convention concerning Minimum Standards of Social Security (No. 102), containing a chapter on provision of medical care to workers, by states ratifying that part of the convention.[2] This convention was adopted in a world where most development theories were tied to the existence of a formal sector.

A new approach, delinking health coverage from individuals' employee status, was the "WHO Declaration Concerning Health for All by the Year 2000," also known as The Alma-Ata Declaration (1978).[3] This declaration was the launching pad for a two-pronged approach: primary health care and universal coverage by the year 2000. "Health for All" was fundamentally a call for social justice as part of overall development. The primary health care platform promoted a top-down "global" strategy on health policy at the country level.

A decade later, the focus shifted from governmental health systems to empowerment of communities through "their ownership and control of their own endeavours and destinies."[4] The Bamako Initiative (1987),[5] adopted in a meeting of ministers of health from Africa,[6] went a step farther. It recognized the importance of behavioral change by households, and bottom-up action by communities, to complement or replace weak public institutions. The Bamako Initiative also recognized that even poor households can, and do, pay modest charges for health care and that their communities can generate income to cover the recurrent, nonsalary costs of basic health units. The Bamako Initiative has promoted substantial decentralization of decisionmaking from central government to district or lower level, community financing of health services, and community control over health system management and the flow of community funds.

The Jakarta Declaration (1997) also calls for health promotion action by community-based organizations (CBOs), nongovernmental organizations (NGOs), the labor movement, the private sector, governments, development banks, and United Nations (U.N.) organizations, among other actors.[7] In addition, all global UN conferences since 1990 have included a resolution recognizing primary health care as a basic human right.[8] As if to confirm developments since it adopted its Convention in 1952, in 2001 the ILC adopted conclusions concerning social security. They recognize that "there is no single right model of social security"; that "of highest priority are policies and initiatives which can bring social security to those who are not covered by existing systems"; that the extension should be achieved notably through insurance; and that the potential of microinsurance should be explored, particularly in access to health care.[9] These high-level political milestones have shifted attention from government operations alone to emphasize community action.[10]

International support for decentralized activity, where government expenditure on health services is insufficient, has stopped short of identifying the specific operative conditions that enable community-based organizations to play that role. These conditions are:

- Local communities need help to launch complex programs such as health care or health insurance. Rarely are such initiatives completely spontaneous. A wide variety of bodies have supported community-funded health insurance schemes: central or local government units, local or international NGOs, charitable societies (for example, churches), cooperatives or mutual societies (for example, microfinance institutions), as well as civic groups organized on a local, ad hoc basis (for example, an association of local health workers). Because each of these external bodies may have its own set of priorities, microschemes may be quite different from one another.

- CBOs can best fulfill their role through voluntary affiliation. To attract members, the community will have to address their specific local health risks, concerns, and living conditions.

Governments can offer political, moral, technical, or financial support even after schemes are launched. For instance, governments can facilitate the purchasing role of community-based health insurance schemes by decentralizing the authority to negotiate the conditions under which services will be supplied to the local government unit or local government-owned health center or hospital.

What Role Do Communities Play in Addressing Exclusion?

When governments create legal exclusion by imposing boundaries and different sets of rights, to handle their health needs, the people left out need alternative solutions, which they often find within their communities. Governments frequently contribute to exclusion through different economic and societal interests: territorial borders, differentiated rights for distinct groups of society (military, civil servants, corporations versus individuals, urban versus rural dwellers, employees versus self-employed, majority versus minority groups). To counteract their own exclusionary rules, governments can provide the funds and the framework to create the supply and influence the demand for health services at the community level. The evidence is building that health services, organized at the community level, reflect both needs and a popular redefinition of "social citizenship" from territorial to some other affinity of interests (chapter 19, this volume).

ROLE OF COMMUNITIES IN PROVIDING FINANCIAL PROTECTION AGAINST ILLNESS

Community initiatives have begun to bridge the wide gap in social protection between people covered by formal schemes and those with no protection at all against the cost of illness (Arhin-Tenkorang 1994, 1995, 2000, 2001; Atim 1998, 1999; Bennett, Creese, and Monasch 1998; Jakab and Krishnan 2001; Musau 1999; and Ziemek and Jutting 2000). What drives the development of community-based health financing mechanisms? Simply put, both governments and markets fail to deliver financial protection against sickness for the poor.

In low-income countries, large segments of the population in informal employment remain without effective collective arrangements to pay for health care or to protect themselves from the cost of illness (Guhan 1994; Midgley and Tracey 1996; van Ginneken 1999; World Bank 1995). Likewise, missing markets and imperfectly functioning markets leave most people without health insurance, and the poor are much more likely to be excluded than are the better-off. The transaction costs (collecting premiums and running the schemes) may exceed premium income, making the insurance unprofitable, even when needed and in demand. Community schemes for financing health care have operated where government failure and market failure have left people without financial protection (Preker and others 2002).

A Lack of Clarity in the Definition of Community-Based Financing Schemes

The term "community financing," as used in the literature, has evolved into a generic expression covering many types of health financing arrangements (Abel-Smith 1988; Dror and Jacquier 1999; Foster 1982; Hsiao 2001; McPake, Hanson, and Mills 1993; Muller 1983; Navarro 1984; Stinton 1982). However, different authors use the term in different ways, and similar, more specific, terms are often used to describe similar financing arrangements. Microinsurance, community health fund, mutual health organizations, rural health insurance, revolving drug funds, and community involvement in user fee management have all been called community-based financing. Yet, each of these risk-sharing arrangements has different objectives, policy, management, organizational, and institutional characteristics—and different strengths and weaknesses.

Community-based health care financing reflects most of these concepts. One common feature of the definitions is the *predominant role of collective action in raising, pooling, allocating/purchasing, and supervising the management* of health financing arrangements, even when they interface with government programs and services in terms of subsidies, supplemental insurance coverage, or access to public provider networks. Some community-financing schemes cover common geographic entities, while others are based on professional affiliations, religion, or some other kind of joint activity. A second common feature of community-financing schemes relates to their beneficiaries—more often than not populations with no other financial protection or access to collective financing arrangements to pay for health care. A third common feature is the voluntary nature of these schemes and the tradition of self-help and social mobilization embraced by the poor in many low-income countries.

Conceptual Underpinnings of Community-Based Action in Health Care Financing

The growth of community-based health financing arrangements rests on developments in three related areas (table 2.1):

- Microfinance (microsavings, microcredits, microinsurance, financial intermediation)

- Social capital (community, network, institutional, and societal links)

- Mainstream theories (welfare economics, public finance, health economics, and public health)

Links to Microfinance Organizations

Microfinance has initially addressed one aspect of poverty alleviation for low-income groups, namely access to credit and savings (Asian Development Bank [ADB] 2000; Brown and Churchill 2000; Otero and Rhyne 1994; and Zeller and Sharma 2000). Poor households are exposed to a variety of events beyond their immediate control that put them at financial risk. These events range from predictable life-cycle events (such as marriage, childbirth, education, and death) to less predictable events (such as droughts, fire, floods, and catastrophic illness).

To cope with these events, nonpoor households, even in low-income countries, resort to savings, credit, insurance, and other financial intermediation mechanisms. The difference between poor and nonpoor households is in the ease of access to such financial coping mechanisms. Until about a decade ago, the poor were considered "unbankable" and "uninsurable." It was assumed that the poor—living on a dollar a day—cannot and do not want to save or contribute to insurance against risks (Zeller and Sharma 2000). Consequently, few formal risk-protection mechanisms

TABLE 2.1   Conceptual Underpinnings of Community-Financing Schemes

		Key conceptual underpinnings
Microfinance	**1.**	**Microcredit**
		Risk taking (take advantage of opportunity, avoid overcautious behavior)
		Current liquidity management (smooth out consumption, increase choice)
		Short-term shocks (drought, famine)
	2.	**Microsavings**
		Predictable life-cycle events (education, marriage dowry, childbirth, death)
		Capital formation (purchase of equipment, downpayment on land, growth)
		Future liquidity management (smooth out consumption, increase choice)
	3.	**Microinsurance**
		Long-term income support (life and disability insurance, pensions)
		Short-term income support (sick pay, unemployment insurance—not well developed)
		Unpredictable health expenditure (health insurance)
		Replacement of loss (fire and theft insurance)
	4.	**Financial intermediation**
		Payment and money-transfer services (facilitate trade and investments)
Social capital	**1.**	**Community links**
		Among extended families, local organizations, clubs, associations, civic groups
	2.	**Network links**
		Between similar communities (horizontal) and different communities (vertical)
	3.	**Institutional links**
		To communities' political, legal, and cultural environment
	4.	**Societal links**
		Between governments and their citizens through public/private partnerships and community participation
Mainstream theories	**1.**	**Welfare of society**
		Income and growth
	2.	**Public finance**
		Taxation and social insurance
	3.	**Social policy**
		Social services and safety nets
	4.	**Health policy**
		Public health priorities and health systems

were accessible to the poor. However, informal risk-protection mechanisms through families, friends, and community networks have always existed. The steady expansion of the role of communities in operating savings, credit, and insurance services by and for the poor has gained prominence in the past two decades and has been recognized in the international statements summarized earlier.

Four microfinance instruments in particular have been developed to improve the productive needs of low-income households. These are: microcredits that help improve the immediate human, physical, and social capital of the poor (for example, small short-term loans to help pay for training, a piece of farm equipment, and access to social networks); savings to be used to build up the medium-term capital of the poor (for example, education, downpayment on a land purchase, or a dowry for marriage promising a daughter upward social mobility); insurance to stave off unpredictable expenses (for example, theft, loss, and illness); and financial inter-mediation (payment systems to facilitate trade and investments). The growing experience with these mechanisms suggests that the poor can be creditworthy, can save, and can buy insurance (chapter 6, this volume).

Many microfinance organizations have gradually moved toward attempting to apply insurance techniques to health risks (Brown and Churchill 2000; ILO 2000a). Extending microinsurance techniques to health care presents a unique set of challenges still being explored (Brown and Churchill 2000; Dror and Jacquier 1999; and ILO 2000b, 2001a). While life and crop insurance deal mainly with the financial cost of income loss, health insurance presents an additional set of issues related to financing tangible services for which the cost is neither fully predictable nor constant. This includes the range and severity of different illnesses, the range and scope of services provided, and the behavior of both patients and providers. (Providers are influenced particularly by the payment mechanism because of moral hazard, including supplier-induced demand, adverse selection, and fraud.)

Links to Social Capital

Why have microfinance organizations reached low-income individuals and house-holds when national systems have not? Clues to answer this question come from the social capital literature of the 1990s, which can be summed up as: What counts "is not what you know, but whom you know" (Platteau 1994; Woolcock 1998; Woolcock and Narayan 2000). When hard times strike poor people, family and friends are often their ultimate safety net.

The four dimensions of social capital include:

- *Community links* such as extended families, local organizations, clubs, associations, and civic groups—people in small communities helping each other (Dordick 1997)

- *Network links* between similar communities (horizontal) and between different communities (vertical) such as ethnic groups, religious groups, class structures, gender, and so on (Granovetter 1973)

- *Institutional links* such as communities' political, legal, and cultural environment (North 1990)

- *Societal links* between governments and their citizens through complementarity and embeddedness such as public/private partnerships and the legal framework that protects the rights of association (for example, chambers of commerce and business groups) and community participation in public organizations (for example, community members on city councils and hospital boards) (Evans 1992, 1995, 1996).

Low-income households already connected with a community credit, savings, or insurance organization are the most likely recruits to micro health insurance programs. Through their experience with those organizations, they are likely to believe that they will be able to exercise some control over the new operation, particularly where the health priorities are local rather than global public health priorities.

But social capital has both benefits and costs. The downside of social capital occurs when communities and networks become isolated or work at cross-purposes to societal collective interests (for example, ghettos, gangs, cartels). Intercommunity ties or bridges are needed to overcome the tendency of communities and networks to pursue narrow, sectarian interests that may run counter to broader societal goals (Narayan 1999). Community-financing schemes are vulnerable to a number of shortcomings associated with social capital:

- Sharing risk only among the poor will deprive their members of cross-subsidies from higher income groups.

- Remaining isolated and small will deprive their members of the benefits of spreading risks across a broader population.

- Staying disconnected from the broader referral system and health networks will deprive their members of the more comprehensive range of care available through the formal health care system.

Links to Mainstream Welfare Concepts, Public Finance, and Social and Health Policy

Community-financing schemes—in addition to their links to microfinance and social capital—can benefit from interconnectivity to the overall welfare of the society in which they exist, to the system of public financing (no matter how weak it may be), and to the broader social policy underpinning the national health system. Establishing such connections early can improve the capacity of communities to evolve in terms of the number of members covered, level of resources mobilized, size of the risk pool, and range of benefits covered. Their members have more to gain through such connectivity than they would through an isolated existence, because of governments' central role in elaborating and financing health policy and delivering care.

Proponents of such public-sector involvement in health care have argued their case on both philosophical and technical grounds. In most societies, care for the sick and disabled is considered an expression of humanitarian aspirations. But in addition to moral principles, collective intervention in health is warranted in the light of failure by the private sector and market forces alone to secure efficiency and equity in the health sector:

- Efficiency is compromised by significant market failure in the health sector: information asymmetries; public goods; positive and negative externalities; distorting or monopolistic market power of many providers and producers; absence of functioning markets in some areas; and frequent occurrence of high transaction costs (Bator 1958; Arrow 1963; Atkinson and Stiglitz 1980; Evans 1984; and Musgrave and Musgrave 1984).

- Equity is compromised by characteristic shortcomings of private health insurance such as exclusion of the high-risk poor, and many individuals and families do not voluntarily protect themselves adequately against the risks of illness and disability because of short-sightedness or free-riding (Barer, Getzen, and Stoddart 1989; van Doorslaer, Wagstaff, and Rutten 1993).

Community-based initiatives manage to overcome principal-agent problems in two ways: by designing a benefit package that aligns the interest of the agent (insurer) with that of the principal (member); and by designing monitoring systems that involve the members (principals) in effective monitoring of the actions of the agent (insurer).

RECENT EVIDENCE OF COMMUNITIES' ROLE IN COMBATING SOCIAL EXCLUSION

The preliminary findings of a large international review of health financing arrangements in low-income countries undertaken for the WHO Macro-Economic Commission on Health shed new light on the role of communities in combating social exclusion (Preker and others 2001).

Based on an extensive survey of the literature, the main strengths of community-financing schemes are the degree of outreach penetration achieved through community participation, their contribution to financial protection against the cost of illness, and the increase in access to health care they afford low-income rural and informal-sector workers (Jakab and Krishnan 2001). Their main weaknesses are the small amounts of revenue that can be mobilized from poor communities, the frequent exclusion of the very poorest from participation unless subsidized in some way, the small size of the risk pool, the limited existing management capacity in rural and low-income contexts, and isolation from the more comprehensive benefits often available through more formal health financing mechanisms and provider networks. The review of the literature also provided some insights into policy and institutional capacity–building measures that could be used to strengthen community-financing schemes in low-income countries. These recommendations are summarized below in this chapter's conclusions.

A parallel review of selected experiences in Asia and Africa supported many of those conclusions. The authors emphasized the diversity of community-financing arrangements in these regions (Hsiao 2001; Arhin-Tenkorang 2001). Many appear to improve financial protection against the cost of illness, allow better access by poor households to essential health care, and improve efficiency in collecting, pooling, managing, and using scarce health care resources.

The existence of risk-sharing arrangements as well as trust and local community control over the schemes appears to increase their enrollment rates. The reviewers emphasized that, although income is a key constraint to participation by the poorest, even they are often willing and able to participate if their contributions are subsidized by public or donor funds and if they gain access to quality services. These schemes were also more likely to enroll members when the household that would later use them was directly involved in their design and management. People were more likely to enroll when the premiums were based on prior assessments of the local willingness to pay and the benefits included access to a network of health providers within easy reach.

Members would like broad coverage that includes access to both basic health services for frequently encountered health problems as well as hospitalization for rarer and more expensive conditions. In the context of extreme resource constraints, this creates a tension or tradeoff between prepayment for basic services and the need for insurance coverage for rare, more expensive, life-threatening events that may occur once in a lifetime or not at all. This observation is consistent with experience in other areas of insurance where people are much less willing to buy protection against rare, catastrophic events (life insurance) than against more common events (crop insurance). This problem highlights an area of market failure related to voluntary community involvement in health care financing.

The reviewers also pointed to measures the governments could take to strengthen community health financing. The measures included subsidizing the premiums of the poor, providing technical assistance to improve their management capacity, and connecting with formal health care networks. Satisfaction with the scheme was often related to the nature of the direct community involvement in design and management. A critical factor was matching willingness and ability to pay with the benefits expected at some later point in time. The reviewers also highlighted several areas of government actions that appear to impair the operations of community-financing schemes. Top-down interference with design and management seemed especially pernicious to their functioning and sustainability.

An econometric analysis of microeconomic household data from four countries (Gumber 2001; Jakab and others 2001; Jutting 2001; Ranson 2001; Schneider and Diop 2001; and Supakankunti 2001) reinforced the conclusions from the survey of the literature and the two regional reviews. According to the analysis, prepayment and risk sharing through community involvement in health care financing—no matter how small—increases access by poor populations to basic health services and gives them at least some protection against the impoverishing effects of illness. Community involvement alone is not enough to prevent social exclusion since the very poorest often do not participate fully in these schemes. However, the study provided evidence that well-targeted design features and implementation arrangements could overcome this constraint to reach this group.

Finally, an analysis of macroeconomic cross-country analysis gave empirical support to the hypothesis that risk sharing in health financing matters in terms of its impact on both the level and distribution of health, financial fairness, and responsiveness indicators (Carrin and others 2001). The results even suggested that risk sharing corrects for, and may outweigh, the negative effect of overall income inequality. Financial protection against the cost of illness may therefore be a more effective poverty-alleviation strategy in some settings than is direct income support.

CONCLUSIONS

For the 1.3 billion poor in low-income countries, community financing provides a critical first step toward improved financial protection against the cost of illness, and toward access to essential health services.

Most community-financing schemes have evolved in a context of severe economic constraints, political instability, and lack of good public-sector governance. Weak government taxation capacity often prevents a mobilization of significant financial resources through general revenues. Large rural populations and their low participation in formal labor markets rule out social health insurance as a viable option in the financing of health care for the poor. And out-of-pocket user charges often further impoverish the poor, especially when they face hospitalization and serious illness. In this context, community financing—despite all its shortcomings—is often the only potentially viable option for providing the poor with some financial protection and access to basic health services.

Finding ways to expand coverage provided by community-financing schemes and to address known policy, institutional, and implementation weaknesses should therefore be a high priority on the reform agenda for both national governments and the international development community. Needed government involvement should be regarded as an important contribution to—not as a substitute for—community involvement in health care financing at low-income levels.

The research done for this book and other works on community financing (Preker and others 2001) brought to light several actions shown to improve the coverage, sustainability, equity, financial protection, and access to basic health services that community financing can provide. Such government action could include: (a) increased and well-targeted subsidies to pay for the premiums of low-income populations; (b) use of insurance to protect against expenditure fluctuations and use of reinsurance to enlarge the effective size of small risk pools; (c) use of effective prevention and case management techniques to limit expenditure fluctuations; (d) technical support to strengthen the management capacity of local schemes; and (e) establishment and strengthening of links with the formal financing and provider networks. The first of these policies will be discussed in chapter 5. The remainder of the policies will be discussed in other chapters of the book.

NOTES

1. The Declaration of Philadelphia, adopted by the ILC on May 10, 1944, chapter III, paragraph (f).

2. ILO: International Labour Conventions and Recommendations, Vol. 2 (1952–1976), Geneva, 1996, pp. 9–35.

3. Alma-Ata 1978, Primary Health Care. Report of the International Conference on Primary Health Care, September 6–12, 1978.

4. The Ottawa Charter, Health Promotion, First International Conference on Health Promotion, Ottawa, WHO, November 21, 1986.

5. Bamako Initiative: Women's and Children's Health through the Funding and Management of Essential Drugs at Community Level, WHO Doc. AFR/RC37/R.1, WHO, 1988.

6. According to UNICEF, by 1999 35 African, Latin American, and Asian countries had implemented programs in line with the principles of the Bamako Initiative, including major components such as immunization, vitamin A supplementation, and community participation. *Adoption* in the Bamako Initiative context refers to an initiative by a country to implement cofinancing or comanagement of health services; it is not a formal signature of a set of obligations.

7. The Jakarta Declaration on Leading Health Promotion into the Twenty-first Century, Jakarta, July 21–25, 1997, WHO Doc. WHO/HPR/HEP/41HP/BR/97.4, WHO, 1997.

8. World Conference on Education for All (Thailand 1990) Article 6; World Summit for Children (New York, 1990), para 9, 10, 11, 20.2, 24 and Appendices I, II; U.N. Conference on Environment and Development (Rio de Janeiro, 1992), para 6.4, 6.5, 6.12, 6.13, 6.18, 6.23, 6.27, 6.33, 6.34, 6.40,6.41; World Conference on Human Rights (Vienna, 1993), para 31, II.41; International Conference on Population and Development (Cairo, 1994), para 6.7, 7.6, 8.3, 8.5, 8.8, 8.13, 8.15, 8.17, 8.20, 8.21, 8.22, 8.29, 8.31; World Summit for Social Development (Copenhagen, 1995), Commitments 2(b), 5(d), 6,6(c), 6(m), 6(o), 6(q), 6(w), para 35, 36,37, 74; Fourth Conference on Women: Action for Equality, Development and Peace (Beijing 1995), Objectives C.1, C.2, C.3, L.5, para 106, 108, 109, 281; Second U.N. Conference on Human Settlement (Habitat II) (Istanbul 1996), para 32, 36, 115, 118, 119, 121, 136, 137; World Food Summit (Rome, 1996), Objective 2.4. *Source:* U.N. Administrative Coordinating Committee, 1997.

9. ILO 2001: Resolutions and Conclusions Concerning Social Security, International Labour Conference, Eighty-ninth Session, 2001, in ILO, *Social Security: A New Consensus* (Geneva: ILO, 2001).

10. While this progression of ideas within the international community has enabled innovative approaches toward developing health systems to be launched at local and community levels and by the civil society, it does not cancel the state's fundamental responsibility for health services.

REFERENCES

Abel-Smith, B. 1988. "The Rise and Decline of the Early HMOs: Some International Experiences." *Milbank Quarterly* 66(4):694–719.

ADB (Asian Development Bank). 2000. *Finance for the Poor: Microfinance Development Strategy.* Manila: ADB.

Arhin-Tenkorang, D.C. 1994. "The Health Card Insurance Scheme in Burundi: A Social Asset or a Non-Viable Venture?" *Social Science and Medicine* 39(6):861–70.

_____. 1995. *Rural Health Insurance: A Viable Alternative to User Fees.* Discussion Paper. London School of Hygiene and Tropical Medicine.

_____. 2000. *Mobilizing Resources for Health: The Case for User Fees Re-visited.* Report Submitted to Working Group 3 of the Commission on Macroeconomics and Health, Jeffrey D. Sachs (Chairman). Geneva: World Health Organization.

_____. 2001. *Health Insurance for the Informal Sector in Africa: Design Features, Risk Protection and Resource Mobilization.* Report Submitted to Working Group 3 of the Commission on Macroeconomics and Health, Jeffrey D. Sachs (Chairman). Geneva: World Health Organization.

Arrow, K.W. 1963. "Uncertainty and the Welfare Economics of Medical Care." *American Economic Review* 53(5):940–73.

Atim, C. 1998. *Contribution of Mutual Health to Financing, Delivery, and Access to Health Care. Synthesis of Research in Nine West and Central African Countries.* Partnerships for Health Reform Project, Technical Report No. 18. Bethesda, Md.: Abt Associates.

_____. 1999. "Social Movements and Health Insurance: A Critical Evaluation of Voluntary, Non-Profit Insurance Schemes with Case Studies from Ghana and Cameroon." *Social Science and Medicine* 48(7):881–96.

Atkinson, A.B., and J.E. Stiglitz. 1980. *Lectures on Public Economics.* Maidenhead: McGraw-Hill.

Barer, L.M., T.E. Getzen, and G.L. Stoddart, eds. 1989. *Health, Health Care and Health Economics: Perspectives on Distribution.* Chichester, West Sussex, England: John Wiley & Sons.

Bator, F. 1958. "The Anatomy of Market Failure." *Quarterly Journal of Economics* 72(3):351–79.

Bennett, S., A. Creese, and R. Monasch. 1998. *Health Insurance Schemes for People Outside Formal Sector Employment.* ARA Paper No. 16. Geneva: WHO.

Brown, W., and C. Churchill. 2000. *Insurance Provision in Low-Income Communities. Part II. Initial Lessons from Micro-Insurance Experiments for the Poor. Micro-Enterprise Best Practices.* Bethesda, Md.: Development Alternatives, Inc.

Carrin, G., R. Zeramdini, P. Musgrove, J.-P. Poullier, N. Valentine, and K. Xu. 2001. *The Impact of the Degree of Risk-sharing in Health Financing on Health System Attainment.* Report Submitted to Working Group 3 of the Commission on Macroeconomics and Health, Jeffrey D. Sachs (Chairman). Geneva: World Health Organization.

Dordick, G. 1997. *Something Left to Lose: Personal Relations and Survival among New York's Homeless.* Philadelphia, Penn.: Temple University Press.

Dror, D., and C. Jacquier. 1999. "Micro-Insurance: Extending Health Insurance to the Excluded." *International Social Security Review* 52(1):71–97.

Evans, P. 1992. "The State as Problem and Solution: Predation, Embedded Autonomy, and Structural Change." In Stephan Haggard and Robert Kaufman, eds., *The Politics of Economic Adjustment; International Constraints, Distributive Conflicts, and the State.* Princeton, N.J.: Princeton University Press.

_____. 1995. *Embedded Autonomy: States and Industrial Transformation.* Princeton, N.J.: Princeton University Press.

_____. 1996. "Government Action, Social Capital and Development: Reviewing the Evidence on Synergy." *World Development* 24(6):1119–32.

Evans, R.G. 1984. *Strained Mercy.* Toronto: Butterworth.

Foster, G. 1982. "Community Development and Primary Health Care: Their Conceptual Similarities." *Medical Anthropology* 6:183–95.

Granovetter, M. 1973. "The Strength of Weak Ties." *American Journal of Sociology* 78:1360–80.

Guhan, S. 1994. "Social Security Options for Developing Countries." *International Labour Review* 33(1):35–53.

Gumber, A. 2001. *Hedging the Health of the Poor: The Case for Community Financing in India.* HNP Discussion Paper. Washington, D.C.: World Bank.

Gwatkin, D. 2000. "Poverty and Inequalities in Health within Developing Countries: Filling the Information Gap." In David Leon and Gill Walt, eds., *Poverty, Inequality, and Health: An International Perspective.* Oxford: Oxford University Press, pp. 217–46.

Hsiao, W.C. 2001. *Unmet Health Needs of Two Billion: Is Community Financing a Solution?* Report Submitted to Working Group 3 of the Commission on Macroeconomics and Health, Jeffrey D. Sachs (Chairman). Geneva: World Health Organization.

ILO (International Labour Organisation). 2000a. *World Labour Report: Income Security and Social Protection in a Changing World.* Geneva: ILO.

_____. 2000b. *Mutuelles de santé en Afrique: Charactéristiques et mise en place: Manuel de formateurs.* Geneva: ILO, Programme Stratégies et Technique contre l'Exclusion sociale et la Pauvreté, Département de Sécurité Sociale (STEP).

_____. 2001a. *Social Security: A New Consensus.* Geneva: ILO.

_____. 2001b. *Mutuelles de santé et associations de micro-entrepreneurs—Guide.* Geneva: ILO. Programme Stratégies et Technique contre l'Exclusion Sociale et la Pauvreté, Département de Sécurité Sociale (STEP), Small Enterprise Development Programme (SEED).

Jakab, M., and C. Krishnan. 2001. *Community Involvement in Health Care: A Survey of the Literature on the Impact, Strengths and Weaknesses.* Report Submitted to Working Group 3 of the Commission on Macroeconomics and Health, Jeffrey D. Sachs (Chairman). Geneva: World Health Organization.

Jakab, M., A.S. Preker, C. Krishnan, P. Schneider, F. Diop, J. Jutting, A. Gumber, K. Ranson, and S. Supakankunti. 2001. *Social Inclusion and Financial Protection through Community Financing: Initial Results from Five Household Surveys.* Report Submitted to Working Group 3 of the Commission on Macroeconomics and Health, Jeffrey D. Sachs (Chairman). Geneva: World Health Organization.

Jutting, J. 2000. "Do Mutual Health Insurance Schemes Improve the Access to Health Care? Preliminary Results from a Household Survey in Rural Senegal." Paper presented at the International Conference on Health Systems Financing in Low-Income African and Asian Countries, Centre d'Etudes et de Recherches sur le Développement International (CERDI), Clermont-Ferrand, France.

_____. 2001. *The Impact of Health Insurance on the Access to Health Care and Financial Protection in Rural Areas of Senegal.* HNP Discussion Paper. Washington, D.C.: World Bank.

McPake, B., K. Hanson, and A. Mills. 1993. "Community Financing of Health Care in Africa: An Evaluation of the Bamako Initiative." *Social Science and Medicine* 3(11):1383–95.

Midgley, J., and M.B. Tracey. 1996. *Challenges to Social Security: An International Exploration.* Westport, Conn.: Auburn House.

Musau, S. 1999. *Community-Based Health Insurance: Experiences and Lessons Learned from East and Southern Africa.* Partnerships for Health Reform Project, Technical Report No. 34. Bethesda, Md.: Abt Associates.

Musgrave, R.A., and P.B. Musgrave. 1984. *Public Finance in Theory and Practice.* 4th ed. New York: McGraw-Hill.

Narayan, D. 1999. *Bonds and Bridges: Social Capital and Poverty.* Policy Research Working Paper 2167. Washington, D.C.: World Bank, Poverty Reduction and Economic Management Network.

Navarro, V.A. 1984. "Critique of the Ideological and Political Position of the Brandt Report and the Alma Ata Declaration." *International Journal of Health Services* 2(14):159–72.

North, D.C. 1990. *Institutions, Institutional Change, and Economic Performance.* New York: Cambridge University Press.

Otero, M., and E. Rhyne, eds. 1994. *The New World of Microenterprise Finance: Building Healthy Financial Institutions for the Poor.* West Hartford, Conn.: Kumarian Press.

Platteau, J.P. 1994. "Behind the Market Stage Where Real Societies Exist" (Parts I and II). *Journal of Development Studies* 30:533–77, 753–817.

Preker, A.S., G. Carrin, D. Dror, M. Jakab, W. Hsiao, and D. Arhin-Tenkorang. 2001. *Role of Communities in Resource Mobilization and Risk Sharing: A Synthesis Report.* Report Submitted to Working Group 3 of the Commission on Macroeconomics and Health, Jeffrey D. Sachs (Chairman) Geneva: World Health Organization.

_____. 2002. "Effectiveness of Community Health Financing in Meeting the Cost of Illness." *Bulletin of the World Health Organization* 8(2):143–150.

Ranson, K. 2001. *The Impact of SEWA's Medical Insurance Fund on Hospital Utilization and Expenditure in India.* HNP Discussion Paper. Washington, D.C.: World Bank.

Schneider, P., and F. Diop. 2001. *Synopsis of Results on the Impact of Community-Based Health Insurance (CBHI) on Financial Accessibility to Health Care in Rwanda.* HNP Discussion Paper. Washington, D.C.: World Bank.

Sen, A. 2000. *Social Exclusion: Concept, Application and Scrutiny.* Social Development Papers No. 1. Manila: Asian Development Bank, Office of Environment and Social Development.

Stinton, W. 1982. "Community Financing of Primary Health Care." *Primary Health Care Issues* 1(4):1–90.

Supakankunti, S. 2001. *Determinants for Demand for Health Care in Thailand.* HNP Discussion Paper. Washington, D.C.: World Bank.

van Doorslaer, E., A. Wagstaff, and F. Rutten, eds. 1993. *Equity in the Finance and Delivery of Health Care: An International Perspective.* Oxford: Oxford Medical Publications.

van Ginneken, W. 1999. "Social Security for the Informal Sector: New Challenges for the Developing Countries." *International Social Security Review* 52(1):49–69.

Woolcock, M., 1998. "Social Capital and Economic Development: Towards a Theoretical Synthesis and Policy Framework." *Theory and Society* 27:151–208.

Woolcock, M., and D. Narayan. 2000. "Social Capital: Implications for Development Theory, Research, and Policy." *World Bank Research Observer* 15(2):225–49.

WHO (World Health Organization). 2000. *World Health Report 2000—Health Systems: Measuring Performance*. Geneva: WHO.

World Bank. 1995. *World Development Report. Workers in an Integrating World*. Washington, D.C.: World Bank.

Zeller, M., and M. Sharma. 2000. "Many Borrow, More Save, and All Insure: Implications for Food and Micro-Finance Policy." *Food Policy* 25:143–67.

Ziemek, S., and J. Jutting. 2000. *Mutual Insurance Schemes and Social Protection*. STEP Research Group on Civil Society and Social Economy. Geneva: International Labour Organisation.

PART 2

Insurance, Microinsurance, and Reinsurance

CHAPTER 3

Introduction to Insurance and Reinsurance Coverage

J. François Outreville

Insurance was created in response to a pervasive need for protection against the risk of losses. It is feasible because it allows many similar individual loss risks to be pooled into classes of risk. Sometimes, however, the underwriting risk is too large to be assumed by any one entity, even if the probability that an event will occur can be accurately predicted. For example, a single insurance company might be unable to cover catastrophe risks such as an epidemic or war damage because catastrophe can strike a huge number of insured parties at the same time.

Reinsurance, simply defined, is the transfer of liability from the primary insurer, the company that issued the insurance contract, to another insurer, the reinsurance company. Business placed with a reinsurer is called a *cession,* the insurance of an insurance company. The reinsurer itself may cede part of the assumed liability to another reinsurance company. This second transaction is called a *retrocession,* and the assuming reinsurer is the *retrocessionnaire.*

Reinsurance contracts are entered into between insurance (or reinsurance) companies, whereas insurance contracts are created between insurance companies and individuals or noninsurance firms. A reinsurance contract therefore deals only with the original insured event or loss exposure, and the reinsurer is liable only to the ceding insurance company. An insurance company's policyholders have no right of action against the reinsurer, even though the policyholder is probably the main beneficiary of reinsurance arrangements.[1]

WHAT DOES REINSURANCE DO?

No single insurance company has the financial capacity to extend an unlimited amount of insurance coverage (contracts) in any line of business. Similarly, an insurance company is always restricted in the size of any single risk it can safely accept. If a risk is too large for a single insurance company, it can be spread over several companies. Insurance companies often use this process, known as *coinsurance.*

Reciprocity is the practice of cession between two primary insurers. It is the exchange of one share of business for another insurer's business of the same type.

The author thanks Patrick Goergen, United Nations Conference on Trade and Development, Geneva, for his comments on a draft of this chapter.

Reciprocity is an attempt to maintain the same premium volume while widening the risk spread.

Reinsurance is more efficient and less costly than having several insurers underwrite separate portions of a loss exposure. It is also a more efficient way to spread the risk among several companies. But an insurer might decide to buy reinsurance for other reasons. Reinsurance offers advantages in financing, capacity, stabilization of loss experience, protection against catastrophe, and underwriting assistance.

Financing

An insurer's limit on the value of premiums it can write is related to the size of its surplus. When premiums are collected in advance, the company must establish an unearned premium reserve. Reinsurance enables a company to increase its surplus by reducing its unearned premium reserve. This mechanism is particularly useful to a new or growing insurance company or to an established insurance company entering a new field of underwriting.

Capacity

Capacity, in insurance terminology, means a company's ability to underwrite a large amount of insurance coverage on a single loss exposure *(large line capacity)* or on many contracts in one line of business *(premium capacity)*. Reinsurance also allows insurers to cover larger individual risks than the company's capital and surplus position would allow or risks that the company's management would consider too hazardous.

Stabilization of Loss Experience

An insurance company, like any other business firm, likes to smooth out its year-to-year financial results as much as possible. However, underwriting losses can fluctuate widely in some lines of business as a result of economic, climatic, and other extraneous reasons, or as a result of inadequate business diversification. Reinsurance enables an insurance company to limit year-to-year fluctuations. It is sometimes compared to a banking operation where the insurer borrows from the reinsurer in bad years and pays back when its loss experience is good.

Catastrophe Protection

The potential impact of a catastrophe loss from a natural disaster, an industrial accident, or similar disasters on a company's normal (or expected) loss experience is the main reason for buying reinsurance. A catastrophe loss may endanger a company's very existence. In that case, a reinsurance contract insures the insurer.

Underwriting Assistance

Reinsurance companies accumulate a great deal of information and statistical experience regarding different types of insurance coverage and methods of rating, underwriting, and adjusting claims. This experience is quite useful, especially for a ceding company that may want to enter a new line of business or territory or underwrite an uncommon type of risk. Reinsurance facilities can provide extremely valuable services for a company entering new markets, but they are also useful when an insurance company decides to stop underwriting in a particular line of business or geographic region.

WHAT ARE THE TRADITIONAL REINSURANCE METHODS?

The two major categories of reinsurance contracts are facultative reinsurance contracts and treaty reinsurance contracts.

In *facultative reinsurance* (single risk), the ceding company negotiates a contract for each insurance policy it wishes to reinsure. This type of insurance is especially useful for reinsuring large risks, that is, those that the insurance company is either unwilling or unable to retain for its own account.

Facultative reinsurance, by nature, involves some degree of adverse selection for the reinsurer. It is expensive for the insurance company and practical only when the risks are few. It is useful when the primary insurer has no experience with a particular risk and turns to the reinsurer for underwriting assistance.

In *treaty reinsurance,* the ceding company agrees in advance to the type, terms, and conditions of reinsurance. Treaty reinsurance affords a more stable contractual relationship between primary insurer and reinsurer than does facultative reinsurance. Most insurers depend heavily on treaty reinsurance because facultative reinsurance is not practical when dealing with a single business class or line. The reinsurer does not examine each risk individually and cannot refuse to cover a risk within the treaty. The treaty method is also less expensive and easier to operate and administer than facultative reinsurance.

Although the reinsurer must accept all business cessions under the treaty, adverse selection is less likely to occur if the insurer wants to establish a long-term business relationship with the reinsurer. In this case, the reinsurer follows the ceding company's good or bad operating results (somewhat as a banker does) over a longer period of time.

The type of reinsurance contract chosen depends on the distribution of risks between insurer and reinsurer. There are two types of reinsurance contract: proportional *(pro-rata)* or nonproportional *(excess)*. Proportional reinsurance can be extended through a quota-share or a surplus-share contract. Nonproportional reinsurance can be issued for risk excess *(working XL per risk),* for occurrence excess *(per catastrophic event: cat-XL),* or for aggregate excess *(stop loss).*

Quota-Share Contracts

Under a quota-share contract, the primary insurer cedes a fixed percentage of every exposure it insures within the class of business covered by the contract. The reinsurer receives a share of the premiums (less a ceding commission) and pays the same percentage of each loss.

Quota-share contracts are common in property and liability insurance. They are simple to administer, and there is no adverse selection for the reinsurer. Quota-share contracts are usually profitable for the reinsurer because both commissions and terms are better.

A quota-share contract is a most effective means for small companies to reduce their unearned premium reserve when taking on a new line or class of business. A quota share is also ideal for reciprocal treaties between insurance companies. For example, two insurance companies with similar business volumes and profitability could each reinsure a 50 percent quota share of the other's business. This could have substantial diversification effects on each, particularly if they are involved in different geographical areas.

Surplus-Share Contracts

Surplus-share contracts, like quota-share contracts, are defined as proportional reinsurance, but the difference between them is in the way the retention is stated. In a surplus-share contract, the retention is defined as a monetary amount instead of as a fixed percentage.

As a result, in a surplus treaty, the percentage varies with the extent of loss exposure and the limit imposed by the reinsurer on the size of the potential loss. This reinsurance limit is usually defined as an "n-line surplus treaty," which means that the reinsurer will accept reinsurance coverage up to n times the retention amount. The surplus can be divided among several companies.

The following example illustrates the application of a surplus-share treaty with a retention of 50,000 monetary units and a reinsurance limit of 500,000. This would be referred to as a "10-line surplus treaty."

Size of loss exposure	Cedent's retention	Surplus cession (percent)
50,000 or less	50,000	0
80,000	50,000	30,000 (37.5)
160,000	50,000	110,000 (68.7)
400,000	50,000	350,000 (87.5)

The reinsurer would pay its share of losses in the same proportion as its share of the premium. The surplus treaty is particularly useful for large commercial and industrial risks. It provides a larger line capacity than the quota-share treaty and does not require the primary insurer to share small exposures that it can carry itself. However, it does not confer any unearned premium relief, which small insurers might need.

In a surplus contract, only the portion of the risk exceeding the company's retention is reinsured, leaving the company with a homogeneous portfolio. The ceding company can keep more profitable business, and the reinsurer takes on a higher share of the less-secure risks. However, the reinsurer pays the ceding company lower commissions than under quota-share treaties, and administrative costs are much higher.

Excess-Loss Contracts

Excess-loss (XL) contracts are different from pro-rata contracts in that the ceding company and the reinsurance company do not share the insurance coverage, premium, and losses in the same proportion. In fact, no insurance amount is ceded under an excess-loss contract. The reinsurer is not directly concerned about the original rates charged by the ceding company. It pays the ceding company only when the original loss exceeds some agreed limit of retention.

Usually, the ceding company pays the reinsurer a premium related to the nature and extent of the coverage assumed by the reinsurer, and no commission is paid to the ceding company. This is called the *burning-cost* system.

The burning cost is a percentage calculated by dividing total losses above the excess point in a period by the premiums for the same period. A maximum rate and a minimum rate are applied, and a deposit premium is paid. As in the retrospective premium, the final premium is adjusted at year end.

Per-Risk Excess Contracts

The retention under a per-risk contract is stated as a monetary amount of loss (not an amount of loss exposure or coverage). The reinsurer is liable for any loss amount greater than the retention stipulated in the contract. This amount is often subject to a limit, for example $200,000 in excess of $50,000. Under this type of treaty, the reinsurer pays all losses exceeding a deductible. As long as they do not overlap, more than one excess-loss treaty may cover the same business.

For example:

$200,000 in excess of $50,000
$500,000 in excess of $200,000
$1,000,000 in excess of $500,000

In this example, losses would be paid as follows:

Loss amount	Cedent's retention	Reinsurers		
		First layer	Second layer	Third layer
50,000	50,000	0	0	0
100,000	50,000	50,000	0	0
300,000	50,000	200,000	50,000	0
900,000	50,000	200,000	500,000	150,000

Per-risk excess treaties are effective in providing large line capacity, since they absorb large losses. They are also effective in stabilizing loss experience. In the short run, a primary insurance company can even improve the results of an inherently unprofitable business through excess reinsurance. However, the reinsurer will probably refuse to renew participation, and the primary insurer will have to pay more for any future reinsurance.

In health insurance, per risk could have several meanings. Insurers may face increasing exposure to major claims arising from a specific medical treatment, which explains the growing demand for reinsurance to cover the risk of very expensive treatments. However, a claim in health insurance is difficult to define because the distinction between a new illness and the consequences of an ongoing illness is problematic. Coverage is often based on all treatment a person receives in one calendar year.

Per-Occurrence Excess Contracts

Property insurers are particularly subject to large accumulations of losses from a single occurrence such as a hurricane or an earthquake. Individually, most claims may be too small for a per-risk excess treaty to apply, but collectively the accumulated amount can ruin a company. A per-occurrence treaty, called a *catastrophe treaty*, is the only type of reinsurance that offers protection from this fundamental type of risk.

Like the per-risk contract, the per-occurrence contract states the ceding company's retention as a monetary amount. However, all losses arising from a single occurrence are added up to determine the loss amount. The definition of a single occurrence is probably the most important part of a catastrophe treaty, but it is very difficult to define in health insurance. Per-occurrence treaties are often combined with per-risk treaties as a means of protecting the insurer's retention capacity.

Aggregate-Excess or Stop-Loss Contracts

Under an aggregate-excess treaty, the reinsurer begins to pay when the ceding company's losses for a stated period of time (usually one year) exceed the retention negotiated in the treaty. The retention may be defined as a monetary amount, as a loss-ratio percentage, or as a combination of the two.

An aggregate-excess contract is the most effective means of stabilizing a ceding company's underwriting results since it puts a limit on the ceding company's losses (or loss ratio). However, the limit is never set at a level that would guarantee the cedent an underwriting profit. Otherwise, the cedent could take on extremely risky business and still make a profit. Only the reinsurer would suffer, and the risk of adverse selection is too great.

A coinsurance factor is usually written into the contract. For example, the loss ratio in health insurance (the ratio of losses incurred over premiums earned) would be computed by using the company's (or market) experience over the previous five years:

year t	=	73.2 percent
t − 1	=	81.3 percent
t − 2	=	82.5 percent
t − 3	=	87.1 percent
t − 4	=	80.9 percent

Average loss ratio = 81 percent

Assuming that, at a loss ratio of 81 percent, the underwriting result for this line of business is zero (after deducting operating expenses), a stop-loss treaty might say: "90 percent of the amount by which the loss ratio of the ceding company exceeds 81 percent, provided always that the maximum amount recoverable shall be limited to $1,000,000 in the aggregate."

Because the balance between premium and indemnity usually is very unfavorable for the reinsurer, stop-loss is combined with a quota-share treaty and often excess-loss coverage for specific risks.

WHAT IS NONTRADITIONAL (FINANCIAL) REINSURANCE?

Instead of limiting their business to traditional methods of assuming and financing risks in isolation, reinsurers have developed financial products that blend elements of reinsurance, insurance, and capital markets. These products are based on alternative risk-transfer solutions with longer-term and more comprehensive forms of coverage. The objective is mainly to protect the financial resources of the business as a whole (balance-sheet protection), as contrasted with conventional event coverage.

Types of Contract

A reinsurance contract can be prospective, retroactive, or both. Under a prospective contract, the ceding company pays the assuming company a premium in return for indemnification against loss or liability relating to events that occur after the contract's effective date. Under a retrospective contract, the ceding company pays the assuming company a premium in return for indemnification against loss or liability resulting from events that have already occurred. This reinsurance practice, called *loss-portfolio transfer,* has become very popular.

By definition, the insurance risk involves uncertainties about the ultimate amount of any claim payments *(the underwriting risk)* and the timing of these payments *(the timing risk).* A *reinsurance contract* is an agreement between the ceding company and the assuming company whereby the latter assumes all or part of the insurance risk. Contracts that do not transfer underwriting risk are referred to as *financing arrangements* or *financial reinsurance.*

Historically, financial reinsurance took the form of retrospective reinsurance covering catastrophe losses and past experience. Today, the primary focus is on prospective products, which are a mixture of banking and reinsurance products. Their characteristics include the assumption of limited risk by the reinsurer, multiline coverage and multiyear term, sharing of results with the primary insurer, and the explicit inclusion of future investment income as a pricing consideration.

Nontraditional solutions, generically referred to as *alternative risk transfer* (ART), meet insurers' needs for long-term planning and balancing cash flow and resources. Coverage is limited over the entire, multiyear term of the treaty, and risk transfer is less significant than the timing of the payments (*timing risk*).

Finite-Risk Reinsurance

Finite-risk reinsurance (FR), one type of financial reinsurance, insulates the primary insurer from the peaks and troughs of volatile underwriting results during the contract period. It is a type of coverage that combines risk transfer with a profit-sharing relationship between reinsurer and client. Finite risk involves a limited transfer because the client ultimately pays for most of the losses through premiums and investment income. The reinsurer's risk lies mainly in the untimely payment of losses (*timing risk*). The multiyear nature of the contract allows the reinsurer to use the time value of the money and to spread losses over several years. This means that the client effectively trades today's underwriting income for tomorrow's investment income.

In finite-risk reinsurance, insurers are reimbursed a substantial portion of the profits accruing over a multiyear period. Coverage under finite reinsurance products is generally broad, without the list of exclusions in traditional products. Among the most popular new forms of ART are *finite quota shares*, which apply to business in current and future underwriting years, and *spread-loss treaties*, which are used to manage financial risks associated with payment time.

Aggregate stop-loss on a prospective basis is becoming a popular form of finite-risk reinsurance. It is used to address a client's exposure to a low-probability, high-severity event. In the case of potential catastrophe risks, the excess loss risk is partially retained by the reinsurer, and the remainder is transferred to the capital markets via securitization through event-linked bonds or derivatives. Risk-sharing partners in capital markets have been attracted to assuming insurance risks because they are uncorrelated with the price movements of the stocks and bonds that comprise a traditional investment portfolio.

WHAT PRINCIPLES GOVERN A REINSURANCE PROGRAM?

The first step in creating a reinsurance program for an insurance company is choosing a correct amount of net retention and the limits of reinsurance coverage.

If net retention is too low, the insurer's capital and surplus are not put to effective use. Low retention probably means lower underwriting results and investment income but also shows a lack of involvement on the insurer's part. The practice of reinsuring large proportions of risks *(fronting)* has been widely criticized as bad insurance practice.

If the retention level is too high, however, the insurer runs a risk of wide swings in the results and, in extreme cases, financial ruin. The retention decision is usually based on the following factors:

- Insurer's own resources, that is, paid-up capital and surplus

- Amount of premiums written expected to be generated by a portfolio

- Portfolio composition (size and number of policies)

- Class of business

- Geographical location and risk spread

- Insurer's experience in the class of business

- Projected underwriting profitability

- Probability of ruin

- Company's investment strategy

- Availability and cost of reinsurance

- Local regulations and foreign exchange controls

The four functions of reinsurance—financing, program-management capacity, stabilization against fluctuations, and protection against catastrophe risks—will all be needed at different times in a company's development. Thus, far from being cast in concrete, the reinsurance program has to adapt as the company's needs change (table 3.1).

TABLE 3.1   The Functions of Reinsurance

Coverage type	Financing	Capacity	Stabilization	Catastrophes
Quota share	Yes	Some	Moderate	No focus
Surplus	Some	Yes	Moderate	No focus
Excess per risk	No	Yes	Yes	No focus
Per occurrence	No	No	Yes	Yes
Aggregate	No	No focus	Yes	Yes
Financial	Prospective	Prospective	Prospective	Retrospective

Insurability

Some insurability problems are peculiar to the health insurance business. To be financially viable, insurance rates must be compatible with projected losses, and the lack of reinsurance or the inability to reinsure often boils down to incompatibility between the reinsurance rate and the direct rate, which is too low to make a profit or to break even.

- The low value–high frequency of some risks may raise premiums to the point where coverage may not be affordable.

- The high loss variance and propensity toward catastrophe losses from specific risks may also make rates unaffordable and increase the insurer's dependence on reinsurance.

- High premiums may discourage participation as well as increase moral hazard and adverse risk selection.

Risks with poor insurability profiles are sometimes initially written at a loss in order to build capacity. Inferior risks are frequently covered for social development or political reasons. This is not an insurance or reinsurance problem, however, and will not be further considered here.

Reinsurance Costs

In pro-rata treaties, the ceding commission paid by the reinsurer to the ceding insurer varies according to the reinsurer's estimate of the loss ratio to be incurred and the premium volume ceded under the treaty. It usually covers the primary insurer's acquisition expenses without providing a long-term commission "profit" or incentive to the insurer to cede a larger amount of business than necessary. Retrospective *(profit-sharing)* commission arrangements are common.

In excess-loss treaties, the rate-setting procedure is more complicated because the reinsurer expects long-term profitability. However, market competition in reinsurance often drives reinsurance rates below the "normal" rate. The rate is usually defined as the expected losses divided by the premium volume (the burning cost) and multiplied by a profit margin. When the primary company's net retention increases (a similarity with the deductible clause), the rate also declines.

In financial reinsurance, an account is established at the start of a finite arrangement that is maintained according to a specific formula throughout the life of the contract. Over time, the account fluctuates according to experience under the contract. Coverage under finite reinsurance is generally broad and, at the beginning of the term, the insurer may pay a higher premium which, in addition to the customary reinsurance procedure, is invested and earns interest over a multiyear period.

Projected investment income is taken into account in calculating the future premium. Over time, in a limited-loss situation, finite insurance can cost much less than traditional products. However, in case of catastrophe risks, when the primary insurer sustains a loss, finite-risk products afford less protection than does traditional reinsurance.

WHAT DO COMMUNITY-BASED HEALTH INSURANCE FUNDS NEED?

Rarely can microinsurance units constitute a perfectly balanced portfolio, either because their business volume is too small or because the relatively large risks they cover acquire a disproportionate influence on the portfolio. Furthermore, sometimes a variety of related insured events cause a chain of losses with cumulative effect on the insurer.

Such adverse events can disrupt the balance of insured risks in the portfolio, so that large discrepancies occur between the initial, probability-based forecast and the actual gross results. The four functions of reinsurance are all needed at different times in a company's development, and the principles of a reinsurance program apply to all community-based health insurance funds (table 3.2).

Different types of contracts offer community-based reinsurance funds different advantages:

Quota-share. Quota-share contracts are suitable for young, developing companies or companies entering a new class of business. Because loss experience is limited, defining the correct premium is difficult, and the reinsurer bears part of the risk of any incorrect estimates.

Surplus. Surplus contracts are an excellent means of balancing the risk portfolio and limiting the heaviest exposures because retention can be set at different levels according to the class of risk (or business) and expected loss. This type of treaty

TABLE 3.2   Community Health Insurance and the Four Functions of Reinsurance

Function	Applicability	Effect
Financing	Yes	Define amount of capital available to direct insurance company to establish retention limits.
Capacity	Yes	Coverage of large sums and highly exposed risks may require limiting size of some accepted risks, by setting up boundaries for each type of risk, scaled down by nature, severity, and experience.
Stabilization of loss experience • Per risk • Per occurrence	Yes	• Calculate risk of fluctuation and risk of error in loss experience. • Calculate probability of company's risk of ruin by assuming catastrophic event.
Underwriting assistance	Yes	Lack of expertise is major factor for failing to establish optimal retention limits.

allows the direct insurer to adjust the acceptable risk to fit the company's financial situation at any time. One of the drawbacks of this type of contract is the considerable administrative work involved in determining retention and amount ceded.

Excess loss. Excess loss *per risk* (WXL-R), almost compulsory in a reinsurance program, is the best way for a company to hold probable claim peaks to an acceptable level. Excess loss *per occurrence* (cat-XL) is useful only for classes of business with a significant accumulation potential. *Per-risk and per-event excess loss* (WXL-E) combines WXL-R and a cat-XL coverage, which is very useful for health insurance risks.

Stop-loss. The stop-loss contract is preferred over all the others for an entire line of business or portfolio. It provides insurers with the most comprehensive protection for the business in their retention, but it cannot be used to guarantee a profit for the insurer. Nonetheless, it is a useful solution where the insurer wants protection against a real threat to its existence as a result of an accumulation of negative influences all in the same year.

Alternative risk transfer. ART, characterized by the provision of funding arrangements for perceived risks, involves the long-term use of traditional reinsurance operations and derivative instruments or capital market operations. This is a primary reason this approach is particularly suitable for small health insurance funds.

Timing risk is at least as important as underwriting risk in finite-risk arrangements. This coverage smooths out current and future premium and claims patterns. For schemes with a high social-welfare component and no demonstrable commercial viability at the beginning of their operations, traditional reinsurance is unlikely to be available. Finite-risk products appear to be a viable solution here because the underwriting result is traded over a longer investment period.

However, traditional reinsurance may still be useful with a very high franchise to cover catastrophe risks. A catastrophe severe enough for a high franchise to be reached occurs only once in a while, and the risk can be commercially assessed.

Substitute for Own Funds

Substantial own funds are traditionally viewed as the mark of a healthy financial position, but using own funds to cover peaks in risk is not recommended. Reinsurance will serve as an aid to financing, especially for newly established insurance companies, because in the case of finite quota-share treaties, for example, the reinsurer shares proportionally both in costs and the formation of actuarial provisions.

Many of the insurance schemes implemented so far in developing countries for small groups and rural populations have not been financially self-sufficient and may require subsidization of premiums, administrative expenses, or both.[2] Again, this is not an insurance or reinsurance problem per se, but subsidies will be discussed later in this book (Busse, chapter 13, this volume). Even if insurance schemes cannot be expected to be economically viable in the short run, a cost-effective reinsurance program should be devised, one that does not rely unduly on reinsurance as a substitute for own funds.

Reinsurance is not a panacea for all the problems of microinsurers in developing countries. The schemes may not be commercially viable, and the private sector has little interest in participating in them. Reinsurance in itself cannot increase productivity or provide financing, although it can enhance both, as it does for microfinance schemes.

Reducing Risk by Equalizing Reserves

By its nature, the business of insuring small community-based health insurance funds can be subject to wide fluctuations in claims. A spread-loss treaty is the most useful instrument for protecting the ceding insurer's portfolio from these swings. As another precaution, an equalization reserve can be set up in fiscal years with light claims.

HOW DOES A REINSURANCE PROGRAM WORK?

Reinsurance assists the functioning of the law of large numbers in two ways. First, reinsuring a large number of primary insurers allows a reinsurance company to diversify risk in a way that a single insurer cannot. This can be done by allowing primary insurers to underwrite a larger number of loss exposures, by improving geographical spread, and by reducing the effective size of insured exposures.

Reinsurance plays a different financial intermediation role from a pure brokerage in several ways:

- It provides a mechanism for allocating funds to the most efficient premium capacity.

- It enables risks to be diversified and transferred from ultimate insurers.

- It enables changes to be made in the structure of insurance portfolios.

These considerations apply equally to national and international transactions, irrespective of the actors' geographical location. The presumption must be that efficiency in reinsurance intermediation is enhanced to the extent that agents have access to a global system of universal information about worldwide options, transaction costs, exchange-rate uncertainty, and any extra risk dimension in sovereign exposure.

"Utmost Good Faith"

Reinsurance contracts belonging to the class of contracts known as *uberrimae fidei* [utmost good faith] require fullest disclosure of all facts considered material to insured risks. This doctrine applies equally to both treaty and facultative reinsurance.

Details of every risk ceded to the reinsurer are forwarded in a bordereau. It includes information on insured risks as well as an estimate of the maximum possible loss, the company's net retention, and the amount reinsured. Because reinsurers are always bound to follow the primary insurer's settlements, reinsurance is an indemnity against the insurer's payment of a claim.

Pools

Under the basic principle of a reinsurance pool, all members create a common fund for a specific risk class and share agreed proportions of the aggregate claim liability. Profits, losses, and expenses are shared in the same way. A pooling system creates the capacity to handle risks of a catastrophic nature or of a special class with large risks (for example, aviation). It does not necessarily improve the underwriting results of the class of business.

Governmental pressure has been the initiating force in the formation of some pools among developing countries in some regions to reduce the flow of reinsurance premiums to reinsurers outside that region. Members must cede to the pool all business that falls within the scope of the arrangement. This pooled portfolio is then protected with a suitable reinsurance treaty. The usual practice is also to retrocede to each member proportionately according to the volume of business ceded by the member.

Although pools are usually formed to cede and redistribute proportional business (quota share), they may eventually operate on an excess-loss basis, that is, they may be liable for losses exceeding a certain amount in respect to each and every event. The proper functioning of any pool clearly requires that all members, although expecting to benefit from their participation, should put the community's interest before their own individual interests.

Reinsurance Companies

Risk sharing among several companies is usually confined to a limited area with similar market conditions. A company accepting reciprocity from other companies is faced with the difficulty of thoroughly investigating the business offered. This is especially difficult for small companies in which management's efforts would be dissipated between the company's prime objectives and the managerial activity necessary to secure and administer adequate reciprocity.

Reinsurance institutions provide an excellent means of serving the interests of participating insurance companies and the proper functioning of reinsurance. The mere existence of a reinsurance institution in a developing country has usually promoted sound market development. A local reinsurance institution can provide local companies with information about risks, tariffs, and claims as well as broad knowledge of market conditions and many other matters that small companies cannot possibly acquire on their own.

In the past, few major markets have been in a position to offer reinsurance on an international scale. However, increased demand for reinsurance all over the world has spurred a rapid expansion in the number of reinsurers, particularly in countries that offer offshore facilities. Captive companies, syndicates such as Lloyds, associations, and pools have also been formed to provide a market. More recently, the entry of large primary insurers has expanded this market (box 3.1).

The reinsurance environment for operating microinsurance schemes is discussed in part 3 of this book, which deals with the implementation challenge.

SUMMARY

Insurance companies everywhere, regardless of type and size, use reinsurance. It is a mechanism that allows an insurance company to share the assumed risks with others, so as to improve the spread and moderate fluctuations in the net results.

BOX 3.1   THE WORLD REINSURANCE MARKET

The volume of international reinsurance today is large, but no one knows exactly how large. According to Standard & Poor's, the first 125 reinsurers, covering more than 90 percent of the world's reinsurance capacity, wrote premiums worth US$72 million in 1999, and the top 30 companies wrote about 75 percent. A few companies rule this market. The top 15 companies wrote about 59 percent of total net premiums in 1995. The top 15 companies hail from only four countries.

Country	Market share (percent)	Number of companies
Germany	35.41	17
United States	27.14	37
Switzerland	9.24	4
United Kingdom	8.06	11
Bermuda	4.96	15
France	3.09	7
Ireland	1.85	7
Japan	1.35	1
Italy	1.25	2
Australia	1.03	3
Other countries	6.62	21
Total	100.00	125

Source: Top 125 companies in 1999, listed by Standard & Poor's 2001.

The reinsurance functions and methods explained in this chapter apply equally to small community-based health insurance funds. The four functions—financing, capacity, stabilization, and catastrophe protection—are all needed to protect a company's development. Nontraditional reinsurance or finite-risk reinsurance are well suited to the company's needs.

NOTES

1. A complete analysis of the principle and functioning of reinsurance contracts is available in the following references: Gerathewohl 1980; Kiln 1981; Outreville 1998; and IAIS Reinsurance Subcommittee 2000.

2. If no provision is made for a reasonable amount of insurance coverage via the price mechanism, subsidization of the reinsurance mechanism is one way to make insurance accessible. While the subsidization of the health care sector is widely accepted, the subsidization of health insurance schemes remains a contentious issue.

REFERENCES

Gerathewohl, K. 1980. *Reinsurance Principles and Practice*. Karlsruhe: Verlag Versicherungs-wirtschaft.

IAIS Reinsurance Subcommittee. 2000. *Reinsurance and Re-insurers*. Working Paper. Basle: International Association of Insurance Supervisors.

Kiln, R. 1981. *Reinsurance in Practice*. London: Witherby & Co.

Outreville, J.F. 1998. *Theory and Practice of Insurance*. Boston: Kluwer Academic Publishers.

CHAPTER 4

From Microfinance to Micro Health Insurance

Bernd Balkenhol and Craig Churchill

The delivery of health insurance services to low-income communities is an exciting opportunity to improve the quality of life of the working poor. This concept is still being tested, but the learning curve can be shortened if microinsurers and reinsurers consider lessons gleaned from the delivery of other financial services to the same market. Since microfinance institutions are potential delivery agents for insurance, it is important to recognize their diversity, strengths, and weaknesses. Toward these ends, this chapter:

- Describes imperfections in the financial markets that microfinance was designed to overcome;

- Introduces a typology of microfinance actors and presents the accomplishments of leading microfinance institutions;

- Outlines the debate regarding subsidies to microfinance institutions;

- Summarizes microfinance institutions' brief experiences in providing insurance;

- Analyzes the characteristics of successful microfinance institutions that may be relevant to microinsurance delivery; and

- Considers the implications of the microfinance experience for the development of microinsurance.

THE EVOLUTION OF MICROFINANCE

Microfinance began as microcredit in Bangladesh in the mid-1970s. Microcredit had a two-pronged development strategy: to reduce poverty through loans for income-generating activities (for example, cattle fattening and paddy husking) and to empower the landless poor, especially women, through education and consciousness raising that was integrated into the credit-delivery system. At about

The authors acknowledge, with thanks, helpful comments on a draft of this chapter from Paul Siegel, World Bank, Social Protection Sector, and Michael McCord, an independent consultant who is creating a global Microinsurance Center to promote the partner-agent model.

the same time in Latin America, microcredit emerged with a slightly different spin: to generate economic growth and create jobs by providing loans, with a limited emphasis on empowerment, to market vendors, street hawkers, home-based manufacturers, and other poor entrepreneurs. Both microcredit varieties used credit for productive purposes: to boost income and reduce poverty. To reach these goals, microcredit had to overcome several market imperfections that prevented the poor from accessing formal financial services (box 4.1).

Collateral Requirements

Banks require security for their loans, but the poor have few assets. Microcredit providers had to rely on collateral alternatives such as social capital, peer pressure,

---

BOX 4.1   WHY DON'T COMMERCIAL INSURERS SERVE THE LOW-INCOME MARKET?

Lenders and insurers, for many of the same reasons, have traditionally viewed poor people as unacceptably risky. The obstacles to serving the poor come from both the customer side and the insurer/banker side. The obstacles include economic, social, operational, and policy issues—some real, some perceived.

BANKING BARRIERS
The operational and economic obstacles are real. High transaction costs on small loans and savings accounts, and the disparate locations of some low-income communities, result in high operating costs. For a commercial bank, other markets offer more lucrative investment opportunities. A prudent policy environment, including large capital and reserve requirements, also creates disincentives for banks to serve the poor.

Traditional bankers have a limited understanding of low-income communities' needs. Because they cannot relate to this market, they do not try to find ways of serving it. This is particularly true in an uncompetitive banking sector such as jurisdictions that restrict the entry of foreign banks. In some competitive environments, the margins on services to the upper-end market are being squeezed, which encourages some banks to consider serving the relatively untapped markets of small and microenterprises and low-income communities in general.

Many poor people do not even think of requesting services from a financial institution. The atmosphere in a bank can be intimidating. A prospective depositor or borrower would have to deal with significant cultural and educational barriers: speaking a business language (often different from the local language) and being sufficiently literate to complete the paperwork. Even if the prospective customer is persistent, tolerant, and educated enough to overcome these barriers, it is unlikely that the financial institution's products are appropriate (for example, savings accounts with large opening balances and loan sizes that exceed the applicant's needs).

(Box continues on the following page.)

BOX 4.1 (continued)

INSURANCE BARRIERS

In the insurance market, all these barriers—and then some—apply to the institutions' relations with poor people. The low-income market is vulnerable to risk, especially health-related problems, and insurable and uninsurable health events are hard to separate. Private insurers that apply risk rating are likely to charge poor people higher rates because of higher expected losses. Frequent small claims also increase transaction costs. Even if the poor could afford the high premiums insurers have to charge to cover costs, the insurer might prefer not to serve the low-end market to avoid the public relations problem of charging the poor more than the low-risk/low-transaction rich.

Since insurance is more complicated than saving or lending, design adjustments to suit the market are also more complicated. With loans, microfinance institutions have had to overcome information asymmetries and collateral problems. Although health insurers need not deal with collateral, they must address information asymmetries, ensure regular premium payments, and reduce exposure to moral hazard, overuse, adverse selection, and fraud.

Another unique obstacle is the market's perception of insurance. Evidence of indigenous mutual support in anticipation of future risks is uncommon. As a rule, poor people pay for health care when they need it by direct spot transaction from patient to healer. Changing from spot transaction to prepayment for a future service is not always accepted or trusted. As a result, it is difficult to explain to this market how insurance works and why it offers better utility and financial protection than spot payments.

Since the poor have limited resources, they want to get the most for their money. If they pay premiums but do not need to make a claim (and they hope they will not), they believe that they wasted their meager resources. Early experience with short-term, voluntary health insurance suggests that the poor who make no claims are much more likely to drop out than are policyholders who do make claims (McCord 2001).

The complicated pricing and operational obstacles to serving a high-risk market have kept commercial insurers from targeting the poor. With no assurance of success, they hesitate to invest in an educational marketing strategy and product adaptations to attract this market. Insufficient actuarial information also makes it difficult to apply sound pricing techniques. However, once effective methods of providing health insurance are developed and it is shown that this market can be served profitably, commercial insurers may think twice about their involvement.

and character lending. Some microcredit providers also require an up-front deposit of part of the loan as a compensating savings balance (typically between 10 percent and 25 percent of the loan amount). Some microlenders accept nontraditional collateral such as personal effects to secure larger microloans.

Information Asymmetries

Banks traditionally overcome information asymmetries by requiring borrowers to submit business plans, credit histories, and other documentation. For the low-income market, these approaches are inappropriate. Some microcredit providers lend to self-selected borrower groups that know each other socially or through work. Alternatively, microcredit providers use cosigners, guarantors, or the endorsement of community leaders.

Perceived Risk

Besides the collateral and information asymmetries, the key design elements in minimizing credit risk include small loans for short terms, frequent repayment periods (often weekly with new borrowers), a personal relationship between loan officer and client, and a zero tolerance for delinquency. With the right lending methodology, the poor are better credit risks than the not-so-poor because they take their obligations more seriously and do not want to lose their best, or perhaps only, source of financial services (Churchill 1999; Stack and Thys 2000).

Efficiencies

The process of issuing many small loans (often below $300) can be labor-intensive, especially considering the design elements required to suppress credit risk. Many microcredit providers rely on borrower groups to improve efficiencies (and serve as a collateral substitute). They also streamline application requirements to fit the small loan size. Further efficiencies are generated with repeat borrowers who have established a strong credit history. The achievement of significant scale, at least 10,000 to 15,000 borrowers, also helps to spread fixed overhead costs (for example, back office, information systems) over an adequate customer base. Additional efficiencies are gained by decentralizing decisionmaking and by paying incentives to encourage loan officers to achieve optimum productivity and portfolio quality with minimal supervision.

Costs

To a banker, the costs of serving this market seem prohibitive, but microfinance has a completely different cost structure, and operational ratios between the two cannot be compared. By offering simple products, microcredit providers keep costs down—they do not need expensive staff to deliver the products. Many microcredit providers also charge high interest rates to cover the costs of providing small loans—sometimes annual effective rates of 30 to 40 percent or higher (box 4.2).

BOX 4.2   CHARGING THE POOR HIGH INTEREST RATES?

It seems counterintuitive that an organization dedicated to helping the poor needs to charge high interest rates and strive for profitability. From a long-term perspective, however, the commercial approach makes sense. Microfinance has the unique ability to provide sustainable development services if they are designed and implemented properly. Clients do not want lending or savings facilities just for the next three to five years. They want—and deserve—a safe place to save their money and a convenient place to borrow funds indefinitely. Only by fulfilling the commercial mission of microfinance can lenders provide this valuable service over time—and generate its important development benefits.

Motivation

Besides all of the valid business reasons that keep banks from serving the low-income market, there are also social and cultural obstacles. Few bankers know or want to know this market. Microcredit providers address this challenge by filling field positions with socially motivated staff from local communities (their local knowledge also helps reduce information asymmetries).

Many efforts to overcome these market imperfections were successful. In the mid- to late 1980s, two new aspects were incorporated into microfinance that made it a more effective and enduring development strategy: the realization that income on small loans could cover costs and the recognition that there was a demand for voluntary savings services. If microlending was done well, it could be part of a *sustainable* development strategy. Microcredit thus became a favorite of donors looking to provide subsidies for a finite period of time to an initiative that would continue to provide low-income communities with development benefits long after the grant spigot was turned off. The introduction of *savings* into the discussion turned microcredit into microfinance and changed the perspective from helping entrepreneurs to providing low-income communities with financial services. This shift in perspective came from the realization that savers and borrowers are usually different people. Entrepreneurs are not noted for their saving habits since they often plough excess cash back into their businesses. Yet, depending on the market, credit unions and other financial intermediaries for low-income communities find an average of five savers for every borrower, with savers depositing enough money to meet borrower demand (Richardson 2000; McDonald 2000).

UNDERSTANDING MICROFINANCE TODAY

This section defines three key elements of microfinance and introduces a typology of microfinance practitioners that reveals a diversity of institutional forms. It then provides data on the financial performance of microfinance institutions around the world that expose important geographical differences in accomplishments, outreach, and motives.

Defining Microfinance

Microfinance is defined as the provision of financial services to the poor on a sustainable basis. This working definition encompasses three elements: the range of financial services provided, a focus on poverty reduction, and sustainability.

Microfinance involves a *range of financial services*, even if loans have been the de facto focus of many microfinance institutions. The provision of deposit-taking facilities, payment services, remittances, leasing, and insurance are part of microfinance. Different financial services are often closely linked. Some microfinance institutions, for example, require clients to purchase life or property insurance as part of a credit transaction.

The focus on *poverty reduction* is a fundamental element of microfinance. Outreach to the poor is the social mission of microfinance, which distinguishes it from normal finance. But this focus is interpreted differently in different regions or between different microfinance institutions. Some insist on serving the poor exclusively, through targeting and motivational methods, and try to push the envelope deeper to serve extremely poor clients. Other organizations are content to serve a broader range of low-income individuals and look to income from larger loans (although still small from a banker's perspective) to subsidize losses on the smallest loans.

Microfinance also has a commercial mission: microfinance institutions should be *sustainable*; they should make at least enough money to cover their cost of doing business—perhaps not immediately, perhaps not completely, but the aim is for poverty reduction to eventually become viable on market terms. Whether microfinance institutions' financial performance matches this claim remains to be seen. In the meantime, the microfinance field is enveloped in a debate about how fast to phase out subsidies (chapter 13, this volume). Microfinance proponents take it for granted that some kind of subsidy is needed during a transition period of unspecified duration.

Typology of Microfinance

The microfinance field is diverse, in constant evolution, with moving boundaries. While the term microcredit has been around for the past 25 years, applied mainly to externally initiated schemes often implemented by nongovernmental organizations (NGOs), other structures also offer sustainable financial services to the poor. Microfinance runs the gamut from informal to formal, with a wide range of ownership and governance structures, sources of capital, levels of external regulation and supervision, motivations, and degrees of success.

ROSCAs. Rotating savings and credit associations (ROSCAs) are indigenous bodies, usually run by volunteer or collective management. Members of these informal associations do not sign loan contracts, and the agreements are not enforceable under civil law. ROSCAs are usually small (5 to 50 members), and all capital is internally generated. ROSCAs do not have to answer to any supervisory authority or respect any externally defined prudential ratios.

Credit unions. Credit unions (savings and credit cooperatives) are larger, more formal versions of ROSCAs in several respects. They are member-owned and -governed financial intermediaries for people who have a common bond such as residence location or place of work. Because of the boundaries of this common bond, outreach for individual credit unions is limited (a hundred to a few thousand members). This type of microfinance institution, however, has shown an amazing capacity to form networks and build pyramids of common organizations. Credit unions reach more customers in most countries than do other formal microfinance institutions (with some notable exceptions such as in Bangladesh and Indonesia). Credit unions are savings-driven organizations, usually with many more depositors than borrowers. Most of their capital comes from member shares and deposits. The extent of external supervision varies by region, sometimes involving a secondary or tertiary credit union association as well as some form of government oversight. Access to external sources of capital varies, but where it exists it can be destabilizing. Some credit unions have achieved mixed financial results; a relationship to a strong tertiary association often makes the difference between success and failure (Balkenhol 1999).

NGOs. The NGO structure is the most widely recognized type of microfinance institution. Because NGO-microfinance institutions usually receive donor funding, they are regularly scrutinized and documented to justify the use of public money. A scan through the microfinance literature therefore finds this type of organization overrepresented. As with credit unions, the degrees of success range significantly. Most microfinance NGOs usually peak at around 20,000 borrowers. Some NGOs are profitable, but many rely on donor subsidies to continue operations. NGOs are credit driven, and they are usually restricted from offering voluntary savings services (as contrasted with compulsory compensating balances sometimes required to access a loan). NGOs do not have owners as such, and governance by volunteering professionals is often weak. These organizations are not externally regulated or supervised, with the exception of NGOs that belong to international networks such as ACCION International or Women's World Banking.

Transformed NGOs. Some of the most successful microcredit NGOs have become regulated financial institutions, usually as a commercial bank or nonbank financial institution (NBFI). The first, BancoSol in Bolivia, is the most prominent example, but 20 or more microfinance banks operating today began as NGOs, including some in Africa and Asia as well as Latin America, where they are more common. There are usually two related motivations for upscaling: to leverage private capital that will enable a dramatic increase in outreach and to provide financial services, especially savings, that an NGO cannot offer. Private shareholders, who typically see their investment in social terms rather than as an opportunity to maximize returns, own this new breed of microfinance institution. These shareholders include development corporations, private foundations, microfinance investment funds, and socially responsible individuals. Transformed NGOs are generally more profitable, more stable, and potentially larger than NGO microfinance institutions (Campion and White 1999; Glosser 1994).

Downscaling banks. A handful of banks around the world are downscaling— either developing products or creating subsidiaries to serve low-income communities. Their motivations vary. Some have a social element in their ownership structure (for example, the government or the Catholic Church). Some are being pushed down-market by stiff competition for traditional banking clients, especially in industrial countries where banks such as Wells Fargo are using credit-scoring technologies to target previously untapped markets. Others enter this market as a public relations strategy to stave off, or in response to, political pressure. As financial institutions, they are probably the strongest type of microfinance institution, but their commitment to the target market may be thin and their outreach limited. Some government-owned commercial banks are exceptions to the thin commitment–limited scale characterization, most notably Bank Rakyat Indonesia (BRI), whose microfinance division serves more than 2.5 million depositors and a million borrowers.

Private companies. Another new entrant into microfinance is private companies that extend credit to low-income individuals. These companies are either social entrepreneurs that want to bypass the NGO as the initial phase and go straight to running a microfinance institution as a business, or institutionalized moneylenders that see low-income individuals as a profitable market niche. Donor money may support the social entrepreneurs, who may intend to create a bank once they have a strong track record. The institutionalized moneylenders usually focus on salaried individuals (for example, low-level civil servants, unskilled laborers) whose employers often deduct repayments from their salaries. Salary-backed lending is a low-risk, high-return service that can quickly reach large volumes of customers. This type of microlending is most prevalent in South Africa where it is receiving an increasing amount of attention from consumer protection authorities rather than from banking officials.

Microfinance is not monolithic. This typology, summarized in table 4.1, reveals the diversity of models, motivations, and shades of success prevalent in this fast-changing industry. Downscaling banks and private companies would not have been included in most microfinance discussions just five years ago, and the movement to transform NGOs into banks is not even 10 years old.

TABLE 4.1   Typology of Microfinance Institutions

Institution	Source of capital	Ownership and governance	Regulation and supervision	Scale (number of members/clients)	Profitability	Motives
ROSCAs	Internally generated	Member-owned and -managed	None	Less than 100	Sustainable but not always durable	Self-help
CUs	Mostly member shares and savings	Member-owned and -governed	Secondary or tertiary CU associations, sometimes government officials	100 to 5,000	Not profit-maximizers but can be profitable	Improve members' economic and social well-being
NGOs	Donors, retained earnings, occasional commercial funds	Voluntary board usually consisting of local professionals and management	No government oversight. Some NGOs are members of international networks that provide limited supervision	1,000 to 1 million (but most commonly between 1,000 and 20,000)	Occasionally, but most are not	Reduce poverty, but increasingly using commercial means to achieve that objective
Transformed NGOs (upscalers)	Private equity that leverages commercial borrowings; some savings mobilization	Socially responsible individuals, corporations, and donor representatives	By banking officials	Bigger than NGOs, usually tens of thousands	Yes	Social and commercial
Downscalers	Deposits; equity and commercial debt	Wholly owned subsidiary of bank; or department within bank	By banking officials	Several thousand to a couple of million	Yes	Public relations, profitable niche market, sometimes social
Private company, socially responsible	Private equity, occasional donor support	Private owners	Not usually, unless they are NBFIs	Several thousand	After start-up phase	Socially responsible entrepreneurs
Private company, moneylender	Private equity	Private owners	Increasingly by consumer protection authorities	Can quickly achieve 10,000 to 100,000 clients	Yes	Profitable niche market

Note: ROSCAs, rotating savings and credit associations; NGOs, nongovernmental organizations; NBFI, nonbank financial institution; CU, credit union.

The State of the Microfinance Industry

The handful of flagship microfinance practitioners includes the Grameen Bank, Bangladesh Rural Advancement Committee (BRAC), and Association for Social Advancement (ASA) in Bangladesh, BRI in Indonesia, and BancoSol in Bolivia. These large microfinance institutions, however, are only part of the picture.

According to a recent survey of network-affiliated microfinance institutions (Lapenu and Zeller 2000):

- 48 percent have fewer than 2,500 members.

- 7.5 percent have more than 100,000 members.

- 3 percent serve more than 80 percent of all clients.

This wide divide in scale is supported by data in the *MicroBanking Bulletin*, a semiannual journal that collects performance information from more than 120 leading microfinance institutions around the world. The bulletin organizes the data into peer groups of institutions on the basis of three characteristics: region, size,[1] and target market.[2] The peer group averages for selected performance indicators in table 4.2 reveal the diversity of the microfinance industry, including striking regional differences.

The most obvious difference involves size. Microfinance institutions in the Asia Large peer group dwarf all others with an average of 2 million customers and US$352 million in loans outstanding. The peer group with the second largest outreach, LA Large, averages fewer than 30,000 borrowers.

TABLE 4.2   Performance Indicators for Microfinance Institutions, by Size and Region

Peer group MFI (country)	Number of borrowers	Outstanding portfolio (US$)	Average US$ loan balance per borrower (percent of GDP per capita)	Real yield (percent)	Adjusted return on assets (percent)	Portfolio at risk > 90 days (percent)
1. Africa Medium	14,668	1,525,339	128	34.5	13.5	0.8
Citi S&L (Ghana), FINCA Uganda, KWFT	*7,286*	*613,677*	*35*	*12.0*	*10.3*	*0.7*
(Kenya), NRB (Ghana), Pamécas (Senegal),			*(33.6)*			
Pride Tanzania, Pride Uganda, Pride Vita			*(14.8)*			
(Guinea), SEF (South Africa), WAGES (Togo)						
2. Africa Small	5,633	512,948	91.8	44.2	−11.4	2.4
ARB (Ghana), Faulu (Uganda), FINCA	*2,802*	*215,068*	*29.0*	*15.9*	*9.8*	*2.4*
Malawi, FINCA Tanzania, FOCCAS			*(31.3)*			
(Uganda), MKRB (Ghana), Piyeli (Mali),			*(11.6)*			
SAT (Ghana), SEDA, UWFT (Uganda),						
Vital-Finance (Benin)						
3. Africa/MENA	15,411	6,445,652	492	21.7	−0.7	4.0
ABA (Egypt, Arab Rep.), Kafo Jiginew	*2,903*	*1,235,647*	*237*	*0.7*	*2.8*	*3.3*
(Mali), Nyésigiso (Mali), PADME (Benin),			*(81.8)*			
UNRWA (Gaza)			*(22.0)*			
4. Asia (Central)/MENA	8,042	1,310,412	166	36.8	−11.2	0.1
Al Amana (Morocco), Al Majmoua	*6,789*	*617,411*	*62*	*3.7*	*10.2*	*0.1*
(Lebanon), Constanta (Georgia), Faten			*(11.9)*			
(West Bank/Gaza), FINCA Kyrgyzstan,			*(3.9)*			
Microfund for Women (Jordan)						

(Table continues on the following page.)

TABLE 4.2 (continued)

Peer group MFI (country)	Number of borrowers	Outstanding portfolio (US$)	Average US$ loan balance per borrower (percent of GDP per capita)	Real yield (percent)	Adjusted return on assets (percent)	Portfolio at risk > 90 days (percent)
5. Asia Large	2,046 752	352,532,707	194	17.6	4.7	2.0
ACLEDA (Cambodia), ASA (Bangladesh),	*835,243*	*430,311,722*	*112*	*4.9*	*3.0*	*1.2*
BAAC (Thailand), BRAC (Bangladesh),			(33.6)			
BRI (Indonesia)			*(13.3)*			
6. Asia (Pacific)	12,974	1,509,701	159	36.3	0.7	2.8
CARD Bank (Philippines), EMT (Cambodia),	*11,424*	*906,275*	*24*	*5.1*	*3.4*	*3.1*
Hatta Kaksekar (Cambodia), Hublag			(14.3)			
(Philippines), RSPI (Philippines),			*(2.3)*			
TSPI (Philippines)						
7. Asia (South)	25,764	2,220,962	82	13.3	−6.8	1.7
AKRSP (Pakistan), Basix (India), BURO	*19,443*	*1,487,520*	*36*	*8.2*	*3.9*	*2.5*
Tangail (Bangladesh), CDS (India), FWWB			(22.0)			
(India), KASHF (Pakistan), Nirdhan (Nepal),			*(8.6)*			
SEEDS (Sri Lanka), SHARE (India)						
8. Eastern Europe High	1,377	2,698,678	2,249	15.3	−2.3	0.1
AMK (Bosnia and Herzegovina), LOK						
(Bosnia and Herzegovina), Moznosti	*504*	*516,150*	*526*	*3.1*	*1.4*	*0.1*
(Bosnia and Herzegovina), Sunrise (Bosnia			(202.8)			
and Herzegovina), WVB (Bosnia and			*(41.8)*			
Herzegovina)						
9. Eastern Europe Broad	2,652	2,352,138	1,088	22.7	−0.3	1.0
Bospo (Bosnia and Herzegovina), Fundusz	*1,916*	*1,253,418*	*301*	*5.2*	*2.1*	*0.9*
Mikro (Poland), Inicjatywa Mikro (Poland),			(66.2)			
MC (Bosnia and Herzegovina), Mikrofin			*(25.3)*			
(Bosnia and Herzegovina), Nachala						
(Bulgaria), NOA (Croatia)						
10. LA Large	29,730	27,175,166	971	29.9	2.3	2.6
BancoADEMI (Dominican Republic),	*9,360*	*8,699,651*	*279*	*3.5*	*1.3*	*0.7*
BancoSol (Bolivia), Caja de Los Andes			(70.3)			
(Bolivia), Calpiá (El Salvador), CM			*(26.0)*			
Arequipa (Peru), FIE (Bolivia), Finamérica						
(Colombia), Mibanco (Peru), PRODEM						
(Bolivia)						
11. LA Medium Broad	7,453	3,427,876	609	33.1	−1.9	2.8
ACODEP (Nicaragua), Actuar (Colombia),	*5,924*	*1,332,599*	*414*	*7.3*	*0.7*	*1.7*
ADOPEM (Dominican Republic), ADRI			(64.3)			
(Costa Rica), BPE (Dominican Republic),			*(29.1)*			
Chispa (Nicaragua), FAMA (Nicaragua),						
Finsol (Honduras), FONDECO (Bolivia),						
ProEmpresa (Peru), Sartawi (Bolivia)						
12. LA Small Low (upper-income						
countries)	2,182	1,669,824	788	40.3	−10.6	2.7
Banco do Povo (Brazil), CEAPE/ PE (Brazil),	*1,207*	*880,531*	*113*	*5.3*	*8.0*	*2.2*
Contigo (Chile), Emprender (Argentina),			(14.9)			
Portosol (Brazil), Vivacred (Brazil)			*(4.0)*			

(Table continues on the following page.)

TABLE 4.2 (continued)

Peer group MFI (country)	Number of borrowers	Outstanding portfolio (US$)	Average US$ loan balance per borrower (percent of GDP per capita)	Real yield (percent)	Adjusted return on assets (percent)	Portfolio at risk > 90 days (percent)
13. LA Medium Low	19,663	3,506,001	197	50.2	4.5	1.0
CAM (El Salvador), CMM Medellín	4,173	1,465,732	93	3.2	8.2	0.9
(Colombia), Compartamos (Mexico), Crecer			(12.4)			
(Bolivia), Enlace (Ecuador), FINCA			(2.8)			
Honduras, FMM Popayán (Colombia),						
FWWB Cali (Colombia), ProMujer (Bolivia)						
14. LA Small Low (lower-income						
countries)	8,975	853,632	91	55.3	−3.4	2.7
AGAPE (Colombia), FED (Ecuador), FINCA	3,127	409,407	17	6.4	6.9	2.2
Ecuador, FINCA Mexico, FINCA Nicaragua,			(6.3)			
FINCA Peru, WR Honduras			(4.0)			
15. LA Credit Unions	5,121	4,105,127	887	−9.5	−2.6	N/A
15 de Abril (Ecuador), 23 de Julio	1,504	1,295,656	420	32.4	4.4	
(Ecuador), Acredicom (Guatemala),			(56.7)			
Chuimequená (Guatemala), COOSAJO			(26.0)			
(Guatemala), Ecosaba (Guatemala),						
Moyután (Guatemala), Oscus (Ecuador),						
Sagrario (Ecuador), Tonantel (Guatemala),						
Tulcán (Ecuador)						
16. Worldwide Small Business	4,934	10,322 826	2,968	17.0	−2.1	1.0
ACEP (Senegal), Agrocapital (Bolivia),	3,348	2,30, 970	775	3.7	1.7	0.9
BDB (Indonesia), CERUDEB (Uganda),			(391.4)			
FEFAD (Albania), MEB (Bosnia and			(175.5)			
Herzegovina), NLC (Pakistan)						

MFI Microfinance institution.

Note: Data in italics are standard deviations. The averages are calculated based on the values between the 2d and the 99th percentile for each peer group. For acronym and program descriptions, refer to the appendix of the *MicroBanking Bulletin* 6 (April 2001).

Source: MicroBanking Standards Project 2001.

A comparison of performance between organizations also has to consider the differences in customer base. The average loan balance per borrower (and its relationship to gross domestic product [GDP] per capita) is a rough indicator of the customer's poverty level. This indicator ranges from 6.3 percent of GDP per capita (LA Small Low–Lower Income Countries) to 391.4 percent (Worldwide Small Business). In general, Asian microfinance institutions serve poorer clients; at the other extreme, East European organizations go farther up market. In another regional difference, interest rates (shown in the table through the proxy indicator yield) tend to be higher in Latin America and Africa than in Asia.

In terms of financial performance, it is certainly easier to be profitable if a microfinance institution serves a broad market instead of only the poorest, but it is not a prerequisite. Surprisingly, the peer group with the best return on assets is LA Medium Low, which has an average outstanding balance per customer of just $197, 12.4 percent of gross national product (GNP) per capita. Although only four peer groups produced an average positive return on assets, 64 of the 124 microfinance institutions are financially self-sufficient. This finding suggests a range of financial performance even within homogeneous peer groups. Extenuating circumstances also affect performance. For example, LA Credit Unions have historically been one of the *Bulletin's* strongest peer groups, but in 2000, high inflation in Ecuador caused the peer group average to reflect a negative real portfolio yield.

MICROFINANCE SUBSIDIES

MicroBanking Bulletin participants are among the world's most successful microfinance institutions. Of the hundreds, perhaps thousands, of microfinance institutions that do not submit data to the *Bulletin*, most are not profitable. The numerous microfinance institutions that do not generate enough income from their loan portfolios to cover their expenses require additional sources of revenue, in the form of donor subsidies (box 4.3).

BOX 4.3   THE ROLE OF DONORS IN EXPANDING MICROINSURANCE

Many organizations want to jump onto the microinsurance bandwagon because they think it looks like a good way to make money through new grant opportunities, premium payments, or both. Unfortunately, many of these organizations do not appreciate the challenges and risks of offering insurance. Insurance is a fundamentally different business from credit and savings, and microfinance institutions should not approach it uninformed. To improve their chances of success, microfinance institutions need technical assistance from insurance professionals. Donors receiving requests to support microinsurance pilot projects and action research initiatives have an important responsibility to guide and temper myopic enthusiasm.

Before offering insurance, a microfinance institution should have a long track record of excellent portfolio quality and financial sustainability. If it is not there yet, it is probably not ready to divert its attention from its core business. The microfinance institution should be interested in insurance for the right reason; it should have clear evidence of customer demand for insurance.

Donors have a range of opportunities for expanding the supply of microinsurance. Besides reinsurance, the following five areas are worth considering.

(Box continues on the following page.)

BOX 4.3 (continued)

- *Optimizing risk-managing financial services.* A holistic understanding is lacking about ways of using financial services to reduce vulnerability to different kinds of risks. Each financial service—savings, credit, and insurance—provides a different type of protection. More has to be learned about the optimal mix of financial products and about the conditions under which one is better than another.

- *Understanding demand for microinsurance.* Microfinance institutions that provide microinsurance as a mandatory part of membership do not have sufficient motivation to explore which services are most attractive to members. But where microinsurance depends on voluntary affiliation, a better understanding is needed of arguments that persuade clients to purchase the product and benefit types that are most attractive. Microinsurers need market research tools to help them develop appropriate products and marketing strategies.

- *Integration with savings.* The purpose of integrating insurance with other financial services is to reduce transaction costs and smooth out members' capacity to pay insurance premiums during periods of income fluctuations. Layering insurance on top of savings gives customers better value than credit/insurance layering (box 4.7). Current experiments with integrating savings and insurance should be better understood; developing new ways of combining these products can improve cost-effectiveness.

- *Improving risk-management knowledge.* Partnering with commercial and cooperative insurers is an important way for microfinance institutions to gain expertise (and financial resources) to develop microinsurance. Projects to increase involvement with these partners could include documenting existing partnerships; writing a business plan to market the microinsurance opportunity to potential partners; drafting guidelines for microfinance institutions on selecting a partner; facilitating discussions between microfinance institutions and insurers; creating incentives for insurers to collaborate with microfinance institutions; and developing apprenticeship and consultancy relationships between microinsurers and experienced insurers.

- *Microinsurance development fund.* Donors can initiate the creation of a centralized fund for microinsurance. This fund could have several roles, including acting as a source of funding for innovative start-ups and for transitional subsidies; documenting and disseminating best practices; providing technical assistance to microinsurers; providing indirect subsidies to microinsurers in the form of a guaranteed return on the investment of premiums; and advocating a regulatory framework for microinsurance practice.

Source: Adapted from Brown and Churchill 2000b.

Microfinance institutions provide a public good, namely access to vital financial services for people who would not have them otherwise and who might pose a financial, economic, social, or political risk. This is one rationale for donations to microfinance institutions. If, as supporters claim, this strategy will eventually pay for itself, external financial and technical support and promotion is time-bound.

Microfinance tries to serve as many poverty-stricken people as possible while achieving full sustainability. Balancing outreach and sustainability is an ongoing challenge and a source of debate within the industry. This debate roughly reflects the roots of microfinance: Southeast Asians advocate a focus on poverty while Latin Americans aggressively pursue sustainability. Depending on their ideological position, some donors put a premium on poverty outreach at the expense of a longer path toward cost coverage. Others make a priority of attaining sustainability as quickly as possible and assume that, once established and mature, an institution will be in a more stable position to cater to the poor.

But the justification for subsidies does not mean that all grants are good. Subsidies distort the market. Bad examples of good intentions litter the short history of microfinance. Some donors, for example, have made subsidized lines of credit available to credit unions for specific purposes such as on-lending to farmers or women entrepreneurs. Credit unions might be attracted by the cheap source of capital, but it gives them a disincentive to mobilize deposits and can undermine a credit union's democratic spirit if some members (for example, farmers or women entrepreneurs) receive special treatment (Morris 1999).

The availability of donor money has encouraged many development and relief organizations to add microcredit projects to integrated development programs. The resulting project approach is a recipe for disaster because managers lack technical expertise in microfinance and do not strive for sustainability, since the project is only supposed to last three to five years. Alternatively, donor money has encouraged some real microfinance institutions to provide nonfinancial services such as business and technical skill training and market linkages. Adding noncore services often impairs an organization's performance by overloading limited management capacity.

And donors have behaved like donors: They have not required microfinance grantees to meet investment-grade standards of transparency and accountability. Traditionally, donors have been less interested in a microfinance institution's portfolio at risk or return on equity than in social results (for example, number of jobs created, percentage of female borrowers). They have also been slow to cut off funding to underperforming microfinance institutions because of its ramifications for clients who might lose their only source of institutionalized financial services. In any case, if one donor did pull out, others might readily fill their shoes, so high is microcredit's profile. Instead of promoting sustainability, donors are often complicit in (although not solely responsible for) creating a dependency that has retarded the microfinance industry's maturation.

MICROINSURANCE AS PART OF MICROFINANCE

Most poor clients, especially women, do not expect spectacular rises in their incomes as a result of participation in a microfinance scheme. Income stabilization, achieved through a modest increase in business sales, is usually their primary motivation. Only after the household has a stable economic foundation do a few clients aspire toward more significant business growth, including hiring employees instead of relying on family labor. This behavior reflects a sense of vulnerability that must be addressed before a person can seriously pursue business growth. Microfinance can reduce vulnerability in the face of a host of economic stresses, including seasonal variations in income, illness or death of a breadwinner, unstable and precarious employment, and expenses linked to life-cycle events such as births, weddings, and funerals. The integrated nature of the household and the business means that any business-related incident has dramatic implications for family income, and vice versa.

Although microfinance can help clients achieve these risk-management objectives, most microfinance products are not specifically designed to do so. Only a handful of microfinance institutions offer emergency loans and, with the exception of credit unions, few offer open-access savings accounts. The microenterprise loan products most commonly offered by microfinance institutions are rigid in structure and not particularly responsive to emergency needs. Slowly, microfinance institutions are recognizing their clientele's risk-management needs, and some are developing appropriate savings and credit products.

Some microfinance institutions are venturing into the world of insurance. Their motivations for offering insurance reflect the social and commercial mission of microfinance. Their customers' vulnerability is becoming increasingly evident to microfinance institutions, especially when health issues interfere with repayments, contribute to loan losses, and hinder institutional growth. At the same time, microfinance institutions see potential institutional benefits from insurance, including cross-selling opportunities, increased client retention, and improved portfolio quality and profitability (box 4.4).

The most common type of insurance offered by microfinance institutions is a credit-life product covering the outstanding loan balance if the borrower dies. This product benefits the institution more than the borrower, but coverage has occasionally been expanded to include life insurance for family members and additional payouts to cover funeral expenses. Credit unions have a long history of providing credit-life as well as a life-savings product that pays a beneficiary a multiple of a savings balance if the account holder dies. Few microfinance institutions offer property insurance, except to protect assets bought with a loan (Brown and Churchill 2000a).

A few microfinance institutions are experimenting with the delivery of health insurance services to their clients, either on their own or, preferably, as agents for a health insurance provider. Experience thus far reveals the enormous challenges of delivering such services sustainably, as they are prone to fraud and overuse. Poor customers' ability to afford commercially priced health insurance policies

BOX 4.4   MICRO CARE: USING A PARTNER-AGENT MODEL TO DELIVER HEALTH INSURANCE

Together, a microfinance NGO and a catholic hospital in Uganda experimented with providing health insurance for the poor that neither could offer individually (see figure 4.1). FINCA Uganda (FU), the microfinance organization, saw many of its borrowers struggle to repay their enterprise loans when confronting illness. It also recognized that it did not have the expertise to offer health insurance, having had difficulties managing health coverage for its own staff. At about the same time, the Nsambya Hospital contracted with a team of professionals to develop a strategy and business plan and to start operating what became Nsambya Health Insurance Plan (NHHP), an insurer for low-income communities.

From their experience with low-income markets, NHHP's management recognized that income fluctuations deterred the poor from purchasing insurance because of uncertainty about being able to pay premiums on schedule. NHHP thought that partnering with a savings facility could help overcome this problem. Instead of dealing with individuals, NHHP also preferred to deal with a single strong policyholder, representing a group.

Thus, a natural synergy emerged between NHHP and FINCA Uganda. NHHP wanted to target clients who were already accumulating savings, and FU offered access to a village-banking program with an established list of clients. The microfinance institution perceived significant indirect advantages from a healthier clientele, including improved attendance and on-time repayment. By offering this additional service, FU hoped to improve customer retention and gain an advantage over competitors.

FU facilitated NHHP's outreach by introducing their clients to the health insurer. FU also helped groups prepare their premium payments (although this transaction was between the individual client and NHHP). The arrangement provided credit officers with informal training as they watched NHHP sales techniques and learned about the health insurance plan by listening to explanations to new members.

A third party, the United Kingdom's Department for International Development (DfID), also played a role by covering deficits from claims and operating costs. The donor guarantee was critical during the start-up phase since NHHP had no reserves. Nor could NHHP access reinsurance, normally the next line of defense for insurers after reserves, for it is not (yet) a regulated insurer. DfID's subsidies enabled NHHP to test systems and methodologies for serving the poor. To limit its own risk, DfID reserved the right to monitor pricing and achievement of business plan objectives.

This arrangement allowed each party to do what it does best. The microfinance institution could concentrate on its credit and savings business, while providing clients with access to health insurance but without bearing the insurance risk or processing claims. NHHP tested the operation of health insurance to low-income communities by tapping into ready-made groups. Nsambya Hospital delivered health care to poor people and increased its client base. And DfID facilitated the collaboration of these three organizations through donor funding.

(Box continues on the following page.)

BOX 4.4 (continued)

After the pilot phase, a core team from NHHP broke away and incorporated as an autonomous body, under the name MicroCare. Several insights gained from the pilot have changed the way MicroCare operates. For one, the client base has been enlarged to four microfinance institutions, and the link with FINCA was ended. The insurer has enlarged its list of providers to include four hospitals, partly to widen customer choice and to encourage competition between providers. Donor funding continues to replace autonomous contingency reserves. Although DfID has ceased its involvement, other donors are expected to provide deficit financing for MicroCare.

Source: Adapted from McCord 2000.

FIGURE 4.1   NHHP/FINCA Uganda Health Financing Product

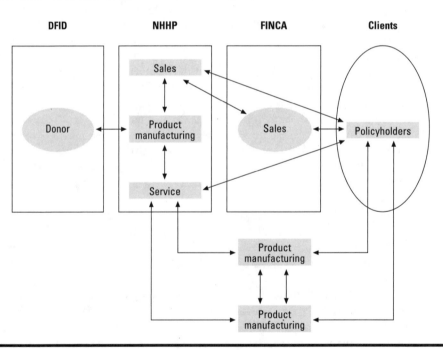

with sufficient coverage is also questionable (Brown and Churchill 2000a; McCord 2000, 2001). But it is too soon to assess affordability because most health insurance experiments are new and small; they have not reached maturity or achieved economies of scale.

SOME LESSONS FOR MICROINSURANCE

Some microfinance institutions manage to serve many low-income borrowers—and generate enviable profits. But for every success story, a host of small, stagnant microfinance institutions survive on donor generosity. Despite the absence of any scientific analysis to determine what causes the differences between the two, some characteristics of success stand out. These lessons carry messages on three fronts: institutional, client and product, and external.

Institutional Issues

Successful microinsurance institutions have a long-term vision that they are building an institution that will generate long-term development benefits. This outlook is more common in private-sector initiatives (including some nonprofits) than in the public sector (government involvement usually spoils a credit scheme).

Institutional type. Of the various types of microfinance institutions, credit unions seem to have the strongest potential to deliver micro health insurance. Many credit unions already have experience offering life insurance, so the transition to health insurance is not too great a leap. Because they are not donor dependent, credit unions are generally more stable than NGOs. In many countries, credit unions reach more persons than other microfinance institutions. And, despite their name, credit unions are savings- rather than credit-driven, which provides promising potential to link insurance with the savings service. Upscalers, downscalers, and other microfinance institutions that offer voluntary savings would also be plausible partners.

Management. Successful microfinance institutions are often run (or founded by) charismatic visionaries who surround themselves with strong managers. This produces two enviable results. First, charismatic leaders elicit above-average performance and loyalty from employees. Second, a strong management team creates and implements systems that strive for optimal performance and continuous improvement. Both results are critical for microfinance institutions because of the ongoing challenge to overcome the high costs of processing many small financial transactions by maximizing productivity and efficiency.

Staffing. Like microfinance institutions, microinsurers can overcome information asymmetries and cultural barriers by hiring people from the communities they serve. To boost productivity and enhance efficiencies, microinsurance providers need highly motivated and trained employees who can do their jobs with minimal supervision. Many microfinance institutions use financial incentives to align goals of the institution with those of the field staff, but that requires a delicate balance between outreach and portfolio quality. It is easy to have many customers if the microfinance institution does not care about loan losses or to have near-perfect repayments if outreach is not an objective. The lesson for microinsurance is that staff incentives should not overemphasize sales at the expense of service, and vice versa.

Institutional culture. The ongoing tension between social and commercial missions taxes many microfinance institutions. Successful microfinance institutions cultivate a balanced perspective among employees (or err on the commercial rather than the social side) through hiring, training, and management techniques. Investments in these techniques must be made early to create an effective corporate culture, one that balances a commitment to the poor with institutional sustainability. An important sign that a microfinance institution has found that balance is the willingness to charge interest rates high enough to cover costs. Other hallmarks of a healthy culture include adaptability to changes in conditions; innovation and openness to new techniques and technologies; and commitment to customer service.

Portfolio quality. Since a microfinance institution's loan portfolio is its primary asset and main source of income, Herculean efforts are justified to protect portfolio quality. Because many microloans are unsecured and delivered through group mechanisms, a small spike in delinquency can quickly spread into a serious portfolio-quality problem. Lessons in how microfinance institutions have extracted timely repayments from their customers have a direct bearing on insurance providers who want to avoid premium lapses.

Capacity challenge. The insurance service must be designed in a way that involves a microfinance institution in health insurance delivery without making great demands on the institution or its field staff, given many microfinance institutions' capacity limitations (box 4.5). A partnership between a microfinance institution and an insurance company can accomplish this objective. The partner-agent model is structured to allow both parties to do what they do best. The microfinance institution's loan officers, in effect, become the insurance company's sales agents by marketing the products to microfinance institution clientele. This arrangement benefits the microfinance institution, since it gets a new income source and has a new product to offer its customers (which may improve the performance of other products), without causing either a significant drain on the microfinance institution's financial and management resources or, most importantly, an insurance risk. The microfinance institution can focus on its core business of savings and loans, and the insurer gains quick and cost-effective access to a large, previously untapped market (Brown, Green, and Lindquist 2001).

Information management. Lack of early focus on the critical role of information systems hampered the development of the microfinance industry. Since health insurers need to manage and analyze considerably more data than a savings and credit scheme, early attention to developing management information systems will pay valuable dividends.

BOX 4.5   CAMBODIA: SHOULD MICROFINANCE INSTITUTIONS OFFER HEALTH INSURANCE?

Illness is a primary destabilizing factor for a borrower's household. Although microenterprise loans can help clients increase incomes and build assets, family health problems often push them back into poverty. To pay health bills, clients sell productive assets, thus curtailing future earning potential. Health financing causes problems with all aspects of household finances—including debt servicing.

These were the main findings of a study conducted in 1996 by Ennathian Moulethan Tchonnebat (EMT), a Cambodian microfinance institution established in 1991 by Groupe de recherche et d'échanges technologiques (GRET) a French NGO. To protect clients from the financial shocks of future illnesses, EMT and GRET decided to develop and test a health care financing system. After market research into clients' knowledge of insurance, their biases, their most common illnesses, and their risk-coping mechanisms, the two organizations launched a pilot product.

At first, they tried adding sales and service of health insurance to two loan officers' lending activities. This did not work because the officers were too busy with their lending jobs. EMT recognized that developing the new insurance business would divert too much time and effort from its core product. EMT then asked GRET to create an autonomous unit to provide insurance in coincident markets. The unit, still in its pilot stage, became the GRET Health Insurance program.

In its health maintenance organization model, GRET acts as both insurer and health care provider, employing a doctor (technically a "medical assistant") who provides limited, door-to-door primary care. This approach was necessary because heath care infrastructure in rural Cambodia was weak. However, government clinics now being established have begun to siphon off GRET policyholders, and the insurer is reevaluating its approach.

One important lesson from GRET's experiences involves pricing. As is common in the industry, GRET's Health Insurance program is having difficulties striking the elusive balance between quality health care and its own viability. The initial pricing was based on optimistic assumptions regarding use and costs. Information gathered during the first year of operations and an improved costing model resulted in a dramatic increase of the premium in the project's second year. This cost increase, without any improvements in the benefit package, caused a strong public relations backlash. The lesson is to price conservatively at the beginning because lowering premiums is much easier than raising them.

Source: Adapted from McCord 2001.

Reinsurance. Critical to the success of any insurance scheme is access to reinsurance. The closest aspect in microfinance to reinsurance is the role of guarantee funds to assume a portion of the lender's credit risk (box 4.6).

Since the health of a reinsurer depends on the financial stability of its subscribing insurers, the financial performance of microfinance institution delivery agents is highly relevant. Microfinance institution performance varies widely,

---

BOX 4.6   LESSONS FOR REINSURANCE FROM MICROFINANCE GUARANTEE SCHEMES

In lending, the closest arrangement to a reinsurance mechanism is the use of guarantee funds to share losses associated with default risk. Guarantee mechanisms backstop creditors against default by allowing them to seek compensation from a third party, the guarantor, in place of the debtor. The mixed experiences of guarantee funds may provide insights for the development of reinsurance.

Lesson 1. When guaranteeing loans, there is no efficient intermediation and risk transformation unless the guarantor has information about the borrower's situation that the lender does not have.

A guarantee mechanism "insures" the creditor against a default loss. Guarantees are meant to overcome an information deficit in the credit market: the creditor does not really know whether the debtor is able and willing to pay back on time. The guarantor, on the other hand, has—or claims to have—this information. If the information advantage is plausible, banks are inclined to accept the risk sharing proposed by the guarantee. If the guarantee fund is managed by civil servants who lack the required technical and professional insights and sit in an office far away from the borrower, the information advantage is less obvious, and banks are less likely to consider this guarantee mechanism.

Lesson 2. Providing second-level coverage against loan losses (in the form of a counter-guarantee, for example) does not necessarily lead to moral hazard problems, provided that there is some risk- and loss-sharing and the conditions are clearly spelled out.

Centrally managed and bureaucratically administered guarantee funds use budget allocations. Usually no counter-guarantee insures them against simultaneous substantial claims by many creditors. However, mutual guarantee associations (MGAs) organized around small and medium enterprises and artisan federations do have that cover. In Germany, public counter-guarantees cover 70 percent (in Switzerland 50 to 60 percent) of the losses that MGAs are called upon to compensate for creditors. The rationale is that keeping MGAs afloat is a public good and that they may be unduly exposed to covariant risk, since they are often organized around a single trade. Attempts to implant MGAs in developing countries have had a mixed record of success (Balkenhol 1990).

---

so a reinsurance scheme needs tools to screen and select appropriate microfinance agents. The tools would rely primarily on quantitative criteria, but their effectiveness would be enhanced if they included a qualitative assessment of management and the institutional culture.

Not all microfinance institutions succeed. Dealing with failing or failed organizations is an ongoing challenge in the microfinance industry. Based on the experience of donors and networks that have had trouble disengaging from weak microfinance institutions, a reinsurer should write contingency plans or an exit strategy into the initial contract with partner insurers on the basis of objective targets. This will allow the reinsurer to extricate itself from organizations that do not fulfill their end of the partnership.

Client and Product Issues

Designers of microinsurance products should look closely at group-lending methodologies to see if groups are appropriate mechanisms to reduce adverse selection and fraud, improve screening, minimize lapses in premium payments, and enhance efficiencies. In credit delivery, groups can quickly reach many people, but their usefulness does not last indefinitely. Some group lenders have high dropout rates because borrowers outgrow their groups or lose patience with them.

Transparency. Integrated service delivery, whereby insurance is layered on top of a savings or credit product, can enhance efficiency (box 4.7). But microfinance

---

BOX 4.7   INTEGRATING INSURANCE WITH OTHER FINANCIAL SERVICES

Microinsurers, like microfinance institutions, must minimize transaction costs to achieve sustainability. Integrating insurance with an existing credit-distribution system can cut these costs. Customers can then pay for two products in a single payment, for example, a loan installment and an insurance premium. Because people should not have to take out a loan to access health insurance, layering health insurance onto a savings product would allow broader coverage. Integrating savings and insurance can produce the following benefits:

- *Limitations of the credit-insurance link.* Some poor households do not borrow because their irregular incomes do not coincide with strict repayment schedules. High desertion rates in microcredit programs also suggest that the credit relationship with customers is temporary or occasional. As a result, the linkage between savings and insurance can provide deeper and more durable outreach than a credit-insurance product.

- *Fewer lapses in premium payments.* Poor households, with variable income, may have trouble keeping up with regular premium payments. A savings-insurance linkage can reduce premium lapses by allowing policyholders to save toward the premium payment. For example, the Self-Employed Women's Association (SEWA) in India has an open-access savings account where members can make deposits until they have enough money to cover annual insurance premiums. This facility can reduce the insurer's risk of client desertion or low compliance, while reducing the insured person's risk of being without coverage because of premium lapses.

(Box continues on the following page.)

BOX 4.7 (continued)

- *Premium payments earned on account.* An alternative is to offer a savings product that automatically pays the premium in lieu of interest. Again, SEWA offers such a product—as long as the account maintains a certain minimum balance, the member receives access to insurance coverage. This arrangement also benefits the microfinance institution because it reduces transaction costs and helps stabilize deposit balances.

- *Increased deposit mobilization.* A savings-insurance combination can boost deposit mobilization and improve client retention in a competitive environment. For example, ACODEP, a Nicaraguan credit union, experienced an increase in average savings balances after introducing a life insurance–savings product. To the extent that health insurance reduces fluctuations in income caused by illness, households should be better able to maintain savings balances, thereby benefiting the microfinance institution by reducing withdrawals.

- *More than peace of mind.* Many low-income persons are reluctant to commit to making premium payments for an uncertain benefit. If the insured risk does not occur, poor households are concerned about having received no tangible return for their premium payments. A savings-insurance link could give policyholders something to show for their accumulated premiums besides peace of mind.

---

institution insurers must disaggregate the revenue, costs, and risks associated with each of their products. Microfinance institutions need information on income and expenses to monitor per product profitability and determine if the rates or prices set are sufficient. In terms of risks, analysts cannot determine the health of an organization unless its credit and insurance risks are separated. In particular, microfinance institutions should resist the temptation to reinvest their premium income in their loan portfolio. Such reinvestment could become a problem for microfinance institution insurers because low-risk, high-return, liquid investment opportunities are hard to come by.

Customer retention. Customer retention counts. Most microfinance institutions lose money on loans to new clients because of the small initial loan balances and high acquisition costs. In fact, an organization may not recoup its losses on an individual customer until he or she has repaid four or five loans (Brand and Gerschick 2000). Moreover, customers who do not remain with the organization cannot derive the social benefits associated with microfinance. Pursuing their dual mission, successful microfinance institutions have found ways of promoting customer loyalty, despite increasing competition (Churchill and Halpern 2001).

One size does not fit all. The development of micro health insurance should start with market research—insurance may not be the financial tool that low-income households want to manage their risks. A key lesson from microfinance is that a single basic loan product is insufficient. The market is more heterogeneous than the microfinance institutions themselves, and customers demand a range of services to suit their needs and repayment capacities. Only recently has the microfinance industry realized that it had to do market research to understand its customers' behavior and preferences. Where health insurance is in demand, offering two or three different service levels is appropriate so that policyholders can select the best coverage for their health care needs and budgets.

Affordability. Early experience with health insurance suggests that affordability is a big challenge. To deepen the outreach of microinsurance providers, some form of cross-subsidization from the better-off to the poor may be worth considering, just as large borrowers subsidize small borrowers. It took the microfinance industry many years to realize that loans should be priced to achieve breakeven or profitability, yet a handful of critics still say that the poor should not have to pay such high interest rates. Sustainable microinsurance schemes will have to find responses to these same criticisms. One response is to focus immediately on maximizing efficiency.

External Issues

Microinsurance should define performance indicators early and design a performance-benchmarking or -rating system to track actual performance. After 25 years, the microfinance industry is just beginning to move beyond opaque reporting and public relations statistics.

Technical and financial aid. The idea of a reinsurer that provides microfinance institutions with expertise and funding to help them deliver health insurance has all the trappings of the donor-driven agendas that hurt microfinance. Ready advice and money could cause more problems than they solve if microfinance institutions smelled an easy way to access donor money and became sidetracked from their core business. Technical and financial assistance should be designed to be demand driven, first by low-income households requesting health insurance from a microfinance institution, and then by the microfinance institution's requesting the same services from a reinsurer. Reinsurers and donors should be wary of opportunists. Only organizations that can demonstrate that health insurance delivery fits neatly into their long-term strategic plan should receive expertise and funding.

A health insurance scheme will need operational subsidies until it serves enough customers to generate economies of scale. The incentive structure built into these subsidies should be designed to avoid the donor dependency that impeded the maturation of microfinance.

Regional differences. The vast regional differences in microfinance motives and performance also have implications for the design of a global reinsurance scheme. Instead of starting at the global level, taking one region at a time may make more sense. If microfinance institutions are a primary delivery agent, Latin America, with more sustainable microfinance institutions than other regions, might be a good proving ground.

Networks and associations. A capacity-challenged reinsurer might work with second-tier organizations, such as affiliate networks of microfinance institutions and national credit union associations, instead of dealing individually with microfinance institutions. This arrangement would make collaboration with many microfinance institutions easier for the reinsurer. Second-tier organizations can also assist with implementation and oversight and provide the reinsurer with additional assurance of the agent's financial health and backing.

Regulatory environment. As microfinance has learned, there is no need to rush into new regulations. Regulations can stifle innovation and erect obstacles that make it difficult for institutions to serve customers who are poor. At the same time, because these services will evolve naturally from the fringes to the mainstream, the ramifications of regulatory involvement have to be considered long before that involvement takes place.

CONCLUSIONS

The diversity of the microfinance industry makes an off-the-shelf health insurance product and a single workable delivery system for every environment difficult, if not impossible, to devise. Yet, attempting to customize services for each microfinance institution could undermine the efficiencies associated with using microfinance institutions as delivery agents.

As a relatively new initiative, microinsurance can learn from its predecessors. Efforts to create sustainable financial institutions that cater to the poor hold relevant lessons for the development of microinsurance as it seeks to overcome some of the same challenges associated with serving low-income communities. By learning from the checkered history of microfinance, microinsurance may avoid repeating the same mistakes.

Demand for affordable health care and health insurance is enormous, but developing an effective system is extremely complicated. Learning to swim in the shallow end may be prudent before jumping into the deep end. With microfinance institution partners, starting with simple products such as life insurance, and then building on a foundation of accomplishment by adding health insurance, would enhance the chances of success.

NOTES

1. Large = > US$8 million; medium between $1 million and $8 million; small < $1 million.

2. Low, broad, and high, based on the average outstanding balance per borrower in relationship to gross national product (GNP) per capita.

REFERENCES

Balkenhol, B. 1990. "L'accès au crédit des petites et moyennes entreprises en Afrique de l'Ouest: quels gages donner aux banques?" *International Labour Review* 129(2): 267–75.

Balkenhol, B., ed. 1999. *Credit Unions and the Poverty Challenge: Extending Outreach, Enhancing Sustainability*. Geneva: International Labour Office.

Brand, M., and J. Gerschick. 2000. *Maximizing Efficiency: The Path to Enhanced Outreach and Sustainability*. Washington, D.C.: ACCION International.

Brown, W., and C. Churchill. 2000a. "Providing Insurance to Low-income Households: Part II—Initial Lessons from Micro-Insurance Experiments for the Poor." Bethesda, Md.: Development Alternatives Inc., USAID's Microenterprise Best Practices Project.

_____. 2000b. "Summary of the Current Market for Insurance in Low-Income Communities and Prospects for Future Development." Prepared for the Ford Foundation. Toronto: Calmeadow.

Brown, W., C. Green, and G. Lindquist. 2001. "Cautionary Note for Microfinance Institutions and Donors Considering Developing Microinsurance Products." Bethesda, Md.: Development Alternatives Inc., USAID's Microenterprise Best Practices Project.

Campion, A., and V. White. 1999. *Institutional Metamorphosis: Transformation of Microfinance NGOs into Regulated Financial Institutions*. Occasional Paper 4. Washington, D.C.: MicroFinance Network.

Churchill, C. 1999. *Client-Focused Lending: The Art of Individual Microlending*. Toronto: Calmeadow.

Churchill, C., and S. Halpern. 2001. *Building Customer Loyalty*. Technical Guide No. 2. Washington, D.C.: MicroFinance Network.

Glosser, A. 1994. "The Creation of BancoSol in Bolivia." In M. Otero and E. Rhyne, eds., *The New World of Microenterprise Finance*. West Hartford, Conn.: Kumarian Press.

Lapenu, C., and M. Zeller. 2000. "Distribution, Growth and Performance of the Microfinance Institutions in Africa, Asia and Latin America—A Recent Inventory." Draft. Washington, D.C.: IFPRI.

McCord, M. 2000. *Microinsurance in Uganda: A Case Study of an Example of the Partner-Agent Model of Microinsurance Provision, NHHP/FINCA Uganda – Health Care Financing Plan*. Nairobi: MicroSave-Africa.

_____. 2001. *Microinsurance: A Case Study of the Provider Model of Microinsurance Provision, GRET Cambodia*. Nairobi: MicroSave-Africa.

McDonald, J. 2000. "Credit Unions: Efficient and Profitable Financial Intermediaries." In *MicroBanking Bulletin* 4 (February).

MicroBanking Standards Project. 2001. *MicroBanking Bulletin* 6 (April).

Morris, K. 1999. "Using Credit Unions as On-lending Agents for External Lines of Credit: The Experience of the International Credit Union Movement." Chapter 2 in B. Balkenhol, ed., *Credit Unions and the Poverty Challenge: Extending Outreach, Enhancing Sustainability*. Geneva: International Labour Office.

Richardson, D. 2000. "Unorthodox Microfinance: The Seven Doctrines of Success." *MicroBanking Bulletin* 4 (February).

Stack, K., and D. Thys. 2000. "A Business Model for Going Down Market: Combining Village Banking and Credit Unions." In *MicroBanking Bulletin* 5 (September).

CHAPTER 5

Health Insurance and Reinsurance at the Community Level

David M. Dror

Microfinance institutions have acquired experience operating certain types of insurance (Balkenhol and Churchill, chapter 4, this volume). Often, microfinance lenders sell life or crop insurance as security for loans in lieu of traditional collateral. Such an arrangement, making the lender both beneficiary and insurer, protects the lender instead of the insured. The basic difference between this type of insurance and health insurance is in the definition of beneficiary or principal. Because health insurance is not a necessary condition for access to credit or other resources, the agent cannot easily impose affiliation on its principals. For that reason, the principal-agent relationship in health insurance is significantly different from the relationship under other forms of community-level insurance. This chapter deals only with community-funded health insurance.

INSURANCE

The term "microinsurance" has been suggested to distinguish community-funded health insurance schemes both from other insurance activities at the level of communities and from noninsurance community-based health schemes[1] (Dror and Jacquier 1999). Bearing in mind that insurance, by its nature, is a macroeconomic tool, is it not a contradiction in terms to combine the two words, "micro" and "insurance"? Theory and debate on microfinance, summarized in chapter 4 (this volume), has already dealt with concerns about drawing a clear dividing line where "micro" ends and "nonmicro" activity begins. Micro refers to the small size of a group or volume of transactions but also to the locus of operations—at the lowest level of social organization, just above the family.[2] To be rightly called insurance, an activity has to satisfy several requirements: pool risks across a group of individuals, collect premiums or contributions in relation to the insurance contract rather

The author acknowledges, with thanks, the insightful comments on this work from Wouter van Ginneken, Senior Social Security Specialist, Planning, Standards, and Development Branch, Social Protection Sector, International Labour Office; and of Charles C. Griffin, Sector Manager, World Bank, Latin America and Caribbean Region, Health Sector.

than the need for insured services, and offer to cover a predefined part of the cost of care (with a link between the contribution and the benefit package).

Insurance is a completely different type of instrument from a savings account or a credit facility.

- *Savings* are a form of intertemporal transfer of current consumption to future consumption. Savings respond only to individualistic preferences and offer no opportunity for interpersonal transfers.

- *Insurance* is a trade across states of nature, from good to bad, and across different individuals or units (Besley 1995, pp. 2123–207). Insurance is an economic interaction linking otherwise unrelated people through mutual selection of risk-averse preferences.

The experience with medical savings accounts in Singapore, the United States, and elsewhere sheds light on the difference between savings and microinsurance.

- A m*edical savings account* is a plan to encourage (or coerce) individuals to save. It includes rules about spending those savings only for health costs of the owner or a limited number of family members. Such intertemporal transfers could probably be used to buy a "health annuity" that would spread risks across the members of the annuity group. But medical savings accounts provide negligible risk pooling, or none, among different income levels, health status levels, or age or gender groups outside the immediate annuity group, and the resources available to this limited group depend on steady and sufficient accumulated savings. Nor do such accounts provide benefits in relation to the cost of the event, since protection is, by definition, limited to the accumulated balance.

- *Microinsurance* is a mechanism for pooling resources and spreading risks across income, age, gender, or health status differences of the entire group.

This difference is cardinal in terms of who bears the responsibility for the health risk. The savings plan puts responsibility for risk exclusively on the beneficiary. Microinsurance, like any other social health insurance, recognizes the complementary responsibility of individuals and their community.

Can Communities Operate Health Insurance?

In a perfect world, insurers would rather deal with a large group, because size adds viability. But, in the reality of most developing countries and their informal sectors, two concurrent forces plead for the development of a decentralized approach to health insurance. First, health insurers have, by and large, been unwilling to include disadvantaged population segments in larger pools. Second, the disempowerment of disadvantaged populations within the social system has excluded people from claiming access to large schemes. If these disadvantaged people are to overcome both constraints, microinsurance units must be adapted to communities' specific living and working conditions. Effective adaptation can occur through a two-pronged mediation process that:

- Gives the target population a voice to express its needs and priorities.

- Shapes public opinion favorably toward insurance.

Community involvement in selecting the covered risks sets microinsurance apart from traditional health insurance (private and social) and from any other type of insurance operated by microfinance institutions (Dror 2000). Unlike social insurance plans that rely on compulsory affiliation or private insurers that actively market their products, microinsurers enhance membership by offering group involvement in self-management and a focus on members' priorities. This is not merely a consultative process but recognition of the members' own legitimate economic options. The community's and its individual members' interests are correlated. A large membership generates more resources than a small one, enabling the group to pay certain expenses that a single individual or small group could not afford. At the second level, community interactions ensure that benefits remain "in the family," instead of responding to an external insurer's profit motives. This process depends on trust building (reassuring the group that the microinsurer will remain solvent when contingencies occur) and on cultural change (modifying a natural dislike of up-front payment for a deferred health care benefit). In both interactions, the community mobilizes familiar social interactions to introduce a new and complex financial concept—health insurance.

Can Microinsurance Attract the Excluded?

Affiliation with a microinsurer is assumed to be voluntary, but it is important to understand what motivates individuals to join. The underlying motivation is assumed to be a desire to seek reciprocity in sustaining risk-sharing arrangements among essentially self-interested individuals. This motivation is sometimes contrasted with altruistic feelings among members who join a "friendly society," based on their belonging to the same social class, neighborhood, or other affinity group.

The difference in approach between the two motivations affects the consequences of an individual's withdrawal from the group after recuperating dues or premiums paid in. In a friendly society (and in commercial insurance), withdrawing after profit taking is tolerated (although the two have different reasons for this tolerance). In sustained risk-sharing arrangements, defection carries the sanction of exclusion from all future insurance benefits by blocking reentry. This severe tradeoff can explain why even poor individuals may prefer to remain insured through periods when they pay premiums but get no benefits in return. And the cost of premiums, even over long periods of time, is more affordable and more efficient than paying for health through savings.[3]

A second motivation affecting affiliation with microinsurers is people's deep-rooted need to seek voluntary and repeated interactions with others. Persons who have a formal employment relationship transfer part of their attachments from family and community to the workplace in return for the rewards of employment. The excluded population cannot do so for lack of access to a workplace and the social protection it offers. For them, the community is an alternative source of support. Members of the same community rely on each other in many ways and refer to each other in the context of roles, values, habits, and customs to satisfy emotional and material needs. Such links can encourage individuals to adhere to collective objectives. Outside pressures may enhance group cohesion, prompting individuals to buy microinsurance. Both sets of motivations to join are mutually supporting, because they respond to economic and societal needs.

The acid test of affiliation is payment of premiums, which is translated into *compliance rate,* or income collected by the organization versus the income due. Economic theory predicts that the incentive to remain within the group will be strongest if individual members face large differences in their incomes, for it is then that they need to transfer large sums to equalize their marginal utilities of income (Besley 1995, p. 2167). Although health insurance does not necessarily depend on large income disparities to thrive, microinsurance gains relevance if it can flatten out income fluctuations resulting from large temporal variations in the flow of income, as is typical for rural or poor populations.

In chapter 2, Dror, Preker, and Jakab made a schematic distinction between needs and demand, which can now be complemented by a more detailed analysis of risks covered by microinsurers. According to available information (Atim 2000, pp. 17–21; Bennett, Creese, and Monasch 1998), microinsurers simultaneously favor two kinds of risks: high-cost, low-incidence catastrophic events (for example, emergency treatment, hospitalization, and some types of surgery) and nonrandom, low-cost events resembling primary care (for example, drugs, laboratory fees, and supplementary care not provided by the government). Because community choices influence the interplay between needs, demand, and supply, the lack of any standard model for designing microinsurance benefit packages is not surprising. Dynamic changes in available resources (from increased membership, surpluses, or external influx of resources) and members' evolving ideas about priorities for risks and benefits also suggest that microinsurers' benefit packages will change more frequently than will those of large schemes.

To attract the excluded, microinsurers must cover their perceived essential needs but also offer an advantageous cost-benefit ratio. A potential inconsistency between these two requirements can be resolved if resources are guaranteed to cover at least the average cost of the benefit package. Where contributory capacity is too low to secure this income, external resources would be required. The alternative of reducing benefits to the level members can afford may annul the attractiveness of affiliating. The perceived utility of affiliating must be at least equal to the spot transactions between patient and healer. Otherwise, changing the existing (unsatisfactory) system of health financing would not stand a chance. Nor could willingness and ability to pay in the informal sector be enhanced without offering a better deal up front than an individual can obtain alone. Thus, targeted subsidies are essential in the first years of operating microinsurance units. Some services with high externalities, for which individuals would not be willing to pay in a spot market but which could be provided on a collective basis, would also have to be financed through subsidies, at least initially (Busse, chapter 13, this volume). Channeling subsidies through microinsurers can provide additional benefits to members and improve the cost-benefit ratio as well as strengthen microinsurers institutionally.

What Goes into Setting Up a Microinsurance Scheme?

Microinsurers deal with people who have little trust in public institutions. To counteract their diffidence, three conditions must be built into the operation from start-up: simplicity, affordability, and proximity.

Simplicity. Most people in the informal sector cannot cope with procedural complexities. Many of them cannot read or write, but even the literate find forms hard to "fill in." They may be unable to provide such seemingly simple details as an address, date of birth, or family name, let alone a bank account. Simplicity is also important to project the image that the scheme is approachable. Simplicity translates into fast and more positive responsiveness without complicated (and potentially unfair) rules of exclusion because of, for example, prior conditions.

Affordability. What makes microinsurance affordable? Both objective and subjective notions come into play. The price of premiums makes a difference, but the perceived return on the premium can be equally important. People tend to view as "affordable" costs they believe are justified. Two features can enhance price acceptance: transparency about expenditures in general and about (low) overhead costs in particular; and knowledge that the same rules apply to all members. Every member has some frame of reference for a perceived cost-benefit because even the indigent spend some resources on health services (Jain 1999, p. 61). Another aspect of affordability is the periodicity of payment. Helping to regularize payments of people with erratic incomes can help, and accepting payment in kind (both goods and labor) in lieu of cash can also enhance affordability.

Proximity. Because distance from service centers is one cause of exclusion, microinsurers need to operate near their client base. Presence is necessary at all periods of operation, not just at recruitment, since rural people have neither the means nor the leisure to travel from their place of residence.

Broad-based community participation is probably the best guarantee of meeting these three conditions. Self-management has several advantages, not least cost savings and administrative right-sizing. All known organizational alternatives, commercial or public, are based on methodologies developed in the formal health sector that favor highly trained, expensive professional management. Replicating such a managerial profile seems incompatible with the management task

at the level of a single community—sizes, quantities, and kinds of services provided. In addition, local management reduces anonymity, which enhances self-
monitoring and transparency, thus reducing the risk of corruption. Closeness
between members also creates intangible but real bonds that augment acceptance
of benefit redistribution according to need instead of solely according to individual utility. Social cohesion around common objectives holds potential for fostering a climate that discourages abuse of the system. Deficient governance, however, limits microinsurers' capacity to operate a risk-management facility. Their
inadequate capacity to record, analyze, and transmit accounting and utilization
data is the basic problem. Microinsurers need help to improve their managerial
capacity, which means more than sporadic courses. The objective is to train
microinsurers to perform three essential functions:

- Prevent free riding by ensuring that only paid-up members receive health services

- Obtain reliable utilization and cost data essential for calculating contributions
  (and subsidies)

- Identify cost escalation and user- or supplier-induced moral hazard

Microinsurers also need help to reach the desired standard, both in terms of
external financing of start-up administrative costs (software, hardware, training)
and in terms of actuarial and managerial "hand-holding" for a period long enough
until they can operate autonomously.

Where Do Reinsurance and Subsidies Fit In?

Microinsurance units can play a valuable role in operating health insurance
schemes for people excluded from national health systems. The strength of
microinsurance is rooted in social capital and communities' capacity to adapt
insurance techniques to specific conditions, thereby overcoming classical problems inherent in the principal-agent relationship. Two key weaknesses relate to
the units' small size, which limits the population across which risks can be spread,
and their members' low income, which limits the amount of financing that can
be mobilized in poor communities. The solution to the first problem lies in reinsurance. The solution to the second problem lies in subsidies and strengthened
links to national programs for health care financing and delivery.

REINSURANCE OF HEALTH INSURANCE FOR THE INFORMAL SECTOR

Governments and development agencies have recognized a role for communities
in extending health insurance in all low- and middle-income countries. The question is no longer whether microinsurance units should exist, but how they can be
sustained financially and how they can improve their operations.

Sharing risks between insurance carriers is common practice in the insurance industry, regardless of the size of insurers. Social health insurers in most industrial countries operate under "pay-as-you-go" financing, which transfers all deficits to the population at large. Microinsurers cannot operate this way because loading deficits onto few members can encourage withdrawal from affiliation because of limited ability to pay. Nor can microinsurers count on unlimited deficit financing from external sources. Hence, microinsurers need a different solution. This section examines the causes of microinsurers' financial instability and looks for ways out of this dilemma.

What Causes Microinsurers' Financial Instability?

Microinsurers' financial instability stems from wide swings in both income and expenditures.

Income-Side Instability

As contributory schemes, microinsurance units must secure enough income to pay for benefits (plus administrative costs). Income-side stabilization depends on accurate calculation of contributions by the microinsurer and on its members' satisfactory compliance rate.

Inaccurate calculation of contributions. Members' contributions must cover at least the expected average cost of the benefit package, minus available subsidies or other steady external resources. Calculation of the average cost depends on the probability that a certain benefit will be claimed and its expected cost. Contributions must also cover administrative costs. Can microinsurers calculate contributions by applying the same methods used by large health insurance schemes in rich countries? Those schemes usually base their income calculations (more often their budgets) on historical expenditure patterns rather than on a needs-based formula (Busse 2000). Because reliable long-term records of benefit utilization are virtually nonexistent at the level of microinsurers, small schemes cannot make projections the way large schemes can. Although microinsurers may have some data on short-term cost and use, estimating the number of future claims from data describing a single microinsurer's experience over a short period may lead to error resulting from high statistical fluctuations (Auray and Fonteneau, chapter 8, this volume). This point is further elaborated below in discussing expenditure-side instability.

In addition to possible errors from statistical fluctuations in the estimated value of the average cost, the underlying assumptions may be weak on the expected local burden of disease. Global burden of disease descriptors are available, but significant variations have been reported between global and local burden of disease estimates for Sub-Saharan Africa, according to a recent study in Burkina Faso (Gbangou and others 2000). Past utilization levels must also be questioned, because they may reflect the diagnostic capacity of local medical attendants as much as a correct range of probabilities. As diagnostic knowledge in many rural areas may be limited to accidents, maternity complications, and a narrow range of prevalent illnesses (in their acute and severe stage), future utilization changes could reflect changes in the diagnostic knowledge of local medical personnel as much as real changes in the local burden of disease.

In reality, premiums have been set less on estimated costs of the benefit package or probabilities of events than by reference to external issues such as outpatient visit fees (Uganda) or the cost of other insurance schemes (PhilHealth, Philippines).[4] Consequently, some margin of error must be acknowledged in assumptions about average cost, expected local burden of disease, and unit cost data used to calculate contributions.

Compliance gaps. Regardless of the method used for setting contributions, a *compliance gap* occurs when a microinsurer cannot collect member contributions and its income falls short of the expected amount. Income instability is an inherent feature of microinsurers, linked to the cyclical income of the people they serve, whether rural and agricultural workers whose income depends on crop cycles or workers in service sectors who are also exposed to cycles (for example, tourism). Other random situations may aggravate income instability such as reliance on a single crop, temporal fluctuations in environmental conditions (drought, floods, typhoons), or political risk (which can affect not only demand factors but also individuals' ability to work).

Cultural factors also influence compliance (Soriano, Dror, Alampay, and Bayugo, chapter 19, this volume) as well as members' sense of utility. The tradeoff between paying for health insurance and paying providers' bills may be perceived quite differently when members face acute health needs and high bills, and when they do not. Attracting members is one challenge; keeping them over healthy periods is another. When membership drops, so too does a microinsurer's contribution income. Accurate data and analysis of either membership or income fluctuation are rare.[5]

Because of their social nature, microinsurers provide services even when they expose themselves to some financial instability. The case made here in favor of stabilization does not imply a desire to change microinsurers' social vocation but to base the consequent policy choices on better knowledge.

Expenditure-Side Instability

Microinsurers' small membership and business volume create unique and endemic problems in the number of claims, unit cost of benefits, estimated risk probability, catastrophic costs, and administrative costs.

Fluctuations in claim numbers. Random fluctuations in the number of claims will always be significant when the number of expected claims is small. Such small claims can occur in two situations: either when the *membership* is small or when the *claim probability* is low, even if the group is not small.

Group size and occurrence distribution. Group size plays an important role in determining the microinsurer's financial viability because group size and occurrence distribution are linked. The distribution of claims around the mean under the binomial law is shown in figure 5.1 in a claim/nonclaim-simulated scenario for one 100-member group and one with 1,000 members, both typical sizes for microinsurers. The graph shows that small groups are more exposed than are large groups to statistical fluctuations in the mean value of the number of claims. Small groups' greater exposure to high-severity *(outlier)* claims translates into higher exposure to insolvency. This statistical linkage between outliers and group size disappears in large groups (more than a few thousand people), because there is a higher convergence around the average value. (That is why this issue is normally ignored in reference to national schemes.)

Impact of low claim probability. High probability of risk exposes the insurer to a high expected claim cost. Less self-evident, when the probability drops, small groups benefit less from the drop than large groups, because the statistical possibility of a higher-than-average claim load is sensitive to group size. Figure 5.2 illustrates this phenomenon, again for 100-member and 1,000-member groups. At a probability of 2 percent, both groups are exposed to the chance that the claim load will be above the expected mean. When the risk that the number of

FIGURE 5.1 Group Size Affects Distribution

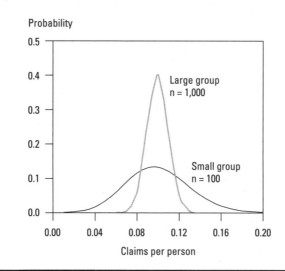

FIGURE 5.2   Variance of Claim and Group Size

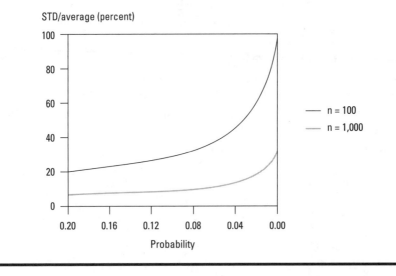

claims will be higher than the mean by 60 percent or more is 1 percent for the large group, it is a significant 16 percent for the small group.

Periodicity of accounting. The length and regularity of an accounting period can also affect these statistical impacts—the longer the time span, the lower the extent of fluctuations. This means that monthly calculations will be less favorable than annual ones. This issue can theoretically be ignored at this stage of the discussion, except where estimates of expected claim load are based on data for a very short period. The point is that one and the same financial period has to be used for all units when comparing microinsurers' operations results.

Fluctuations in unit cost of benefits. Microinsurers are not intrinsically exposed to fluctuations in unit cost, a parameter negotiated between buyer and seller of health services. The stronger the buyer's negotiating position, the more likely is standardization of unit cost. However, if the microinsurer's volume is low or its bargaining position weak, it may be unable to negotiate a standard tariff for all claim liabilities. Also, the cost of different prescriptions is expected to vary significantly (for example, a simple painkiller will cost less than an antibiotic). Similarly, hospitalization costs vary with the length of stay. Figure 5.3 provides an example of variations in the cost of diagnostic procedures paid by the ORT Health Plus Scheme (La Union, Philippines). Although 80 percent of the diagnostic procedures cost up to 200 Philippines pesos, the remaining 20 percent cost up to six times more for a single diagnostic procedure.

Underestimation of risk probability. Most microinsurers have no reliable historical data on utilization for estimating their average number of claims. Considering

FIGURE 5.3   Distribution of Unit Costs

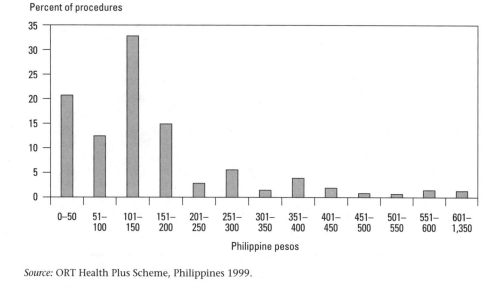

Percent of procedures

Source: ORT Health Plus Scheme, Philippines 1999.

that service use usually increases when people are insured, underestimates are more likely than overestimates—and with severe consequences. Overestimates do not heighten the risk of insolvency for the microinsurer but underestimates do. By extension, the impact of underestimating probability (P) depends on group size and on the level of P itself because both the average number of claims and the variance in the number of claims depend on P. Therefore, underestimating P can cause miscalculation in the funds needed to pay not only the average number of claims but also the risk for a higher-than-average number (figure 5.4). The graph shows that, when an income estimate is based on the assumption of one probability, an error in P can dramatically increase the likelihood of insolvency— way beyond the level admitted in the original calculation.[6] This simulation shows why reliable probability data are indispensable. Without them, neither microinsurers nor reinsurance could forestall deficits, no matter how balanced the benefit package. However, when data are unavailable, alternative methods have to be used to assess risk (Auray and Fonteneau, chapter 8, this volume).

Catastrophes. Although rare, catastrophes carry the risk of colossal costs when they do occur—an earthquake is a classical example. This random, low-probability event, completely inelastic in demand, causes damage most individuals cannot absorb without assistance. Microinsurers might be exposed to both predictable and unpredictable health catastrophes.

Low-probability, high-cost events such as certain life-saving surgeries are known as *"predictable" health catastrophes*. The data collected during a mission to Kisiizi, Uganda, showed that a single case of surgery could bankrupt a microinsurer for

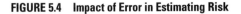

FIGURE 5.4   Impact of Error in Estimating Risk

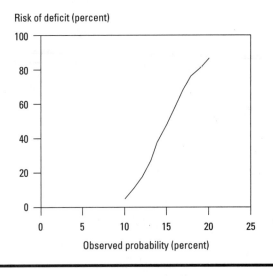

the entire fiscal year. Such an example suggests that the smaller the microinsurer and the smaller its financial volume, the more catastrophic proportions such events take on. Epidemiological studies could provide much help in assessing the probable cost of such events, as the probabilities should, theoretically, be related to the local burden of disease.

Local events that cause a sudden, unforeseen, large increase in the number of claims are *"unpredictable" catastrophes*. They may result from natural calamities (for example, flooding, water contamination) or from other situations that cause a local epidemic or a major accident with widespread injuries. It would seem that such situations can be dealt with through classical insurance or reinsurance, where the microinsurer's and other primary insurers' situations are comparable.

Administrative costs. Microinsurers' expenditures do not stop with paying claims. Their administrative costs are an ongoing part of expenditures, and sometimes they devour contribution income. One important lesson of experience from microfinance is that administrative right-sizing plays a big role in building members' trust. Microinsurance is a more complex operation than microsavings or microcredit, but it interacts with a similar target group. Hence, stabilization of microinsurers' finances requires a close eye to hold down administrative costs.

Stabilizing Microinsurers through Reinsurance

The literature on microinsurance units focuses mainly on their relations with *suppliers of care* and with *members* (for example, the way the benefit package is put together and members' contributions are set) (Normand and Weber 1994; ANMC/

BIT/ACOPAM/WSM 1997; Whitaker 1999, pp. 151–59; Kiwara and van Ginneken 2000; ILO 2001; Atim 2000). Here, we view microinsurers as *insurance entities*.

Virtually all insurers cede part of their portfolio to reinsurance. Social health insurance schemes are a notable exception in that their deficits are passed to the state or the public at large (where coverage is mandatory). Microinsurers do not have the same financial safety net and must therefore take different steps to ensure their financial viability. Reinsuring part of their risk seems the insurance industry's usual way of doing so. Now that microinsurers' specific problems have been reviewed, we can examine some possible solutions through a reinsurance-based approach.

What Can Be Reinsured?

Reinsurance allows first-line insurers to transfer risk beyond their underwriting capacity or to modify risk exposure and composition.[7] Reinsurable risks include those against random fluctuations in the number of claims, unexpected fluctuations in unit costs, and high-cost, low-probability catastrophes.

By transferring risk, losses can be balanced *(homogenized)* collectively over large groups that are united only through the reinsurance link.

Since microinsurers usually rely on outside resources (WHO 2000; Bennett, Creese, and Monasch 1998), they have an incentive to hone their competitive edge over other microinsurers to obtain external help. This interferes with information sharing and other ways of developing intrinsic capacity to organize risk transfers with other schemes. One of the objectives of reinsuring microinsurers is to structure the opportunity to pool risks across microinsurers.

The relationship between microinsurers and a reinsurer would be based on a clear definition of the premium payable by the microinsurer to the reinsurer in return for a defined retrocession of risks. A basic feature fashioning this relationship is the specific method of reinsurance used to stabilize microinsurers' liability (or loss). This relationship is also shaped by the regulatory environment for the operation of both microinsurers and reinsurers.

Fluctuations in claim numbers. Random fluctuation in the number of claims is one of the main problems identified earlier. Large health schemes frequently operate on the assumption that high claim load from expected statistical fluctuations could be financed in the short term through contingency reserves and, in the long term, by increasing contributions in subsequent financial cycles. Both solutions require an increase in contribution rates. The question is whether increasing contribution rates is the best way for microinsurers to avoid insolvency because of random fluctuation in the number of claims (Dror and Duru 2000). This was explored by simulation of 10 microinsurers (figure 5.5).[8]

Even when contributions were raised 50 percent above the level needed for average cost recovery, the risk of insolvency was still 5 percent. At lower contribution levels, the situation was much worse. Reinsurance was the only solution that offered 100 percent survival.[9]

FIGURE 5.5 **Reinsurance Compared with Higher Contributions**

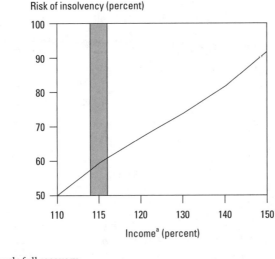

Risk of insolvency (percent)

Income[a] (percent)

a. 100 percent equals full recovery.

These results provide some important insights:

- High income does not remove the risk of insolvency—even when surpluses are carried over across years.

- The cost of ensuring against insolvency through reinsurance was much lower than any other alternative.

- The only option for 100 percent protection against insolvency was reinsurance.

The virtual and simplified representations of the relations simulated may differ from real-life situations, but the ground rules are much the same in both cases. *The conclusion from this analysis is that reinsurance offers a more viable and a cheaper solution than contingency reserves to pay for high variance in the claim load.* Moreover, unlike contingency funds, reinsurance does not put pressure on the microinsurer to enhance the package simply "because there is money in the bank." Thus, the risk of financial mismanagement is probably also reduced.

Fluctuations in unit costs. Where no ceilings are put on the cost of benefits included in the package, the microinsurer bears the risk of unit-cost fluctuations, which can be quantified and reinsured. Frequently, this risk is controlled by a gatekeeper or by transfer to the provider by such payment arrangements as capitation or fixed prices per procedure.[10]

Catastrophes. Microinsurers can insure or reinsure relatively easily against catastrophes. The key to doing so is in the definition of "catastrophe." One option would be to focus on probability. Alternatively, the threshold could be defined by the number of claims, for example, twice the average number of claims from a specific cause.[11] This approach could easily provide the solution to epidemic-like events.

An Integrated Reinsurance–Based Approach to Sustaining Microinsurers

At this point, a description of the overall approach to reinsuring microinsurers might be useful (the technical aspects are covered, by Outreville, chapter 3, and Bonnevay and others, chapter 7, this volume). Stated simply, operating reinsurance would entail not only developing the financial instrument but also enhancing considerably microinsurers' capacity to register, analyze, and transmit data. The two-way transfer of knowledge between local interlocutors and the reinsurance facility would take a concerted and ongoing effort. Microinsurers themselves could not defray the cost of this knowledge transfer and the necessary infrastructure to manage information. Hence, someone else would have to bear the initial costs.

Furthermore, microinsurers might decide to pay for benefit enhancement instead of reinsurance if forced to choose between the two options. After all, they cannot be expected to demonstrate greater understanding of risk management than insurance companies, which are legally required to reinsure. Therefore, introducing reinsurance would require enhancement of the benefit package to compensate microinsurers for the added cost of reinsurance. This strategy opens up possibilities for introducing public health interventions where demand may be low even if the need is evident. This is a four-pronged, integrated approach of reinsurance, package enhancement, knowledge transfer and consulting services, and linkages with formal health-financing institutions.

Component 1: Reinsurance

Reinsurance activity covers four domains: financing, program-management capacity, stabilization against fluctuations, and catastrophe protection (Outreville, chapter 3, this volume). *Financing* entails calculating and accumulating the reserves (surplus) an insurer must retain to guarantee its insurance risk. Traditionally, substantial own-funds are regarded as the mark of a healthy financial position. But newly established microinsurance units have no contingency reserves, and it is dubious whether the use of own-funds to cover peaks in risk is more effective than financial reinsurance, which can be designed to cover actual costs and actuarial provisions. *Capacity* refers to the size of a single type of risk the insurer can accumulate. *Stabilization* describes the ability to reduce year-to-year fluctuations in risk (or loss) exposure. *Catastrophe protection* simply means insuring a microinsurer against a loss that might jeopardize its very existence.

A major prerequisite for a reinsurance contract is the selection of risks that can be considered and those that cannot (Vaté and Dror, chapter 6, this volume).

Insurable benefits. In principle, only health benefits that satisfy the tenets of insurance theory regarding insurability of events can be covered. To be insurable, an event must be random and future, identifiable and measurable—and nonspeculative (disallowing a profit generated from ill health). The premium must also be affordable.

Uninsurable benefits. A brief juxtaposition of some common benefits included in most health insurance schemes shows that the rules of insurability are not always met in health insurance. For instance, preventive care or investments in creating the supply of services are planned, deliberate, and nonrandom expenses. As such, they cannot be insured. The cost of random and inelastic demand can be insured and reinsured, but not "uninsurable" events. These would have to be financed through subsidies not only because they are not reinsurable but also because it is unfair to expect the poor to pay for infrastructure for which the state usually pays through general taxation.

Component 2: Package Enhancement

The technical complexity of reinsurance and the difficulty of explaining its advantages to the public make winning acceptance of this tool difficult. Nevertheless, an effort should be made to offer the reinsurance service because of its great potential for stabilizing microinsurers' financial situation by applying the law of large numbers. One way forward might be to develop a synergy between reinsurers and donors that may want to promote certain "uninsurable" services (for example, vaccinations, micronutrient supplementation, antenatal care). A symbiotic relationship might be cultivated between donors interested in assisting a vertical health-promotion program and those wishing to strengthen the risk-management approach at the community level. Working together, each donor could deliver its own program more successfully than it could without the other. For example, health-promotion plans can benefit from microinsurers' infrastructure and their already established penetration into the rural, agricultural, and informal sectors. Similarly, proponents of risk-management through reinsurance can win the trust of microinsurers when they provide a mix of long-term stabilization and short-term additional benefits.

Component 3: Knowledge Transfer and Consulting Services

To provide the basis for estimating probabilities, microinsurers need to record, analyze, and transmit information on the expected business results. Microinsurers' capacity to do so has to be reinforced if this is to happen. The reinsurer needs this information to decide which benefits to reinsure and what premium to charge. This component recognizes that, to operate a successful reinsurance facility, the backbone of an ongoing working relationship between microinsurers and the reinsurer is a local cadre of experts, as that can improve information management. With time, underwriting and managerial assistance offered by the reinsurer would allow microinsurers to gain otherwise unaffordable information, statistical expertise, and managerial experience

Component 4: Linkages with Formal Health-Financing Institutions

Ranson and Bennett (chapter 11, this volume) elaborate on the wide range of options through which governments can facilitate the development, viability, and impact of microinsurance. This section explains that governments may encourage linkages between microinsurers and formal health financing schemes, but these linkages need not await government initiative.

Linkages can coordinate and may transfer some microinsurance risk to other schemes to the extent that risk transfer improves the microinsurer's financial viability. A similar case can be made for transferring risks that the membership is entitled, by law, to have covered. This process, never simple, is often too complex for a single microinsurer to negotiate without assistance.

Linkages may also entail some technical or regulatory support, including research that microinsurers can rarely assume or afford on their own. For example, to operate in the black, microinsurers sorely need local risk profiles. These profiles should include information on sociocultural influences on peoples' propensity to seek or avoid risk, and on the society's basic approach to social justice and the poor and to balancing individual and collective responsibilities for dealing with the financial consequences of illness.

So far, the literature has barely touched on the linkages between grass-roots and top-down health schemes. This is one domain that should be developed as part of the legitimization of microinsurers' role in the effort to provide health care in the informal sector. And reinsurance can hardly be conceived outside the wider context of regulation, health financing, policy, and management.

Social Re: From Concept to Pilot Project

Community social action has proved effective in channeling familiar social interactions into action among people who are excluded from top-down health systems. This is one of the few options for mobilizing financial contributions from the poor and the informal sector for their own social protection. However, extending access to health services through microinsurance requires a paradigm shift from established thinking about social health insurance, which functions autonomously from the top down. Of the several support groups that have been helping communities organize the provision of health services, few have recognized that this help should be given in the form of health insurance. Still fewer have accepted that microinsurance should be sustained from inception as a viable alternative to unstable external financing.

This book is the first detailed analysis of the unique difficulties that expose microinsurers to higher financial volatility than large health insurance schemes.[12] These difficulties include small group size, the target population's low and irregular income, higher exposure to the impact of local catastrophe, and added risks from poor information on risk probability. All these causes lie outside the control of small communities, which cannot be expected to remedy these problems on their own. Because these communities often operate among the poorer and less-educated segments of the population, technical help, and the cost of this knowledge transfer, must come from the outside.

The reinsurance facility proposed here as a tool for stabilizing microinsurance units does not yet exist. A project for conceptualizing, modeling a solution, piloting it, and assessing its viability has been developed. Called *Social Re*, it is being financed by an award from the World Bank's Development Marketplace 2000 and the International Labour Office. Implementation of the four-pronged development strategy would include setting up a reinsurance facility, extending the benefit package to include some fundamental preventive and health-promoting services, developing an extensive module for knowledge transfer, and providing on-site or on-line consulting needed to build the capacity of microinsurers to become full counterparts for reinsurance. Last, the reinsurance facility would also provide advice and facilitation in establishing links to national health insurance schemes.

Social Re promises many payoffs:

- With better knowledge of their health risks, individual communities can improve their capacity to plan remedial services.

- More stable risk management can enhance community members' willingness to participate in voluntary health insurance.

- Financially stable microinsurers could expand the supply of services and would improve their negotiating positions to obtain attractive prices for these services.

- Building local capacity for self-management is the first step toward a win-win linkage between individual communities and larger (national) health systems. Over time, this relationship should provide a framework for flows of funds and other resources between bottom-up and top-down health systems. The fundamental economic process established through reinsurance will increase the volume of pooled resources, promote monetarization of barter transactions, spread risk more efficiently, and reduce the exposure of the poor to the financial cost of illness.

- Last, but not least, this development approach offers a tangible option for linkage between existing social protection institutes and individual microinsurers that provide health insurance to the informal sector. This linkage can benefit both partners.

Yet reinsurance is not a panacea for microinsurers' every problem. Reinsurance cannot increase productivity or be a source of funding, although it can play a role in developing both. However, if microinsurers are to act as health insurers in the informal sector in developing countries, they need access to the same tools that insurers elsewhere use to sustain their operations.

NOTES

1. A more accurate (but also more cumbersome) labeling would probably be "micro health insurance."

2. Discussions of whole countries would be at the national level.

3. Shaw and Griffin (1995, p. 145) have the following to say about saving as an alternative to insurance: "Insurance aims to protect people from a low-probability, catastrophic loss. To illustrate, suppose that a typical African adult between the ages of 15 and 60 years has 1 in 10,000 chances of experiencing severe illness or injury, resulting in a US$3,000 hospital bill in any given year. If this hospital bill were spread over all 10,000 people, then on average, each person's expected annual cost would be (.0001) x (3,000) = $0.30 a year for insurance that covers such a catastrophic loss, thus transforming the low-probability $3,000 loss into a certain but small $0.30 annual loss… If an insurance company could assemble 10,000 people with this loss probability and collect $0.30 from each of them, it would be prepared to incur the hospital expenses of one $3,000 loss a year… [and] if each person were to pay $0.60 per year… the insurance could probably survive on a profit making basis…"

4. These observations were made during exploratory missions in Uganda in April 2000 and in the Philippines in October 2000 and February 2001.

5. Free riding was observed during the exploratory missions both in Uganda and in the Philippines.

6. In the graph, contributions were set at a level limiting the risk of insolvency to 5 percent at an assumed $P = 10$ percent. Several other simulated observations were noted to examine the impact on insolvency of different levels of P (assuming that income remains steady). When the observed value of P is 15 percent, the risk of insolvency jumps from 5 percent to 50 percent; and when the observed P stands at 20 percent instead of the estimated 10 percent, the risk of insolvency escalates to 90 percent instead of 5 percent!

7. Two basic types of reinsurance are usually recognized: *traditional* and *financial* (nontraditional), described in detail by Outreville (chapter 3, this volume).

8. All microinsurers were assumed to have a risk portfolio of 10 percent probability and a time line of 10 years. The microinsurers were required to operate with current income plus carryover surpluses but cease to operate if insolvent. The survival over the 10-year period was explored at different contribution levels (100 percent was the one required to cover average costs. The premium for reinsurance was set at 15 percent of the average. Then, the survival rate over the same period was compared under the reinsurance alternative.

9. A 15 percent premium was assumed to provide the income needed by the reinsurer to ensure its own solvency.

10. Providers may be equally interested in reinsuring the above-average (or above capitation-rate) cost of high-severity cases. The option of reinsuring providers, not discussed here, would require different adjustments in the reinsurance facility.

11. A more likely option to define the threshold would be in terms of standard deviations (for example, 2 STD).

12. For a partial treatment of this problem, see Dror 2001.

REFERENCES

ANMC/BIT/ACOPAM/WSM (Alliance Nationale de Mutualités Chrétiennes de Belgique, Bureau International de Travail, Programme d'Appui Associatif et Coopératif aux Initiatives de Développement à la Base, Solidarité Mondiale/World Solidarity). 1997. *Mutuelles de santé en Afrique: Guide pratique à l'usage des promoteurs, administrateurs et gérants*. Brussels: WSM.

_____. 1998. *Rural Health Insurance: A Viable Alternative to User-Fees? A Review and Evidence from Three Countries*. Public Health and Policy Departmental Publication No. 199. London: London School of Hygiene and Tropical Medicine.

Atim, C. 2000. *Training of Trainers Manual for Mutual Health Organisations in Ghana*. Bethesda, Md.: Abt Associates Inc., Partnership for Health Reform.

Bennett, S., A. Creese, and R. Monasch. 1998. *Health Insurance Schemes for People Outside Formal Sector Employment*. Current Concerns ARA Paper No.16. WHO/ARA7CC/98.1. Geneva: World Health Organization.

Besley, T. 1995. "Savings, Credit, and Insurance." In *Handbooks in Economics, No. 9, Handbook of Development Economics*, Vol. 3A. Geneva: World Health Organization.

Busse, R., with A. Riesberg. 2000. *Health Care Systems in Transition—Germany*. Edited by A. Dixon. [Available in German.] Copenhagen: European Observatory on Health Care Systems.

Dror, D.M. 2000. "Reforming Health Insurance: A Question of Principles?" *International Social Security Review* 53(2):75–99.

_____. 2001. "Reinsurance of Health Insurance for the Informal Sector." *Bulletin of the World Health Organization* 79(7):672–78.

Dror, D.M., and G. Duru. 2000. "Financing Micro-Insurance: Perspective and Prospective." *Proceedings*. Seventh International Conference on System Science in Health Care, Vol. 1. International Society on System Science in Health Care (ISSSHC), Budapest.

Dror, D.M., and C. Jacquier. 1999. "Micro-Insurance: Extending Health Insurance to the Excluded." *International Social Security Review* 52(1):71–97.

Gbangou, A., R. Sauerborn, C. Schmidt, and R. Würthwein. 2000. "Measuring the Local Burden of Disease—A Study of Years of Life Lost in Rural Burkina Faso." Discussion Paper 1/2000. Heidelberg: Ruprecht-Karls-Universität.

ILO (International Labour Organisation). 2001. *Mutuelles de santé et associations de micro-entrepreneurs—Guide*. Geneva: ILO, Programme Stratégies et Technique contre l"Exclusion Sociale et la Pauvreté, Département de Sécurité Sociale (STEP), Small Enterprise Development Program (SEED).

Jain, S. 1999. "Basic Social Security in India." In W. Van Ginneken, ed., *Social Security for the Excluded Majority: Case Studies of Developing Countries*. Geneva: International Labour Organisation.

Kiwara, A., and W. van Ginneken. 2000. "Manual for Mutual Health Insurance: The UMASIDA Experience." Geneva: International Labour Organisation. Processed.

Normand, C., and A. Weber. 1994. *Social Health Insurance*. Geneva: World Health Organization.

Shaw, P.R., and C.C. Griffin. 1995. "Financing Health Care in Sub-Saharan Africa through User-Fees and Insurance." *Directions in Development*. Washington, D.C.: World Bank.

Stiglitz, J.E. 1988. *Economics of the Public Sector*. New York: Norton. Quoted in A.B. Atkinson, *Income and the Welfare State: Essays on Britain and Europe*. Cambridge: Cambridge University Press, 1995.

Whitaker, T., ed. 1999. *Social Health Insurance*. Geneva: International Labour Organisation and International Social Security Association.

WHO (World Health Organization). 2000. *The World Health Report—2000, Health Systems: Improving Performance*. Geneva: WHO.

CHAPTER 6

To Insure or Not to Insure?
Reflections on the Limits of Insurability

Michel Vaté and David M. Dror

*There exists then, a necessary cause of inequality, of dependence and even of misery...
We can destroy a large part of this by opposing chance to itself.*

—Condorcet 1793

How can social reinsurance sustain community health financing when governments cannot fund universal coverage? The answer to this question is the overriding focus of this book. "Appropriate insurance" is one option (Musgrove 1999, p. 55), but what kind of insurance is appropriate?

The realm of insurance is ever-changing. When new risks are identified—or as new forms of risk transfer are formulated for known risks—the question about the limits of insurability comes up again and again. In the ordinary framework of casualty and liability insurance, routine technical analyses usually suffice to determine whether or not a given risk is insurable. Such calculations are performed routinely before an insurer agrees to underwrite a risk or renew a contract.

But here the focus of debate is intrinsically different from the casualty and liability context. It is rather unusual because it concerns health costs, low-income countries, and microinsurance. The basic question is: Can insurance play any role at all in covering microinsurers' health risk and, if so, what is it? To answer this question, we draw on a set of basic concepts as well as modern problematic subjects from three parts of the literature: theory of insurance (Briys 1990; Ewald and Lorenzi 1998; Henriet and Rochet 1991; Outreville 1998), social protection and health care finance (Charpentier 2000; Cichon and others 1999), and health insurance in low-income countries (Atim 2000; Dror and Duru 2000; Fonteneau and Dror 2000; Gertler and Solon 2000; Meesen 2000). This chapter explores a method for establishing a coherent and simple-to-operate distinction between cost-generating health events that can be insured and those that cannot.

Health risk, as used here, designates any situation in which the health status of an individual—or group of individuals—is exposed to possible deterioration. When this risk occurs, expenses are incurred either from treatment to improve the health status or from compensation for its deterioration. We analyze several examples to separate insurable from uninsurable health events.

For his helpful comments on a draft of this chapter, the authors thank Philip A. Musgrove, Lead Economist, World Bank, Human Development Network, Health, Nutrition, and Population Team.

Human development is both a process and an end (World Bank 1993; UNDP 2000). This general affirmation also applies to the health risks of populations in low-income countries insofar as the related costs can both contribute to, and result from, such development. For this reason, health systems seek to improve the health of individuals (as measured by accepted indicators) and, at the same time, to adapt mechanisms to protect the overall development process. For example, insurance can provide protection against random poverty-generating events, but if similar results can be achieved by pooling resources, no matter how small, by alternative mechanisms (such as savings and prevention), they should not be ruled out. A combination of insurance and prevention can be just as effective in poor countries as it has been in rich countries.

Finally, we are talking about *microinsurance units*, that is, community-funded health insurance schemes that are neither commercial nor national (Dror and Jacquier 1999). These microinsurers do not have access to the resources and financial techniques of commercial insurance and are not constrained by general policy considerations of governmental insurance. For these reasons—and no doubt more than with other types of insurance—the viability of microinsurance depends to a large extent on a coherent distinction between insurable and uninsurable risks.

THE PROBLEM OF INSURABILITY

Where is the borderline of insurable risks? Condorcet might have suggested the answer more than two centuries ago: A risk is uninsurable if it does not allow "opposing chance to itself" (Condorcet 1793, p. 273). Stated in modern terminology, and bearing in mind the limits of microeconomic theory, the following implicit insurability axiom would apply:

> Insurance is a contract under which, in return for payment of a fee (or premium), a specialized body (the insurer) agrees to pay the contract holder (the insured party), a defined benefit if a predefined event occurs to which the insured may be exposed.

This definition excludes random losses resulting from financial speculation or games of chance, because the insured is not exposed unwillingly to the risk. The definition also implies that the insured risk is legal. But taken literally, it also excludes risks whose probability, or the scope of the potential damage, cannot be evaluated, because the indispensable elements for a contractual definition of the event are missing.

The history of insurance is replete with examples of coverage of new risk categories and a broadening of the scope of insurable risks, resulting from a concurrent need for new types of insurance and the technical possibility of responding to these requests through more advanced technical risk-transfer instruments. Yet, many risks are uninsurable if their occurrence is potentially exposed to moral hazard. For instance, a bad driver can be insured against car accidents, including those for which she or he is responsible, but a student would not normally find insurance against the risk of failing an exam, even if the exam question is randomly drawn from a large number of subjects. A puncture in a bicycle tire or the loss of cash may be random risks, or similar to other events that may by common sense be viewed as insurable, yet they are not normally insured for the same reason. Natural catastrophes and industrial risks, long considered uninsurable, have become insurable. These events, once excluded from insurance because their cost exceeded the insurer's capacity, have become insurable as a result of new reinsurance techniques.

Both theoreticians and practitioners would welcome practical, objective criteria for defining clear limits for insurability. Such criteria would enable risk takers to select the risks they can transfer and insurers to choose the risks they will cover. In practice, however, establishing such criteria is difficult. The following discussion shows why.

MULTIPLYING CRITERIA OR DIVIDING THE CONCEPT

Contemporary studies deal with insuring risks that could be qualified as atypical compared with the traditional range of casualty and civil (third-party) liability insurance (Vaillier 2001). Some theoreticians have studied natural and industrial catastrophes (Moatti 1989; Maréchal 1991), development risks, therapeutic risks (Ewald 1993), health risks carried by microinsurance in poor countries (Dror and Jacquier 1999), and so on. As the purpose is to establish selection methodology, two approaches may be considered: an exhaustive list of conditions that, if met, would *include* an event as "insurable"; alternatively, a conceptual framework of conditions applicable to each type of risk that, if satisfied, would *exclude* an event from insurability.

Theoreticians following the first approach define as *insurable events* only random risks that occur in the future, are not exposed to moral hazard or free riding, can be pooled, can be insured by law, and which at least one insurer is willing to insure (that is, the insurer thinks this is economically viable (Yeatman 1998, p. 15). Another theoretician added that the maximum loss must be limited, that the event cannot be too rare (to allow homogenizing), and that the premium should be affordable (Berliner 1982). There is no way of knowing whether this list of conditions is so exhaustive as to cover every new case that might arise.

The second approach is to formulate a meta-law, containing four essential elements—the risk, the insurer, the insured party, and the contract—in relation to which an event can be insured only if it is not excluded by one (or more) of the following conditions:

- *Risk characteristics* (RC). A risk that is not random cannot be insured, for instance, because it is an unavoidable consequence of events that have already occurred or because it depends entirely upon the choice of the insured party.

- *Obligation of the insurer* (O). A risk is uninsurable if no insurer agrees to cover it under conditions considered acceptable by at least one insured party.

- *Affiliation of the insured party* (A). A risk is uninsurable if nobody accepts the conditions at least one insurer considers acceptable.

- *Social utility of the contract* (SU). Taken literally, the contract implies the insurer's future obligations toward the insured, because insurance is not a monetary spot transaction. In addition, the legal environment and the broader social environment within which insurance contracts are made incorporate the notion of social utility. In other words, a risk is uninsurable if the law forbids its coverage, if such insurance does not improve social welfare, or if it contributes to its deterioration.

The conditions of obligation and affiliation refer to the feasibility of the insurance contract irrespective of the technical characteristics of the risk itself. This feasibility depends on assessments of the economic viability of the contract between two contracting parties, each with its own interests in mind. These conditions, separately and together, imply that the economic foundation of the boundary between insurability and uninsurability is "built on intention and capacity" (Vaillier 2001). This also implies searching for reasons insurance markets are ineffective (Gollier and Kessler 1994; Gollier 1996).

As the contracting parties may be groups as well as individuals, the paradigm of "insuring everything" or "insuring nothing" may be equally undesirable for the general interest. The development of insurance has contributed to economic growth over the past centuries, but too much insurance can foster irresponsibility, bankrupt insurers, and destroy social protection systems.

Thus, the problem of insurability can be categorized by three distinct yet complementary limits: actuarial (RC), economic (O and A), and sociopolitical (SU) limits. Figure 6.1 illustrates this method:

Each of these limits—actuarial, economic, and political—is discussed in the following three sections.

FIGURE 6.1   Insurability Analysis Grid

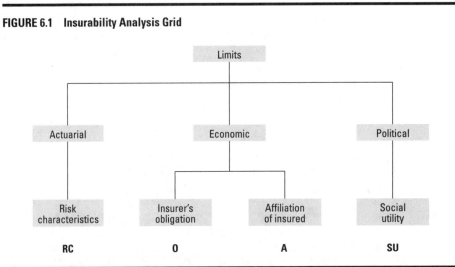

ACTUARIAL LIMITS

Following the meta-law explored above, a risk is uninsurable if its statistical characteristics do not conform to actuarial calculation requirements that:

- Risk-generating events must be random.

- These risks are both observable and diversifiable.

    Meeting these two conditions allows the insurer to set a statistical compensation.

The Random Nature of Events

The etymology of *aléa* [game of dice] suggests that a random event is as predictable as throwing dice. At the moment the die starts to roll, no one can predict which face will appear when it stops. On the other hand, anyone can make a list of possible results and attribute probabilities, under assumptions about how perfect the die is. The only certainty at that point in time is that only the solutions compiled are possible. But things are rarely this simple in insurance, much less in the case of health risks.

    A broken bone, a snakebite, or an infectious disease—none of these examples can be compared to a perfect die and yet they can be qualified as random. For theoreticians and insurance professionals alike, the random nature of events contains—more or less explicitly—five conditions, to which we propose adding a sixth (*nonpresumed*).

- The event is *possible*: it is neither certain nor impossible.

- The risk is *nonspeculative*: occurrence of the risk will not benefit the insured party (unlike bets or speculation).

- The event is *imaginable*: the damaging consequences (both the nature of the damage and its cost) can be imagined, if imperfectly.

- The risk is *exogenous*: the event is unexpected and therefore its occurrence cannot be predetermined before signing the insurance contract. Furthermore, the occurrence of the risk cannot depend upon the sole intention of the insured party, but may occur as a consequence of an action taken by the insured party without malice or intention.

- The risk is *future*: insurance cannot cover a risk that has already occurred (at least known to have occurred) at the time of signing the contract.

- The risk is *nonpresumed*: in addition to the two preceding conditions, chronic risks or those correlated to causes that have occurred, as well as risks that have been forecast according to a conjunction of indicators, are also excluded. Insofar as this category deals with correlation and forecasts, such risks are also exogenous, in the broad sense of the term.

Examples of excluded risks: pathologies that are incompatible with the age and sex of the individual; lump-sum benefits that could exceed expenses incurred; the appearance of an unknown pathology; self-mutilation; diagnosed disease; a chronic condition.

Statistical Compensation of Risks

The statistical compensation of risks—the foundation of all insurance activity—includes two aspects: first, pooling and diversifying risks; second, calculating compensations and determining a corresponding premium.

The risks are diversifiable. Insurance exists when risks can be diversified. This means that, hypothetically, many people are willing to pay to insure themselves against a risk that will strike only a few individuals.

By pooling risks, the insurer applies the law of large numbers. Insurance activity makes sense when risks can be transferred from a risk-averse insured party to the insurer whose risk aversion is lower, as it can "pool" such risks, that is, aggregate a sufficiently large number of independent occurrences (clients). The insurer can calculate an actuarial premium, which can be assumed to be close to the mean amount of compensation paid out, and use the law of large numbers to determine a safety margin to limit its own bankruptcy probability.

The hypothesis that risks are independent is very important, because pooling correlated risks will multiply instead of diversify them. Where chances of risk clustering are high, the insurer may be exposed to systematic risks, as in epidemics.

Example of undiversifiable risks: epidemics

For an insurer of health risks, a client concentration in a single region is dangerous because geographic proximity can increase risk correlation in the case of epidemics or other clustering of communicable diseases. In insurance terms, this translates into a large number of almost simultaneous claims. Theoretically, in this case, risks can be diversified in two ways:

- Intertemporally. Years with epidemics are statistically compensated by years without epidemics—assuming that a sequence of epidemic years is rare and short. This solution presupposes that the insurer has sufficient reserves to pay the cost of claims in "epidemic years."

- Geographically. Through reinsurance, the insurer transfers its risk to a larger pool of insured in other regions with a different exposure to risks. At the level of the reinsurer, the risk no longer has the same systematic character as it did for the direct insurer.

The risks are observable. The condition was set earlier that insurable random events must be imaginable. Quantification of payments relative to potential events is indispensable, as actuarial calculation can be applied only to quantitative data.

The two types of observable characteristics are first, the list of benefits covered and therefore their cost (for the insurer); and second, the probability of events that are likely to trigger the cost.

- *Estimating the cost of insured damage.* An insurer that agrees to cover a specific risk needs to know the approximate (not necessarily the exact) sums it might have to pay. Generally speaking, this excludes risks for which the cost is totally unknown or unlimited, above and beyond the insurer's capacity to pay (including hypothetical recourse to a larger reinsurance system).

- *Estimating probabilities.* To begin with, the probability of the insured events—and more important, their probable cost—have to be known. In effect, the insurance covers the insured person's damage, expenses, or losses resulting from an event. The event's occurrence is not meaningful, as insurance is neither a gamble nor a bet.

  Example: In microinsurance, the useful estimate is not so much the probability of being infected with malaria but the probability of a mild or severe flare-up, with the corresponding cost for care $X or $Y. For this estimate, some basic information is needed about the frequency and severity of malaria cases.

To improve the accuracy of estimates, epidemiology or mathematical techniques can be used (Haggerty and Reid, chapter 18, and Auray and Fonteneau, chapter 8, respectively, this volume). Estimating errors can also be treated as a random variable, that is, as a risk the insurer can transfer to a reinsurer. If no information (not even incomplete) can be gathered about a risk, it is technically uninsurable. When coverage cannot be based on actuarial calculations, other decision criteria must be used such as social or philanthropic considerations.

If the insurer does not know the probability of a risk, it might refuse to cover it, choosing to avoid the possibility of a high unknown probability. In this same state of uncertainty, a risk-averse individual might wish to seek insurance (which could reinforce the insurer's initial reticence). The risk becomes technically uninsurable because the probability is unknown (ambiguous setting), not because of the nature of the risk itself.

In recent insurance history, coverage has been extended to new risks such as natural catastrophes, major industrial risks, and satellite launchings. The novelty here is not the occurrence of the risk but its coverage despite uncertain observation criteria. In the absence of statistical data, the evaluation of these risks relies on proxy notions such as the scale of potential events or their likelihood.

Microinsurance and observability

Microinsurance is confronted with difficulties figuring out risk-exposure probabilities because the statistical capacity is underdeveloped and because the persons involved are unfamiliar with the concept of insurance, which makes reliable observations doubly elusive. In these circumstances, microinsurance could cover health risks for an "acceptable" price. Since actuarial calculations cannot be applied to this type of risk, premiums can be determined initially by assessing the insured's willingness to pay and comparing this income to the insurer's capacity to support errors in the claim load (which could be considerable in relation to available reserves). If the initial contribution amount is incorrectly estimated, it can be adjusted later on the basis of actual experience. Microinsurance units starting with low reserves would do well to reinsure their business for protection against initial risk-estimating errors.

ECONOMIC LIMITS

Too low a premium exposes the insurer to insolvency if the risk occurs and income does not cover the cost. Insurers might be tempted to lower premiums to enlarge their market share, but potential clients have a vested interest in the insurer's solvency, because they have to be reasonably certain that the insurer can pay a claim. Shareholders also have an interest in collecting a dividend on their capital, which requires positive operating results. By signing an insurance contract, the insured transfers to the insurer the risk specified in the contract but takes on another risk, that the insurer will be unable to meet its obligations (a risk not normally mentioned). Stated in economic terms, the insured is interested in as low a premium as possible but also in the economic viability of the insurance transaction. Each transaction has to offer both parties an acceptable solution. If it does not, the prospect of insuring a risk is economically unviable.

The Insurer's Obligation

Under condition O, it was stated that "a risk is uninsurable if no insurer agrees to cover it under conditions considered acceptable by at least one insured party." Put differently, a risk is uninsurable if no prospective insured party agrees to sign an insurance contract at a price that is economically viable for the insurer. Because the insurer cannot maximize profit without attracting clients, the economic constraints under which an insurer can offer a viable insurance contract have to be explored. We assume that the benefit package is clearly defined. For the microinsurer, the monetary cost of the events covered is a random variable $\tilde{X}$, with a mean of $E(\tilde{X})$ and a variance of s^2. The *actuarial premium* to cover this package could be set at $pr = E(\tilde{X})$. In addition, a *loading factor* is added to the premium, composed of two parts: a safety loading (at rate $-\alpha$), and a loading for administrative costs and capital reimbursement (at rate μ). Thus, the effective (or *commercial*) premium π is equal to: $\pi = (1 + \alpha + \mu)\ pr$.

It is assumed that μ covers costs exactly. The sum of the actuarial premiums, equal to the mathematical expectation of the sum of cost-generating events, is noted as PR. The annual results of the insurer is a random $\tilde{R}$ for which the mean is:

$$E(\tilde{X}) = (1 + \alpha + \mu)\ .PR - PR - \mu\ PR = \alpha\ PR$$

and the variance is S^2. As the maximum annual loss that can be borne, M, is equal at most to the insurer's own capital, the insurer agrees to cover the risk only if the probability is negligible that his final business outcome (M+ $\tilde{R}$) will be negative. In some cases, this means that for insurance to exist, worst-case scenarios that would bring the insurer beyond the limit have to be covered from another source (for example, a subsidy [Busse, chapter 13, this volume]). Since the variance S^2 provides a measure of how far the final business result can be below the expected average, the insurer will choose to operate with a safety loading rate .(α) that will ensure that the available funds M + α PR would cover at least a possible loss going down to βS. This condition is expressed by the following equation:

$$\beta = \frac{M + \alpha . PR}{S}$$

β is referred to as a *safety coefficient* (see glossary, this volume). The statistical distribution of β is linked to the random variable $\tilde{R}$: the larger the value of β, the smaller is the risk of insolvency. For a random probability of insolvency, computation of the corresponding critical value β^* depends upon the shape and parameters of the distribution of $\tilde{R}$. As a minimum, estimates of E($\tilde{R}$) and S are needed (quite likely for microinsurance unit scenario) to approximate the value (see glossary, this volume). In the case where the insurer covers n persons who face, independently, an identical risk (with the same mean *pr*, and the same variance s^2), the mean and variance are PR = n.*pr* and S^2 = n.s^2. Thus, the safety coefficient depends on the number of *insureds*[1] n, and is expressed by the following equation:

$$\beta = \frac{M + \alpha . n\,pr}{s\,\sqrt{n}}$$

Figure 6.2 illustrates the relationship between the safety coefficient β and the number of insureds n for a given set of values for M, α, pr, and s. As M (insurer's capital) is independent of the size of the insured group n, when M is large enough, the safety coefficient β will exceed a critical value β^* regardless of the number of insureds. It can be inferred from the above equation that β(n) increases as M, *pr*, and α increase, but decreases with increasing variance s^2. Assuming that the value of M is independent (and cannot usually be changed), it is used here as a control variable. For a given M, the insurer has two courses of action to operate above the critical value of β^*: it can increase the premium to attain a sufficient safety loading (α); or it can select the risks to ensure a low s relative to *pr*.[2]

When the insurer's capital M is low, insurance operation will be possible either with few members (under point n_1 in figure 6.2), where the constraint $\beta > \beta^*$ is satisfied, but then the law of large numbers no longer applies; or with many more members (exceeding point n_2), which allows for risk pooling and homogenizing of risks (and therefore reduces the need for large reserves), but enlisting a large membership could be difficult to achieve in small community-based health systems.

For a given value of β^*, the safety loading α becomes a control variable. Figure 6.3 describes the critical curve α(n), for a given value of β^* and of M. The rate α has to be high enough to satisfy $\beta \geq \beta^*$, but not too high to raise the price of insurance beyond the household's reach. This is possible in some cases but not in all, as α is like a price variable (save the loading factor at rate μ): the function of

FIGURE 6.2 Safety Coefficient β and Number of Insureds
(for two levels of maximum loss M)

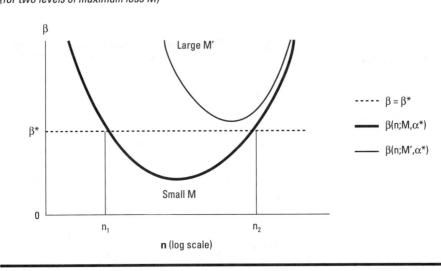

demand for insurance is a decreasing relation $n = \varphi(\alpha)$ between the membership n and the "price" α. Figure 6.3 shows an unfavorable example, where the demand for insurance stands on the left side of the graph (small n, even for small values of α). Microeconomic analysis would suggest that this is likely to happen when the household's income is low, or the consumers are few. With a wider market, or a higher income, the demand curve could stand at the right of, or above, the critical curve $\alpha(n)$ for β^*.

Reinsurance can increase β by covering worst-case scenarios, thus reducing S (that is, the denominator of β). This measure will be effective provided that the net cost of reinsurance is lower than the expected gain. In mathematical terms, the cost of reinsurance needs to remain smaller than β^* times the absolute expected reduction of the standard deviation.

Microinsurance, safety margin, and minimum number of insureds

In the case of microinsurance, unlike traditional commercial insurance, one can consider that $M = 0$ (or even $M < 0$, provided that no loading is added to cover administrative costs). If $M = 0$, the solution of $\beta(n) = \beta^*$ is unique, and represents the critical number of insureds n^*. If the microinsurance cannot attain the critical number of insureds n^*, it cannot operate under normal safety margins.

If, at the anticipated rate α, the demand for insurance is less than n^*, a decrease in price will be ineffective if the demand is inelastic. Such situations can result, for example, from a demographic barrier (the maximum population concerned is too small in relation to the solvency threshold) or from a "poverty wall." To be viable in

FIGURE 6.3   Safety Loading Rate α and Number of Insureds
(for two levels of maximum loss M)

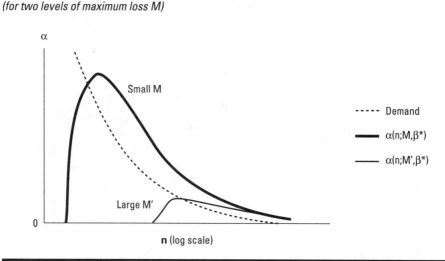

such a case, the microinsurance must either acquire a financial capacity M > 0 or modify its coverage to reduce the variance of risks. If it is unable to increase resource mobilization from the members, the microinsurer needs to explore other solutions such as subsidies or a grant. Without this, the only solution is to adjust coverage toward a lower risk or, alternatively, to raise membership.

Affiliation of the Insured Party

As mentioned, an insurance market exists only when people agree to pay the premium (or contribution) due. Based on the discussion in the preceding paragraph, it can now be said that the number of insureds has to be large enough to enable the insurer to reach the necessary critical mass. If this cannot be done, the premium will increase to levels that, in the economic and social context, will be considered excessive, not only by individual consumers but also by most of the catchment population, signifying that at the given price the insurance transaction is inoperable.

What then is the right price to avoid this circular situation? The price of a good or service cannot be determined to be "acceptable" in absolute terms. According to the utility theory, the price is acceptable if the marginal utility added by acquiring the good is greater than the marginal loss of utility from its cost.[3] This fundamental logic, applied to the decision to accept an insurance contract, is based on the dual risk theory model (Yaari 1987; Cohen 1995; glossary, this volume) and illustrated in figure 6.4 (Vaté 1999, p. 148). This theory is of special interest in the field of insurance because, unlike the standard theory of expected

FIGURE 6.4   Cost/Benefit of Insurance

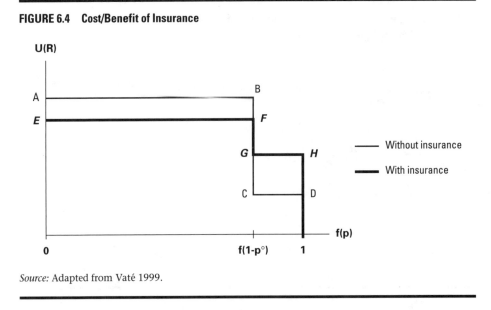

Source: Adapted from Vaté 1999.

utility, it represents separately the attitude of the individual toward the probability of damage and the perception of its magnitude.

According to the usual microeconomic concept, the utility function U(R) is a utility index associated with the level R of the individual's wealth. Any expense or loss has a negative effect upon U, and it is generally assumed that the marginal utility U'(R) does not increase with R. For example, U(R) can be reduced by BC (satisfaction lost because of uninsured damage); by AE (payment of a premium); and by FG (deductible payable by the insured party).

The function f(p) is a distortion function applied to decumulative probabilities, starting from the worst result with probability 1, up to the best result that can be exceeded with probability zero (Quiggin 1982; glossary, this volume). Denoting by p° the probability of a random damage, f(1-p°) is the transformed value of the probability of no damage. Any distortion function can be compared with the identity function f(p) = p; it is pessimistic if f(p)<p everywhere, and optimistic when f(p)>p. Quiggin (1982) suggests that f(p) could combine the first type for p > 0.5 with the second one for p < 0.5. A strong curvature of f in the first case expresses a strong risk aversion.

The amount of the premium is acceptable if the loss of utility (ABFE) is compensated by the gains (GHDC). The situation depicted in figure 6.4 is not favorable to insurance. If all other factors (including the utility function) remain equal, three possible changes in existing parameters could swing the balance in favor of insurance: decreasing the premium (lower AE), eliminating the deductible (FG = 0), or increasing aversion to risk (function f is more curved, -then f(1-p°) decreases).

Doing away with deductibles may increase exposure to moral hazard. Decreasing the premium could compromise the microinsurer's solvency; however, this option may become feasible through reinsurance. Finally, the aversion to risk can perhaps be increased by means of a well-targeted educational campaign.

An actuarial premium that is considered acceptable may become unacceptable after adding transaction costs and a loading factor to compensate for the imperfect insurability of the risk. Transaction costs also increase when real-life situations preclude strict verification of actuarial criteria, (for example, imperfect or imprecise information, elusive contractual fit). This widens the gap between the cost of insurance and the actuarial premium. Without necessarily being aware of it, all individuals manage a "risk portfolio," including domestic risks, health risks, liability, and professional and financial risks. An individual can influence this global risk by preventive actions, prudent behavior, or by purchasing insurance against risks that can be insured. The amount of the premium will seem readily acceptable if the insurance covers risks that contribute heavily to the overall liability, particularly if there is a positive correlation with other forms of loss or damage.

> Good examples of this are illnesses causing chronic disability that impair an individual's professional capacity, compromise future income, endanger the education of his or her children, or lead to social exclusion.

But unfavorable economic and social conditions can lead an individual to view a premium as unacceptable. This is the case when willingness to pay (price effect) prevails over the ability to pay (income effect), notably when health costs' share of average income increases (pushing up the actuarial premium). The likelihood of buying insurance improves when the insured's assets increase, when the premium is subsidized, or when the risks are vital (lower acceptability threshold). However, in the case of health, the tradeoff is not only between the utility and the cost of insurance but also between the benefits in terms of health impacts at different stages of the disease (and at different ages) for an identical amount of money paid.

> Even the very poor spend money on health care, but this money provides a low ratio of cost to benefit, which insurance can improve. Insurability may nevertheless seem compromised either when a "poverty wall" makes paying any insurance premium radically unacceptable or when cultural reasons make signing up for insurance unimaginable or incomprehensible. In this case, regardless of the actuarial characteristics, health risks are outside the economic scope of insurance but can be brought back by providing free health insurance.

If, however, the insured can choose the coverage, and the package covers the insured's perceived priorities, payment of a premium can become acceptable.

And finally, the boundary for insurable risks is also set through *truncated elasticity*. The insurable nature of a random risk (in the actuarial sense) is reinforced when medical consumption remains rigid as prices drop. In the case of emergency surgery or other completely inelastic demand (indicated in figure 6.5 by a specific

FIGURE 6.5   Truncated Elasticity and Other Cases

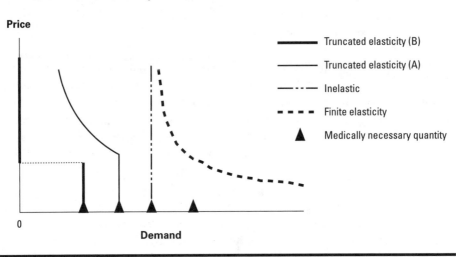

Price

———— Truncated elasticity (B)

———— Truncated elasticity (A)

—··— Inelastic

— — — Finite elasticity

▲ Medically necessary quantity

0

Demand

symbol[4]), the sick person and family must find the necessary resources. When the price exceeds those resources, demand drops to zero. Reducing the price will not increase demand, since nobody will undergo such a procedure unless it is absolutely necessary. For instance, nobody will seek an amputation just because it is cheap or even free of charge. Conversely, price decreases will increase elastic demand (for example, cosmetic surgery), but again, not endlessly. Demand will increase as the price drops up to the point where most prospective users consider it affordable. Below that point, demand will not increase further since the good or service is not useful for the entire population. Figure 6.5 illustrates this concept, where demand is measured in units (for example, hospitalization day, ultrasound imaging), and the price variable c is the cost of one unit. *Truncated elasticity* (the change in demand as a function of price) is non-zero above a certain price level c^*; it becomes zero for all prices under c^* (figure 6.5, case A). Exceptionally, where benefits are an indivisible unit (for example, surgery), elasticity may also be zero above c^* (figure 6.5, case B). The values denoting the limits of elasticity are marked by the small triangle. In the ordinary case of finite elasticity, this specific point makes medical sense but has no particular economic significance.

Nonetheless, demand rigidity/elasticity does not provide a criterion for determining the boundary between random insurable and uninsurable risks. The argument might be true when prices decrease (where overconsumption is similar to ex-post moral hazard), but not when prices increase, which can bring about a drop in consumption even in necessary and urgent treatments.

Corollary: The mere fact that expensive health risks are excluded from insurance does not provide any useful clue about the insurability of those risks.

Thus, in summary, the *solvable* nature of the insurance transaction and *truncated elasticity* constitute, jointly, a concise way of defining the economic limit of insurable risks. This definition suggests that economic limits define a subset of the actuarial rule to identify insurable risks. This is generally correct, but there are exceptions, for example, risks that are not insurable in the economic sense, but which become insurable by their inclusion in an inseparable benefit package. From the insurer's viewpoint, such packaging reduces adverse selection. From the insured's perspective, the higher price of the package reduces the cost-benefit ratio, but it may still be acceptable if it covers a wider range of risks. A single, comprehensive policy is more attractive than a combination of partial insurance policies, even though it is more expensive. This is known as the *portfolio effect*.

Information Asymmetry

The consequences of asymmetrical information (moral hazard, adverse selection) occupy an important place in the theory of imperfect markets (Weber, chapter 9, this volume). This is inherently linked to the essential role of information in determining the insurability of risks and in operating insurance transactions, discussed earlier. Yet this problem is omnipresent in insurance.

Asymmetrical information and health risks: (Arrow 1963; Ehrlich and Becker 1972; Rotschild and Stiglitz 1976; Eeckhoudt and Gollier 1992; Newhouse 1996; Couffinhal 2000).

A short reminder may be useful that adverse selection occurs when high-risk individuals, whose condition is unknown to the insurer, can buy insurance.

Moral hazard manifests itself in three ways:

- *Ex-ante demand-side moral hazard* affects the random nature of the risk, because it incites persons to decrease their preventive efforts simply because they are insured.

- *Ex-post demand-side moral hazard* affects the elasticity of expenses, because it incites persons to overconsume health care that is free or cheap, as a result of insurance.

- *Supply-induced moral hazard* affects the financial balance of the health care system, and thus its ability to deliver public goods, for it pushes providers to oversupply and increase additional costs, if they know the patient is insured.

The information asymmetry issue, despite its importance, cannot serve as a rule for declaring that a risk is uninsurable simply because it may be open to adverse selection or moral hazard. As long as this effect is merely possible and not certain, the remedy to lowering its likelihood could be careful selection of the composition of the package or precise definition of the qualifying conditions in the contract. Only when the magnitude of these insurance failures exceeds actuarial and economic insurability criteria and poses a structural threat to the insurer's solvency, would they become uninsurable.

Linking Economic and Actuarial Limits

In theory, a risk that fulfills the actuarial requirement of insurability would not encounter economic obstacles strong enough to eliminate the offer or demand. But in reality things are not always so clear-cut. Actuarial and economic insurability criteria are rarely binary, and when either actuarial or economic inclusion conditions are imperfectly satisfied, the boundary of their intersection becomes imprecise. This may result in the exclusion of benefits that would have been included under one criterion alone.

Examples of extensions:

- A microinsurer agrees to cover health risks without prior medical examination. It thereby implicitly agrees to cover preexisting or already diagnosed risks, for instance, because the prime objective is to increase the covered population, and this is an economic motive for coverage that appears stronger than those for exclusion (for reasons explained in the previous section on the impact of group size on solvency).

- A particularly costly pathology is not economically insurable because of the risk of adverse selection and the disproportion between the actuarial premium and the insured's ability to pay. This pathology could nevertheless be included if it is bundled in a larger package.

POLITICAL LIMITS

To be insurable from the political point of view, an event must represent a licit risk that can also be transferred legally. The risk transfer also has to conform to the regulatory framework, including its interpretation through jurisprudence (Berliner 1982; Gollier and Kessler 1994). As these limits are the expression of choices made by public authorities, they can be either restrictive—disallowing the insurance of certain risks that are contrary to the public interest (for example, insuring against the payment of fines, losses from games of chance, speculative risks)—or proscriptive, identifying risks that must be insured in the interest of society at large. Such mandatory/universal insurance may apply even to risks that would not be considered insurable under actuarial or economic criteria. One example (from the public sector) is universal health insurance coverage. Public authorities may also decide to operate as an insurer (sometimes operating a monopoly).

Political criteria for insuring health risks

Checklist 1. *Restrictive* political limits would operate when the responses to one of the following four questions are positive (and material) for a given risk:

- Is insuring this risk *forbidden by law*?

- Is the risk *covered elsewhere*, notably by national insurance?

- Does the health care—and other benefits—occasioned by this risk fall into the realm of *public property* (nonexcludable and indivisible)?

- Is there supply-side *moral hazard* for this type of health care and benefit?

Checklist 2. *Expansive* political limits would operate when the responses to one of the following four questions are positive for a given risk:

- Is there a risk of *social exclusion* for the uninsured patient?

- Does the health care—and other benefits—occasioned by this risk fall into the realm of *private property* (excludable and divisible)?

- Does the insured event (for example, illness, accident) occasion negative externality in the form of *collective economic damage*?

- Does the consumption of health care and other benefits create *positive externalities*?

The difference between the third and fourth conditions in Checklist 2 is whether the externality results from the health problem itself, or from the insurable intervention against it. (Public health discussions usually consider only the former kind of externality.)

Political limits are especially relevant when they seem to conflict with actuarial and economic rules, just as they are redundant when they postulate the same logic. Hence, Checklist 1 excludes risks that could theoretically be covered by economically viable insurance. Checklist 2 would enable coverage of otherwise uninsurable risks. Only the powerful intervention of public authorities can achieve this result, for example, by imposing compulsory coverage for all or part of these risks, or by paying subsidies (directly to insurers, health care providers, or insureds), or by providing a reinsurance system.

A PRACTICAL DELIMITATION OF THE SCOPE OF INSURANCE

This section reviews the issue of insurability from an operational rather than a theoretical perspective. Each risk requires a single response to the question: Is this risk insurable? The ideas developed earlier can be summarized in four queries about insurability: Is the risk random and the covered event possible? Is the transaction *solvable*? Is elasticity *truncated*? What is the social *utility*?

Replies to these considerations are illustrated in the *insurability analysis grid* (Second Stage) for a list of events. Figure 6.6, composed from some 30 items discussed so far, shows factors contributing to insurability. Possible redundancies have been eliminated.

The analysis is done from the microinsurer's point of view. Hence, the grid is structured to respond to the specific needs of this kind of insurer, rather than in the order suggested by theoretical analysis. We shall proceed in four stages: preliminary

FIGURE 6.6   Factors Contributing to Insurability

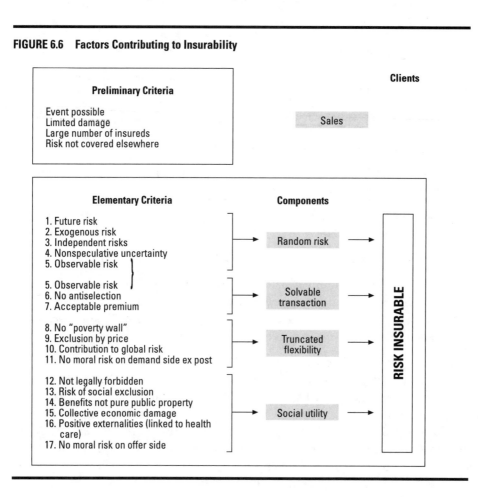

criteria, "external" risk analysis, "internal" analysis of risk transfer, and moving the boundaries.

First Stage: Preliminary Criteria

The following four preliminary conditions provide a framework without which the question of insurability would not make sense:

- The occurrence of the risk is *possible*.

- The damage, or the microinsurer's monetary consequences, is *limited* when the triggering event occurs (for example, illness or accident).

- A *sufficiently large number* of persons sign up for coverage of the risk, enabling the law of large numbers to apply. (Alternatively, the microinsurer can transfer risks to reinsurance, thereby compensating for small membership.)

- The risk *is not covered elsewhere* (for example, social security or governmental programs).

The following analysis assumes that all these conditions have been satisfied.

Second Stage: "External" Risk Analysis

Three of the four characteristics of insurability—random nature, truncated elasticity, and collective utility—are external to the microinsurer's capacity to intervene. Therefore, if these conditions are *not* met, the microinsurer cannot assume the costs related to events that do not respond to the three primary criteria (table 6.1).

Third Stage: "Internal" Analysis of Risk Transfer

This stage looks at the insurance transaction. Here, the microinsurer is directly implicated: It is the unit that knows if—and how—it can respond to its environmental restrictions. But the unit shares the end response with the population, the final judge of the acceptable cost of the insurance, as measured by willingness and ability to pay.

Example

This example is very simplified. It does not take into account, for example, administrative costs ($\mu = 0$), which are necessary in real-life applications. The maximum loss is limited to $M = 0$, in which case costs are exactly covered by loading rate μ or by a subsidy; otherwise $M < 0$.

TABLE 6.1   "External" Risk Analysis

Event	Random risk	Truncated elasticity	Social utility	Insurability
Accident by voluntary exposure to danger	Yes	Yes	No	NO
Accidental wounds	Yes	Yes	Yes	YES
Alcoholism	No	No	No	NO
Chronic disease	No	Yes/No	Yes	NO
Viral disease	Yes	Yes	Yes	YES
Malaria (mild)	Yes	No[a]	Yes	NO
Malaria (severe)	Yes	Yes[a]	Yes	YES
Snake bite	Yes	Yes	Yes	YES
Vaccination	No	Yes	Yes	NO

a. A mild case of malaria differs from a severe case in the cost of treating the flare-up. When the cost is too high, treating a mild case without insurance is cheaper. This is not so with a severe case.

Following the second stage, a benefit package is elaborated that is the basis of the family contract. The following information applies: the level of the actuarial premium is pr = \$5, with a standard deviation of \$20. The target population comprises 4,000 families. Half of them (n = 2000) would enroll if fees equal π = \$5 (that is: α = 0); none would enroll if fees equal $\pi \geq \exists 10$ (that is: α = 1), presuming that the relation between π and n is linear.

As a safety measure, microinsurers make it a rule not to go below, say, β = 5, but this result is unattainable. It is possible to come close, with β = 4.3 for α = 2/3, or π = \$8.3, which enables the microinsurer to insure around 650 families. A decrease in price (by reducing α) serves no purpose, because an increase in the covered population will not compensate for the increase in risk taken by the microinsurer. Hence, this benefit package constitutes an uninsurable economic risk. If the microinsurer cannot find a subsidy, it must eliminate from the package the benefits with the highest variance in utilization rate or cost. We observe that by bringing pr to \$4 and s to \$12, we can cover almost 1,100 families for a fee of \$5.8 (safety coefficient: β = 5).

Fourth Stage: Moving the Boundaries

Two mechanisms can modify the situation described in the preceding analysis: reinsurance and the intervention of public authorities. These mechanisms cannot be disassociated from the insurability issue that the microinsurer must resolve: they are an integral part of decisionmaking and negotiation.

Reinsurance. Reinsurance enables microinsurers to lower their contributions, which improves their capacity to attract demand for insurance among the population. For high risks (those representing considerable damage or a high probability), the actuarial premium is probably out of reach for poor people. By leveling off high risks through reinsurance, the price can be reduced, and usually also broadening the population that can afford coverage. Another important facet of reinsurance is that it enables microinsurers to operate under a lower value of β while transferring the added risk to reinsurance. This opens the way to include in the benefit package risks that have a high variance either in utilization or in cost. These risks are not necessarily the most costly benefits, but the ones with high variability. Lowering the requirement for β will automatically render the proposed benefit insurable.

From the microinsurers' perspective, reinsurance has two conflicting effects: It lowers the variance and thus improves the safety coefficient, but it also increases the cost, which weakens it. As long as the balance is positive, the insurer can cover certain risks previously judged uninsurable for economic reasons.

Moreover, including uninsurable benefits (for example, prevention and vaccination) in the package from the beginning lowers the safety coefficient β. Including these benefits later (that is, financing them from surpluses) makes them dependent on results, which are random. Hence, reinsurance can very likely have a perceptible stabilizing impact on the results, and thus also on the ability to include some uninsurable costs in the package.

Interventions by public authorities. This section summarizes expansive and restrictive interventions by public authorities and their effect on insurable risks (table 6.2).

Hypothetically, whenever insurance is offered, a risk may be considered uninsurable on economic rather than actuarial grounds. The absence of any offer could be for both reasons. The second column illustrates (except in the first line) the kind of interventions that are uninsurable on technical (actuarial) or economic reasons but which the public authorities decree insurable. The third column describes risks that are forbidden for insurance by public order.

The public authorities' role is decisive for at least three reasons: unlike ordinary goods and services that anyone can sell, insurance contracts can be issued only by government-licensed insurance companies; the insurer's solvency falls into the realm of public order; and government social preferences—with or without insurance—can differ from those of the insurers. Public authorities would normally discourage imprudence and would not allow a situation of paralyzing insecurity to persist (Vaillier 2001). In the interactions between the players, each party (the actuary, the insurer, the insured party, and the state) has a different

TABLE 6.2   Public Interventions and Their Effect on Insurable Risks

Situation	*Intervention makes risk insurable*	*Intervention makes risk uninsurable*[a]
Case 1 Offer exists Demand exists Price of balance	Null	Forbidden
Case 2 Offer exists Demand exists Unacceptable premium	Subsidy to insurer or aid to individual	Forbidden
Case 3 Offer exists No demand exists	Aid to individual or compulsory insurance	Forbidden
Case 4 No offer exists Demand exists	Subsidy to insurer or social security[b]	Null
Case 5 No offer exists No demand exists	Benefit funds or social security[b]	Null

a. In every case, the implementation of a public health insurance system (for example, social security, government programs) makes the corresponding risk uninsurable for it is "already covered elsewhere." Here we refer to the uncovered part of the risk. b. In Cases 4 and 5, the implementation of a public health insurance system responds to a shortage of insurance offers. This does not make the risk insurable, but here a noninsurance type transfer covers it.

notion of what is insurable according to different criteria. In reality, necessity rather than choice oblige all four parties to make the same response, which does not satisfy any one of them in every respect. The state can forbid the insurance of a risk accepted by the other two; it can also—through subsidies, legal obligation, or reinsurance—decree that uninsurable risks should be insured. The state—and the state alone—is able to establish rules or provide resources for contingency funds to deal with emergencies.

CONCLUSIONS

The sequence of actuarial-economic-political criteria has moved the debate about the limits of insurability away from a single, objective, technical definition. In reality, the search for a dichotomy between insurable and uninsurable events clashes with a gray area in which the classification of risks depends on economic, legal, ethical, and cultural circumstances instead of solely on the intrinsic characteristics of the risk or on an objective criterion such as actuarial calculations. In addition, actuarial considerations must give way to a fuzzy classification, for several reasons: first, elementary criteria are multiple and often gradual rather than binary (yes/no); second, information is incomplete or imprecise; and finally, measuring risks is more often a question of judging likelihood than applying a true probability law.

The actors' positions also count: the insured party (who determines whether or not there is demand), the insurer (who decides if there is supply), and public authorities (who need to verify that the market created by the responses of the two actors conforms to the general interest). The analysis has attempted to demonstrate reasons and means by which the state might, in effect, reverse the decision of the market. Such a reversal is particularly likely where risks affect human capital or public health, not merely income and financial assets.

The distinction is also rendered complex by diseases that may be insurable at one stage but uninsurable at a later stage. There is no certainty about these events, about when they will first occur or about whether their incidence will be above or below the expected frequency for any given year. But once they occur, they become chronic conditions, and thus uninsurable. For instance, the initial onset of diabetes, asthma, or high blood pressure is random, but the treatment of the individual afflicted by these disorders is nonrandom, vital, and characterized by inelastic demand. In all financial exercises after the initial diagnosis, these conditions will be classified as chronic. This kind of distinction is difficult to explain to lay persons and, in any case, the moral imperative is that the microinsurer must provide continuing treatment for such conditions once diagnosed. Hence, the matter has to be resolved by estimating not only the probability of the initial discovery of the disease, but also the cost of treating the subsequent chronic condition.

Risks are often doomed to be treated as uninsurable not because of their intrinsic characteristics, but simply because information is missing about their probability, variance, or unit cost. Overcoming this problem is a necessary and urgent challenge. Yet, so far nobody seems to have taken on the responsibility for funding this research. Poor people or individual microinsurers cannot be expected to bear these costs as a precondition to implementing insurance. Nor can any single reinsurer carry this cost, as it would increase the administrative load too much. The logical conclusion is that this critical activity must rely on social or philanthropic priorities.

A different situation prevails with events that are uninsurable such as vaccinations of infants. The precise cost of such activity can be foreseen, and success would normally be measured by a high rate of utilization. The value of vaccinations is linked to their far-reaching consequences on reducing infant mortality or morbidity and the local burden of disease.

Classifying a certain benefit as uninsurable should in no way be construed to imply that it should not be covered or that it has a lower priority than an insurable benefit. This classification is nonetheless necessary to identify the limits that can be financed by applying risk-management techniques, applicable only to insurable events. Uninsurable events would thus have to be financed through other sources that have to be secured up-front, for example, subsidies, surpluses from previous years, or external funding. Because they are financed from different sources, the two types have to be kept separately, for policy and for accounting and actuarial purposes.

All these obstacles point toward the possibility that, in the absence of information allowing identification of risks as insurable or uninsurable, the premium required to provide a sufficiently high safety margin to protect microinsurers against underestimation of risk is likely to be unaffordable by the target population. Three conclusions arise from this analysis:

- There are sound criteria for deciding what is insurable, but they are not by themselves enough to define a benefit package.

- There is a sizable gray or fuzzy area where decisions have to be made because of and despite insufficient guidance from the criteria.

- Microinsurers probably have to learn by doing, which implies extra risk in the early years and therefore a need for extra protection via reinsurance or subsidy.

This strongly suggests that public subsidies should be granted for an initial learning period, and then reduced or withdrawn (and shifted to another microinsurer just getting started) as the scheme matures and its risks are better known (Busse, chapter 13, this volume). This could both reduce the level of public subsidy needed at any one time and give microinsurers incentives to learn fast against the day when the subsidy would be reduced.

The way to acquire the knowledge about risk characteristics relatively fast during start-up is to use whatever field information is available to develop solutions by pragmatic rather than theoretical methods such as simulations (Busse, chapter 13, this volume). Clearly, this option is not free of a risk of error. However, this approach is the most accessible option for a gradual improvement in accuracy of risk estimates, which in turn will result in a decrease in the margin of error in microinsurers' projected financial results. As long as microinsurers base their premiums on insurable risk calculations, a decrease in variance from better risk estimates will lower the price of insurance, thus reducing the risk of insolvency and making insurance affordable to a larger segment of the target population. And—with the transfer of some of the risk to reinsurance—the danger of insolvency can be further reduced. Much of this promising prospect hinges on the ability to distinguish between parallel sources of financing for the two types of cost-generating events. This justifies a continued effort to distinguish between insurable and uninsurable risks covered by microinsurers.

The following annex provides a more detailed discussion of several theoretical issues.

ANNEX 6A DUAL THEORY OF RISK AND THE SAFETY COEFFICIENT

The following section looks at dual theory of risk and the safety coefficient.

Dual Theory of Risk

An extensive literature has been devoted to the paradoxes posed by several empirical experiences with *expected utility (EU) theory,* developed by von Neumann and Morgenstern (1944) and Savage (1954). Among the problems raised, one is of particular interest for insurance theory. In the EU theory, the convexity of the individual's utility function expresses two different things at once: the marginal utility of wealth is decreasing, and the individual is risk averse. Consequently, if two individuals have the same utility index for certain wealth, they cannot have a different degree of aversion to risk (and conversely).

By combining the concept of decumulative utility with the dual theory of risk (Quiggin 1982; Yaari 1987), decision theory under conditions of uncertainty was further developed in the 1980s and 1990s (Cohen 1995). From this work, a simple model of the insurance decision emerged, based on two separate tools:

1. Random results are ranked in the order of growing utility, the utility index u(R) of - wealth R being of a classical type (u'>0, u"<0).

2. A distortion function f(p) applies to decumulative probabilities (p) starting from the worst result with certainty, up to the best result that can be exceeded with probability zero. The f function is a continuous, increasing function from [0;1] to [0;1] satisfying f(0) = 0 and f(1) = 1, and it expresses the individual's pessimism (if f(p)<p) or optimism (if f(p)>p). Considered a psychological characteristic of the decisionmaker, it does not depend upon his or her utility function. Notice that the expected utility theory is a special case of the dual theory where f(p) = p, $\forall$ p.

Let us consider an individual, whose initial wealth is R°, who is exposed to a monetary loss L with probability p*. His final level of wealth is R° unchanged (with probability 1-p*) or R°-L (with certainty p = 1). Any one of the future prospects (R°; 1-p*) and (R°-L; 1) is associated with a utility index (through u, in the upper left quadrant of figure 6.7; see Vaté 1999) and a modified probability (through f, in the lower right quadrant). The synthesis is the area S, which gives the "value" of the uninsured situation (upper right quadrant). Buying an insurance policy has a cost (the premium π), but in any case, the final wealth will be R°-π (assuming no deductible). The corresponding "value" is the area S' in the upper right quadrant of figure 6.7. The individual will affiliate and pay the premium π if S<S'.

Two possible modifications could swing the balance in favor of insurance: decreasing the premium π, or increasing aversion to risk (distortion function f is more curved). It can be noticed that, even with an identical utility function (that is to say, identical feeling toward monetary loss L), individuals would likely adopt different attitudes toward insurance because their feeling is different toward the probability of L: the more curved is the function f, the more attractive is the insurance.

Safety Coefficient

The simplest expression for the annual result of the insurer is as follows:

$$\begin{bmatrix} \text{annual} \\ \text{result} \end{bmatrix} = \begin{bmatrix} \text{premium} \\ \text{earned} \end{bmatrix} - \begin{bmatrix} \text{payment} \\ \text{of claims} \end{bmatrix} - \begin{bmatrix} \text{management} \\ \text{costs} \end{bmatrix}$$

FIGURE 6.7   Dual Theory of Risk
(Applied to insurance decisions)

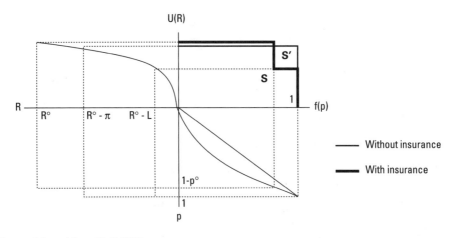

Source: Adapted from Vaté 1999.

Let us assume that :

1. The effective commercial premium includes the pure premium, a safety load-ing (at rate α), and an extra loading for management costs (at rate μ);

2. The rate μ covers costs exactly;

3. The maximum annual loss that can be borne is a given amount M of money.

The sum of the actuarial premiums is noted as PR. The total payment of claims is a random variable of which the variance is noted S^2. By definition of the pure premium, PR is equal to the mathematical expectation (mean) of the payment of claims. Therefore the annual result is a random variable $\tilde{R}$ - for which the mean is:

$$E(\tilde{R}) = (1 + \alpha + \mu) .PR - PR - \mu \, PR = \alpha \, PR$$

Given the solvency condition (R > -M), the insurer faces the following ques-tion: What is the probability of failure? The Bienaymé-Chebichev inequality (Boursin and Duru 1994) teaches that, for whatever distribution with mean $E(\tilde{R})$ and variance S^2, the following holds :

$$\text{prob}[E(\tilde{R}) - \beta.S \le R \le E(\tilde{R}) + \beta.S] \ge 1 - 1/\beta^2$$

In other words, for a given value of β, the probability is at most $1/\beta^2$ for staying out of the considered interval. This probability is divided into the left- and the right-hand side of the distribution, and in the case of symmetry, the probability of failure is at most $1/2\beta^2$.

Example: To avoid a probability of failure greater than p = 1 percent, the insurer must choose $\beta \ge \sqrt{1/2p}$ = 7.1. That means that it must choose α in such a manner that the sum M + α PR is at least equal to 7.1 times S. This is why the ratio:

$$\beta = \frac{M + \alpha . PR}{S}$$

is the so-called *safety coefficient*. The critical value of β (here $\beta^* = 7.1$) depends upon the maximum probability of failure that has been selected (here p = 1 percent).

In more favorable situations, one has more information about the statistical dis-tribution of claims. In the case of continuous, symmetrical, and single-mode distri-bution, the lower limit of probability is more precise (Camp-Meidel inequality):

$$\text{Prob}[E(\tilde{R}) - \beta.S \le R \le E(\tilde{R}) + \beta.S] \ge 1 - 1/(2,25.\beta^2).$$

In the previous example, with the same left-hand side probability p = 1 per-cent, this relation gives the smaller value of $\beta^* = 4.7$. The more precise the knowl-edge of the distribution, the more accurate is the computation of β. Near normal distribution, β^* drops to 2.3. Even outside the normal case, this result can also be used when the conditions hold for the central limit theorem (any distribution, continuous or not, whose mean and variance exist, and the number of insureds approaches infinity). In this case, for example, $\beta^* = 4.7$ would correspond to a probability of failure p = 1,3.10^{-6} (quasi certainty).

NOTES

1. The word "insureds," although grammatically incorrect in English, has taken root to describe more than one insured person.

2. This can be done by selecting risks with high enough probability (for a given n, the variance as a fraction of the average is larger with smaller probabilities) and small variability in unit cost. Both parameters cause an increase in S compared with *pr*.

3. The question whether the utility theory can be applied in all cultural contexts is dealt with in chapter 19, this volume.

4. Precise information about the quantity that is considered medically necessary (small triangles in figure 6.5) is difficult to obtain, but a rough estimate is necessary to illustrate this concept.

REFERENCES

Arrow, K.J. 1963. "Uncertainty and the Welfare Economics of Medical Care." *American Economic Review* 53:941–73.

Atim, C. 2000. "Participation and Adverse Selection in a Voluntary Community Health Insurance Scheme." International Conference on Health Systems Financing in Low-income African and Asian countries. *Colloque du CERDI* (Centre d'Etudes et de Recherches sur le Développement International). Clermont-Ferrand, November 2000.

Berliner, A. 1982. *Limits of Insurability of Risks*. Englewood Cliffs, N.J.: Prentice Hall.

Boursin, J.L., and G. Duru. 1994. *Statistique*. Paris: Gibert-Gestion.

Briys, E. 1990. *Demande d'assurance et microéconomie de l'incertain*. Paris: Presses Universitaires de France.

Charpentier, F., ed. 2000. *Encyclopédie de la protection sociale*. Paris: Economica, Editions Liaisons.

Cichon, M., W. Newbrander, H. Yamabana, A. Weber, C. Normand, D. Dror, and A. Preker. 1999. *Modelling in Health Care Finance*. Geneva: International Labour Office.

Cohen, M.D. 1995. "Risk-Aversion Concepts in Expected- and Non-expected-Utility Models." *The Geneva Papers on Risk and Insurance Theory* 20:73–91.

Condorcet, A.N. de. 1793. *Esquisse d'un tableau historique des progrès de l'esprit humain*. Réédition 1988. Paris: GF-Flammarion.

Couffinhal, A. 2000. "De l'antisélection à la sélection en assurance santé: pour un changement de perspective." *Economie et prévision* 142:101–21.

Dror, D., and G. Duru. 2000. "Stabilising Community Health Insurance Schemes Through Reinsurance." International Conference on Social Security, September 2000, Helsinki.

Dror, D., and C. Jacquier. 1999. "Micro-insurance: Extending Health Insurance to the Excluded." *International Social Security Review* 52(1):71–97.

Eeckhoudt, L., and C. Gollier. 1992. *Les risques financiers*. Paris: Ediscience.

Ehrlich, I., and G.S. Becker. 1972. "Market Insurance, Self-insurance and Self-protection." *Journal of Political Economy* 80(4):623–49.

Ewald, F. 1993. *Le problème français des accidents thérapeutiques*. Paris: La Documentation française.

Ewald, F., and J.H. Lorenzi, eds. 1998. *Encyclopédie de l'assurance*. Paris: Economica.

Fonteneau, R., and D. Dror. 2000. "Les enjeux de la coopération sanitaire (aider ceux qui s'aident)." *Colloque du CERDI*, November 2000, Clermont-Ferrand, France.

Gertler P., and O. Solon. 2000. "Who Benefits from Social Health Insurance in Developing Countries?" *Colloque du CERDI*, November 2000, Clermont-Ferrand, France.

Gollier, C. 1996. "Vers une théorie économique des limites de l'assurabilité." *Revue d'économie financière* 37:59–79.

Gollier, C., and D. Kessler. 1994. "Limites de l'assurabilité." *Risques* 17:89–92.

Henriet, D., and J.C. Rochet. 1991. *Microéconomie de l'assurance*. Paris: Economica.

Maréchal, J.P. 1991. *Le prix du risque*. Paris: Presses du CNRS.

Meesen, B. 2000. "Quelles stratégies de couverture pour les risques liés à la santé?" *Colloque du CERDI*, November 2000, Clermont-Ferrand, France.

Moatti, J.P. 1989. *Economie de la sécurité*. Paris: La Documentation française.

Musgrove, P. 1999: "Public Spending on Health Care: How Are Different Criteria Related?" *Health Policy* 47(3):207–23. Quoted in World Health Organization, *World Health Report 2000: Health Systems: Improving Performance*. Geneva: WHO.

Newhouse, J.P. 1996. "Reimbursing Health Plans and Health Providers: Efficiency in Production Versus Selection." *Journal of Economic Literature* 34:1236–63.

Outreville, J.F. 1998. *Theory and Practice of Insurance*. Boston, Mass.: Kluwer Academic Publishers.

Quiggin, J. 1982. "A Theory of Anticipated Utility." *Journal of Economic Behavior and Organisation* 3:323–43.

Rotschild, M., and J. Stiglitz. 1976. "Equilibrium In Competitive Insurance Markets: An Essay on the Economics of Imperfect Information" *Quarterly Journal of Economics* 90:629–49.

Savage, L.J. 1954. *The Foundations of Statistics*. New York: Dover Publications.

UNDP (United Nations Development Programme). 2000. *Human Development Report 2000: Human Rights and Human Development*. New York: UNDP.

Vaillier, P. 2001. *Les limites de l'assurance*. Paris: La Tribune de l'assurance.

Vaté, M. 1999. *Leçons d'économie politique*. 8th ed. Paris: Economica.

Von Neumann, J., and O. Morgenstern. 1944. *Theory of Games and Economic Behavior*. Princeton, N.J.: Princeton University Press.

World Bank. 1993. *World Development Report 1993: Investing in Health*. Washington, D.C.: World Bank.

Yaari, M. 1987. "The Dual Theory of Choice under Risk" *Econometrica* 55:95–105.

Yeatman, J. 1998. *Manuel international de l'assurance*. Paris: Ecole nationale d'assurances de Paris. Economica.

CHAPTER 7

A Model of Microinsurance and Reinsurance

Stéphane Bonnevay, David M. Dror, Gérard Duru, and Michel Lamure

R einsurance offers insurance companies many advantages, including stabilization of losses and surplus enhancement, according to Outreville (chapter 3, this volume). Can reinsurance therefore ensure the financial stabilization of multiple microinsurance units? This question can be approached in two ways: empirically or theoretically.

The *empirical approach* consists of carrying out repeated field studies in real-life settings and observing the results. However, since there are no field data on reinsurance transactions with microinsurers, whether reinsurance can work for small health schemes needs to be assessed through theoretical reasoning. The *theoretical approach* is based on identifying qualitative information concerning possible solutions, through simplified representations of the problem *(the model)*, and then defining a calculation protocol to validate (or invalidate) the model's underlying hypothesis through the results (Lesage 1999). This chapter describes the theoretical approach followed in the model.

This model tests the hypothesis that microinsurance schemes, operating on their own, are financially less viable than they would be if they pooled their risks through reinsurance. This proof entails consideration of three subissues:

- Demonstration of the positive effect of reinsurance on microinsurers' financial viability

- Exploration of the utility of reinsurance for microinsurers and the variables affecting their decision to reinsure

- Elaboration of a protocol for calculating the reinsurance premium, based on analysis of scenarios that are likely to occur in reality

THE PROBLEM

Reinsurance involves two sets of contracts, between each microinsurer and its members and between each microinsurer and its reinsurer.

For their invaluable contributions to this chapter, the authors thank Michael Cichon, Chief, Financial, Actuarial and Statistical Branch, Social Protection Sector, International Labour Office; Ivan Lavallée, Professor of Informatics, University of Paris 8; and Ruth Koren, Professor, Faculty of Medicine, Tel Aviv University.

The Contract between Microinsurer and Its Members

Under the basic contract between each microinsurer and its members, each member pays the microinsurer a periodic contribution. In return, the microinsurer agrees to pay specified medical costs for the insured. The viability of the basic contract depends on the microinsurer's ability to pay its obligations in full at any future time. Because its ability to do so depends on its financial stability, the microinsurer's profit (or loss) at the end of each accounting period has to be projected. To make these projections, parameters are needed for determining the financial outcome.

Anticipating each microinsurer's business results depends on the number of times events covered by the insurance contract occur and on the costs associated with these events. Both variables fluctuate randomly.

For example, a microinsurer may agree to cover members for up to five days' hospitalization. When the insurance policy is signed, how often each individual will be hospitalized during the term of the contract is unknown. However, within a given target population, the probability distribution can be estimated for the random variable: "number of hospitalizations of up to five days during a certain period." The cost of one event of hospitalization is not constant, because the length of stay and the cost per day may vary. Nonetheless, if the distribution functions of both unit cost and incidence are available, the probability distribution of the overall cost for this type of event can be deduced for the entire microinsurance unit over a given period. The same process can be applied to all benefits included in the insurance package.

The balance at the end of an accounting period is therefore random. How, then, can the probability distribution of this balance be determined? As the balance reflects a difference between income and expenditure, its probability distribution depends on income-side values (including members' contributions, external resources funneled into the microinsurance unit, and the microinsurer's available reserves) and on expenditure-side values (including administrative costs and the composition of the benefit package), and the number of members covered by the microinsurer. With knowledge of the distribution of the microinsurer's business results, its chances of bankruptcy or survival can be estimated.

The microinsurer's financial stability will be measured here in terms of its risk of becoming insolvent (*failure rate*), as the membership has a self-explanatory interest in eliminating or reducing the risk of insolvency. The hypothesis (as defined earlier) can therefore be rephrased to state that transferring part of the risk to reinsurance reduces the microinsurer's failure rate.

The Contract between Each Microinsurer and Its Reinsurer

Under the basic contract between each microinsurer and its reinsurer, the microinsurer pays the reinsurer a periodic premium. In return, the reinsurer pays the microinsurer for costs exceeding a specified *reinsurance threshold*. The fundamental assumption here is that the client microinsurers' business results can fluctuate around a mean value. Thus, in "good years" (when costs are below the mean), the microinsurer will run a surplus (compared with the mean), and in "bad years" (when the costs exceed the mean) the microinsurer will run a deficit (compared with the mean). These fluctuations stem, to a great extent, from the microinsurers' small membership and claim load. The extent of fluctuations can be estimated by applying statistical laws, if the probability of events and their average cost are known. However, no one can know whether the surplus in good years will cover the deficit in bad years, or that good years will precede bad ones, such that the microinsurer always has enough reserves to cover deficits. Therefore, if the microinsurer wishes to lower its financial risk exposure to the mean cost, which is much more predictable and affordable, it has to obtain an alternative source to cover these mean costs. This is what the reinsurance offers to do (figure 7.1).

Reinsurance offers the microinsurer a dual advantage. First, it avoids the risk of bankruptcy in bad years. Second, by freeing the microinsurer from unexpected fluctuations in expenses, reinsurance also removes the microinsurer's obligation to maintain contingency reserves and enables it to use surpluses generated in good years at its own discretion.

This relationship is based on the assumption that the reinsurer remains solvent at all times. Yet, the reinsurer also faces a risk of bankruptcy, as its business results, too, are determined by income (premiums collected) and expenditures (benefits payable to microinsurers plus administrative costs). Therefore, the reinsurer's probability of bankruptcy has to be calculated at the end of each period. The reinsurer's estimated risk of insolvency depends on the probability distribution of client microinsurers' business results, the contract terms, and

FIGURE 7.1   The Dual Advantage of Reinsurance

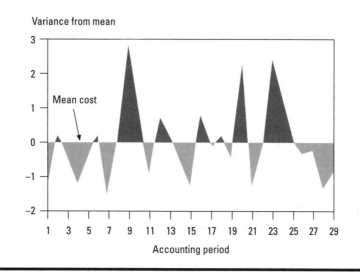

administrative costs. Additionally, the number of reinsured microinsurers (the size of the pool) may influence the reinsurer's business results.

This set of parameters will be structured into a model, described below.

THE PRINCIPLES UNDERLYING THE REINSURANCE MODEL

The reinsurance model proposed here is based on two major principles.[1] First, as the reinsurer's role is to shield its client microinsurers from the risk of insolvency arising out of the cost of random fluctuation of insurable events, the reinsurer takes account only of the microinsurer's insurable activities (for a distinction between insurable and uninsurable events see Vaté and Dror, chapter 6, this volume). Second, in exchange for a premium, reinsurance covers the microinsurer's costs that exceed the reinsurance threshold.

For each insurable activity at the beginning of each accounting period, the microinsurer estimates the resources it will need to pay the benefits. This amount is based on the microinsurer's forecasts of its income and its exposure to cost-generating events during the period. As the actual cost may vary from the estimated cost because of random fluctuations, the exact amount will be known only at the end of a period when the microinsurer finds out whether it has incurred a profit or a deficit. In the model, a deficit is considered a bankruptcy situation (because of the underlying assumption that microinsurers do not maintain contingency reserves to cover fluctuations in the cost of their insurance activity). In the model, the reinsurer covers deficits resulting from higher-than-expected expenses. At the outset, their calculation requires a definition of the level of benefits payable by the microinsurer to the members before the reinsurer takes over (*unceded risk*, called here the *reinsurance threshold*), and the costs for which the reinsurer is responsible (*ceded risk*). The contract (*treaty*) also sets the premium microinsurers must pay for reinsurance.

The two principles mentioned above are necessary to model a comparison of the microinsurer's failure probabilities with or without reinsurance. In addition, the model allows identification of the minimum resources that each microinsurer must secure to cover its unceded risk and pay the reinsurance premium.

FORMULATION OF THE MODEL

The mathematical formulation of the relationship between a reinsurer and microinsurers is elaborated in annex 7A.

The model is formulated to answer the fundamental question: When will a microinsurer want to purchase reinsurance? The reply seems to be: When the reinsurance contract reduces the resources needed to secure at least the same level of solvency for a defined level of expenditure (linked to a defined benefit package). This calls for a comparison between two quantities, which would be straightforward if both amounts were known at the same time. However, the values determining the microinsurer's expenses (for example, number of events, unit cost, length of hospital stay) are random and can fluctuate within a certain range according to the distribution probability. Therefore, the microinsurer's precise payout liability for the entire accounting period is unknown in advance. On the other hand, the maximum cost can be estimated if the distribution is known (as is assumed under the model). The level of solvency also has to be determined, bearing in mind that 100 percent survival (without reinsurance) can be guaranteed only when resources to cover the worst-case scenario are available at the beginning of the period. An example for this comparison is a situation where a microinsurer without reinsurance needs resources equal to its mean benefits, plus a safety margin proportional to the variance of its benefits.[2] Assuming that the reinsurance threshold is equal to the mean benefits, reinsurance would be advantageous for the microinsurer if the reinsurance premium were cheaper than the safety margin. This comparison is pertinent in so far as both options secure the same level of solvency.

When reinsurance is considered, one of the two amounts (the cost of the reinsurance premium plus the microinsurer's reinsurance threshold) ceases to be an estimate and is defined in the reinsurance treaty. The other amount is an estimate of the maximum capitalization needed to guarantee full self-insurance. In reality, as expenditures fluctuate, some years the microinsurer will need less than the maximum, and the challenge is to operate with as little capital as possible at the beginning of the period without increasing the failure rate.

The reinsurance premium has to cover the reinsurer's solvency, which, like that of the microinsurer, is defined up front. A lower solvency rate of the reinsurer would translate into a lower premium, but such a reinsurer may fail to provide adequate levels of solvency for the microinsurer. Hence, in all the examples elaborated here, the reinsurer's solvency rate is assumed to be 95 percent. The conditions that satisfy this requirement will depend on the number of microinsurers in the pool and on each pooled microinsurer's risk profile. An example of an analytical calculation of the reinsurance, applying the model (but for a simplified scenario of 30 microinsurers[3] with identical mean and variance and a simple statistical distribution law for the benefit cost) is illustrated below, based on equations elaborated in annex 7B.

Let us consider a simplified example where more than 30 identical microinsurers sign an identical reinsurance contract for one time period. A uniform distribution of benefits payable by microinsurer to members is assumed,[4] on an interval of [0, 10] monetary units (₪).[5] In this case, without reinsurance, the microinsurer needs 10 ₪ at the beginning of each period to ensure its solvency. With reinsurance, the microinsurer would need to secure, in addition to the premium, only the mean cost, in this case 5 ₪, the reinsurance threshold, because the reinsurer bears all costs above it.

As an illustration, two groups (one with pool size of 36 microinsurers and the other with pool size of 100 microinsurers) are compared, and two scenarios are presented for each group. Under *Scenario 1*, the reinsurer's initial capital is equal to the administrative costs, and all other expenses are covered only from premium income. Under *Scenario 2*, the reinsurer's initial capital is equal to the administrative costs plus 0.5 ₪ per microinsurer (the equations and details of the calculations are provided in annex 7B).

As can be seen in table 7.1, in any of the four permutations, the microinsurers would need less than 7 ₪ to ensure 100 percent survival with reinsurance, compared with 10 ₪ without reinsurance. Put another way, with the same resources, the microinsurers would incur a risk of insolvency ranging from 48 percent to 33 percent without reinsurance, but 0 percent with reinsurance. The conclusion is that in this example, for any level of resources, reinsurance reduces microinsurers' failure rate. Furthermore, for 0 percent failure rate, the level of resources needed is reduced considerably.

Now we have to recognize that, in the example discussed so far and in annex 7B, an analytical approach could be followed, but to do so, some assumptions had to be simplified. However, the mean benefit cost for a microinsurer and the variance of this parameter can be calculated under more realistic scenarios even when their statistical distribution function is not known, by making an assumption regarding the statistical distribution of the incidence of benefits (for instance Poisson distribution law[6]) and of unit cost (Chi-squared distribution law[7]). The method for this calculation is elaborated in annex 7C.

This calculation requires an estimate of the probability of each benefit and its mean unit cost. As in other cases of statistical sampling, the better the data, the more reliable the extrapolated figures will be. The data for these calculations originate from the microinsurers themselves, and may initially be somewhat weak. It is hoped that the quality of such estimates will improve when data are collected over a longer period of time and in line with a methodology proposed by the *Social Re Data Template.*[8]

However, even when the mean benefit cost of each microinsurance unit is known and the variance in this value can be calculated as described above, the statistical distribution function of the overall cost for each microinsurer turns out to be too complex for an analytical solution under most realistic scenarios.[9] As explained earlier, the decision to sign a reinsurance treaty requires a lower reinsurance premium payment than the safety margin the microinsurer must maintain to ensure the same level of solvency that the reinsurance guarantees. But when the statistical distribution function of each microinsurer's business results are unknown or

TABLE 7.1   Reinsurance Results under Two Scenarios

Reinsurer's constraints	Scenario 1 Reserves = Administrative costs Bankruptcy < 5 percent		Scenario 2 Reserves = Administrative costs + 0.5/microinsurer Bankruptcy < 5 percent	
Number of microinsurers	36	100	36	100
Microinsurer's reinsurance threshold + reinsurance premium (₪)	5 + 1.69 = 6.69	5 + 1.52 = 6.52	5 + 1.19 = 6.19	5 + 1.02 = 6.02
Failure rate without reinsurance (percent)	33	35	38	48
Failure rate with reinsurance (percent)	0	0	0	0

unsolvable, its business results cannot be estimated for a general solution over several periods and at different income levels, nor can the reinsurance premium be calculated. The premium calculation becomes even more difficult when the reinsurance pools fewer than 30 microinsurers with a heterogeneous risk profile (as is the case under most realistic scenarios), because the law of large numbers cannot be applied either. This is why it is necessary to resort to simulations (Monsef 1997) in an effort to determine the reinsurance premium. The results of the simulations under selected scenarios are described in the next section.

SIMULATION OF THE RELATIONSHIP BETWEEN MICROINSURERS AND REINSURER

Like analytical calculations, the simulation requires an estimate of the laws of distribution of cost-generating events[10] and their unit cost.[11] To recapitulate the methodology for analytical calculation of the effects of reinsurance, an example is provided as annex 7D, in which all microinsurers are assumed to be identical, and it is also assumed that their number is large (more than 30) to allow the application of the law of large numbers. The weakness of the example is that it does not allow drawing a decision rule for the general case, including the case where the microinsurers are not identical or are fewer than 30. If this is the reinsurer's reality, then the algebraic expression of the distribution of these random variables becomes too complex for an analytical solution. The alternative way to proceed then is to simulate the estimated business results of the applicant microinsurers.[12] To probe the reinsurance model through simulations, the Monte Carlo simulation method[13] has been applied.

One assumption of the simulations is that cost-generating events are independent of each other.

The results of the simulation provide information on:

- The failure rate for microinsurers that did not reinsure over several periods, but used the premium amount as additional income;

- The reinsurance premium payable by each microinsurer for each period;

- The advantages reinsurance provides microinsurers: distribution (mean, standard deviation, minimum, and maximum) of each microinsurer's expected surplus, protection against insolvency, and parameters influencing the microinsurer's utility;

- The distribution of the reinsurer's business results at the end of each period (mean, standard deviation [SD], minimum and maximum) and the reinsurer's survival probability; and

- The impact of external funding on reinsurance.

The simulations were run with computer software, elaborated in Delphi, programmed to respond to these specifications and called the *Toolkit* (described in appendix B).

SIMULATION RESULTS

In the following section we present the answers obtained through simulations corresponding to the five bulleted points above, representing different aspects of the interactions between the microinsurers and the reinsurer.

Question 1: What is the failure rate of microinsurers that are not reinsured?

The microinsurer's survival is secured so long as it is solvent. In large schemes, there is a prevalent assumption that solvency is secured when income covers costs *(recovery rate)*, which is usually estimated to equal the average cost over time. A similar logic has been applied to the microinsurer's solvency as a function of its income over five accounting periods. The question was explored first in relation to a concrete example of one microinsurer with 500 members, covering one risk, with probability of 1 percent (one event per 100 members per period), with average unit cost of 15 ₪. Hence, the average benefit cost for the microinsurer was 75 ₪ per period; the SD (obtained by simulating this microinsurer's business results in 2,500 replications) was 35.70 ₪ (47.6 percent of average cost).

In figure 7.2, four income levels were compared: 100 percent recovery rate,[14] 120 percent, 130 percent, and 140 percent (representing the recovery rate and, respectively 20, 30, and 40 percent above full recovery). The microinsurer is

FIGURE 7.2   Risk of Insolvency as a Function of Available Resources
(percent)

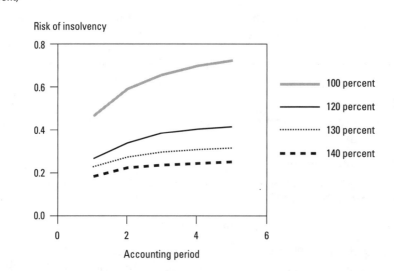

exposed to a high failure rate at every income level examined. Even when its revenue is 40 percent above recovery, the microinsurer can reach a failure rate of 19 percent at the end of one accounting period and 25 percent at the end of five periods. When the income is fixed at the more likely level of the recovery rate, the microinsurer's failure rate is 47 percent at the end of one accounting period and as high as 73 percent at the end of five periods.

This simulation provides two main insights. First, small microinsurers are vulnerable to insolvency, which cannot be remedied simply by increasing contribution levels. Second, this risk of failure worsens over time.

This figure does not offer any insight as to the reason for this vulnerability. However, seeing that microinsurers are usually small, could this vulnerability be linked to group size? This was explored in a second simulation, designed to see whether the same pattern applies to microinsurers of different sizes. Three microinsurers were compared: 200 members, 1,000 members, and 5,000 members; risk probability and unit cost were kept unchanged. The results of this simulation, shown in figure 7.3A, suggest that larger groups are less vulnerable to insolvency for a comparable income level. At an income level of 114 percent of recovery rate, the risk of failure was 22 percent, 44 percent, and 61 percent, respectively, for groups with 5,000, 1,000, and 200 members.

The three microinsurers exhibit almost identical results when income is expressed in terms of SD of the mean cost (figure 7.3B). As each microinsurer has a different simulated value of SD, expressing the microinsurer's resources in terms of multiples of its SD-enabled comparison. For this purpose, we define a coefficient Ω as a multiple of the SD of the total benefit cost. The income for all microinsurers was expressed as their recovery rate (100 percent) plus Ω multiplied by SD. The risk of failure under this representation, at $\Omega = 0.5$, was 45 percent, 44 percent, and 47 percent, respectively, for the microinsurer with 5,000, 1,000, and 200 members. This result suggests that the difference in failure rates between these microinsurers (figure 7.3A) is solely the result of the difference in their variance in benefit cost, which is very sensitive to group size (Dror, chapter 5, this volume).

In conclusion, the reply to the question "What is the failure rate of microinsurers that are not reinsured?" is that the failure rate is too high to ignore. The high risk of failure applies in all cases but will be accentuated by small group size, higher risk profile, and lower income.

This leads to a search for a sustainable and affordable solution. If reinsurance might be such a solution, its affordability needs to be assessed, which is the topic of the next section.

Question 2: What level of premium should be set for the microinsurer's reinsurance?

Under the reinsurance contract, the reinsurer agrees to pay benefit costs exceeding the expected average (75 ₪), whereas the microinsurer agrees to pay benefit

FIGURE 7.3A   Failure Rate of Microinsurance Units

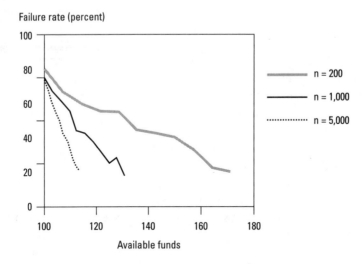

Note: Failure expressed in terms of recovery rate.

FIGURE 7.3B   Bankruptcy Rate of Microinsurance Units with and without Reinsurance

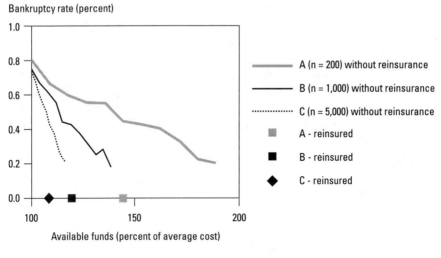

Note: Five accounting periods.

costs up to that level, plus a reinsurance premium. This contract guarantees that the microinsurer would never become insolvent as a result of above-average costs. The premium is set at a level that guarantees the reinsurer's solvency at 95 percent. The objective of the simulation is to explore the lowest value that can satisfy this requirement.

As in the discussion of the previous question, we revert initially to one microinsurer with 500 members, with the same risk profile used above (p = 1 percent, unit cost = 15 ⃠, SD = 35.70 ⃠). And as the reinsurer operates a pool of several microinsurers, six pooling options were simulated (5, 20, 30, 40, 50, or 75 identical microinsurers in the pool).

As the risk of each microinsurer is proportional to the variance of its benefit cost, the reinsurance premium is also a function of the variance, and expressed as Ω multiplied by the SD. The range of acceptable solutions has been calculated for values of Ω between [0,1]. The results are illustrated in figure 7.4.

As can be seen in the figure, the size of the pool makes a moderate difference: when only 5 microinsurers are pooled, the premium to ensure the reinsurer a 95 percent survival rate is at least 0.6*SD (28.6 percent of the average cost). When the pool includes 20 microinsurers, the premium drops to 0.5*SD (about 23.8 percent of the average cost of the stereotypic microinsurer described above[15]). When the pool increases further, the premium does not decrease below $\Omega = 0.5$. The simulation was performed for many scenarios, with different microinsurer sizes and risk profiles. In every case, the lowest premium (at an optimal pool size) was consistently 0.5*SD.

As the variance determines the reinsurance premium, and the size of the microinsurer's membership has an impact on its SD, the premium would be expected to cost a microinsurer with a larger membership less than a microinsurer with a smaller membership. This conjecture was verified in another simulation, the results of which are illustrated in figure 7.5. As can be seen in the figure, when the microinsurer has only 200 members, it must pay 37.6 percent of its contribution income as reinsurance premium; but when the number of members increases

---

FIGURE 7.4   Levels of Reinsurance Premium Securing 95 Percent Survival of Reinsurer

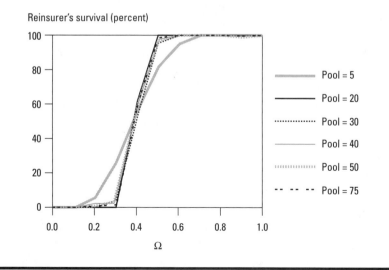

FIGURE 7.5   Effect of Group Size on Premium

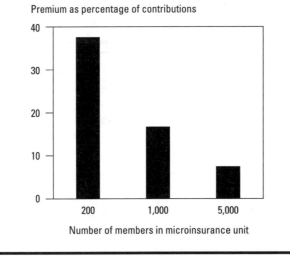

Premium as percentage of contributions

Number of members in microinsurance unit

to 1,000, the premium represents 16.8 percent of contribution income, and it drops to only 7.5 percent when the group size is 5,000, for an identical risk profile in every instance.

So far we have dealt with a homogeneous pool of microinsurers, all sharing the same group size and risk profile. In reality, we may expect heterogeneity of both parameters. The impact of such heterogeneity will be explored using a pool of five microinsurers with different profiles as an example (table 7.2). The same distribution laws used before are used here, too: Poisson law for occurrence distribution and Chi-square for unit cost distribution.

Table 7.2 provides the mean cost of benefits, but not the indispensable information about variance of this value. These values, obtained by applying the general mathematical expression (annex 7C) are provided in table 7.3.

Table 7.3 provides the SD of the mean benefit cost for the five microinsurers, in nominal terms and as a function of the mean. Contrary to the homogeneous microinsurers, these microinsurers differ greatly from each other in terms of the value of their mean (from 2.5 to 36) and in their SD (48 percent to 213 percent of mean). The premium that would be required to satisfy the reinsurer's solvency rate of 95 percent has been simulated for this group. The striking result is that for this pool, the minimum premium required is 0.9*SD (compared with the 0.6*SD required for a pool of five microinsurers with a homogeneous risk profile). Note that the total number of individuals covered by the two pools is similar (2,300 versus 2,500), and the claim load is also almost identical (25 versus 25.1). The results, shown in figure 7.6, should be compared with those in figure 7.4.

In conclusion, the reinsurance contract, as defined above, assumes that the premium is proportional to the risk ceded to the reinsurer. It has been shown that this risk is proportional to the SD of each microinsurer's total benefit cost. As also is

TABLE 7.2   Microinsurers' Characteristics in the Simulation

| | Number of members | Cost-generating event 1 | | Cost-generating event 2 | | Reinsurance threshold = Mean benefits (ru) |
		Mean occurrence (cases per period)[b]	Mean unit cost (ru)	Mean occurrence (cases per period)[a]	Mean unit cost (ru)	
Microinsurer-1	100	1	1	0.1	15	2.5
Microinsurer-2	1,000	8	2	2.0	10	36
Microinsurer-3	150	2	3	0.5	12	12
Microinsurer-4	300	4	4	0.5	30	31
Microinsurer-5	750	6	3	1.0	10	28

a. This represents the number of events for the microinsurer, which also depends on the number of members, to express mean occurrence per member. This number would be divided by the number of members in the microinsurance unit.

Note: The numbers are the mean of three runs. The data used here are theoretical, and it is assumed that the two cost-generating events, their unit cost, and the incidence are independent. This assumption of independence between events is a technical one, allowing random numbers to be generated in a simple way. Introducing correlation between cost-generating events, although possible when necessary, would vastly complicate the process of random number generation.

TABLE 7.3   Distribution of the Benefit Cost

	SD of benefits (ru)	SD (percent of mean)
Microinsurer-1	5.33	213
Microinsurer-2	17.44	48
Microinsurer-3	10.68	89
Microinsurer-4	24.00	77
Microinsurer-5	14.49	52

shown, the SD decreases (per person) when group size increases, all else remaining unchanged. Hence, the reinsurance premium decreases in terms of its share of total expenses as membership increases. An increase in the number of microinsurers pooled through reinsurance also reduces the premium, as the risk is spread over a larger population. However, even when the pool is large enough, the premium does not decrease below half the SD of each microinsurer's total cost. Finally, the vulnerability of small pools increases dramatically when the risk profile is heterogeneous.

Now that the cost of the premium has been identified, the question is whether it is worth paying. Stated differently, the decision to reinsure or not will depend on two considerations: on the premium and on the return microinsurers can expect for this payment.

Question 3: What Do Microinsurers Get Out of Reinsurance?

Reinsurance gives microinsurers both protection against insolvency and some discretionary budget.

FIGURE 7.6   **Reinsurance Premiums for a Heterogeneous Pool of Microinsurers**

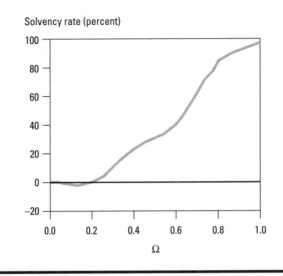

Protection against insolvency. Reinsurance reduces the microinsurer's risk of insolvency. This is its fundamental advantage. Figures 7.2, 7.3A, and 7.3B show that, without reinsurance, the risk of failure is very high, even with enough resources to secure a full recovery rate.

As the reinsurance contract guarantees that the reinsurer pays all costs above the reinsurance threshold, the microinsurer's risk of failure is eliminated. The microinsurer has to decide whether the cost of the premium compares favorably to the safety margin it must preserve (which is proportional to the variance of its benefits). In the following set of simulations, we compared the use of the premium amount (assuming an optimal pool size) to the use of an identical amount as a safety margin. The results are shown in figure 7.7.

The figure shows the same groups depicted in figure 7.3. As can be seen now, for group n = 1,000, the premium was 16.8 percent of the recovery rate. Using this amount as a safety margin would reduce the risk of failure from 73 percent to 44 percent at the end of five periods. Using the same amount to pay the reinsurance premium would reduce the failure rate from 73 percent to 0 percent from the first period. The same utility, observed for all three microinsurers, is related to setting the premium at 0.5*SD (as shown in figure 7.3B), even though its nominal level differs because of each microinsurer's particular features. Therefore, reinsurance presents a clear advantage for all microinsurers, regardless of their specific features.

Discretionary budget. As mentioned earlier, in good years, microinsurers would run a surplus because their actual costs would be lower than the mean. Although the probability of good years is unaffected by reinsurance, this financial safety releases

FIGURE 7.7   Comparison of the Premium to the Safety Margin

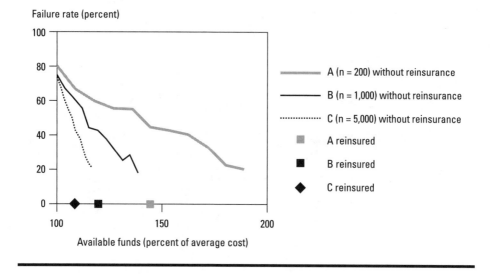

microinsurers from the need to maintain contingency reserves, thus allowing them to use these surpluses as discretionary budgets without taking any additional risk of failure. It seems fair to assume that the larger this financial resource, the more attractive microinsurers would find reinsurance.

The size of the discretionary budget has thus been simulated for each microinsurer and period. Bearing in mind that the premium level is influenced by the microinsurer's membership size, this simulation also looked at three levels, with n = 200, n = 1,000 and n = 5,000. The discretionary budget was shown as a proportion of the premium paid. The results of the simulation are shown in figure 7.8.

Quite unexpectedly, the discretionary budget seems to represent about 80 percent of the premium in every case, regardless of group size and of the period covered. As can be seen in the figure, the likelihood of accumulating a discretionary budget increases over time, because its SD, although high initially, drops over time. These simulations were run on the assumption that the pool size was optimal (premium = half the SD). Incidentally, this simulation was repeated with other variables (risk levels, number of risks in the benefit package), and in every case, the accumulation was, on average, around 80 percent of the premium paid.

The practical implications of this finding have been explored further by looking at four microinsurers with different characteristics (table 7.4).

In terms of perceived utility, microinsurers look at two aspects: first, the premium they need to pay to avoid failure and secure full solvency; second, the amount of discretionary budget they can obtain.

Microinsurers A and B share the same risk profile, but the difference in their membership is tenfold. This membership differential accounts for their respective

FIGURE 7.8   Discretionary Budget

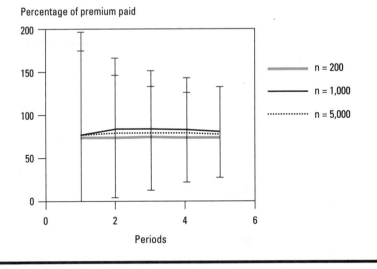

Percentage of premium paid

SD values of 47.6 percent and 15.1 percent of mean cost, respectively, which also explains the more-than-threefold difference in the premium. On the other hand, the discretionary budget also dropped, from 0.14 ₪ to 0.05 ₪ per member.

Microinsurers B and C differ in the number of members and in risk probability but have the same claim load. Both pay the same premium in terms of percentage of mean cost, but C's discretionary budget is 10 times higher per member than that of B. C's perceived utility would thus be higher than B's.

TABLE 7.4   Premium and Discretionary Budget for Different Microinsurers

Microinsurer's characteristics	A	B	C	D
Members	500	5,000	500	500
Number of benefits	1	1	1	3
Risk probability (percent)	1	1	10	$P1=P2=P3=1$
Mean claim load	5	50	50	15
Unit cost	15	15	15	15
Premium and discretionary budget data				
Mean total cost of benefits	75	750	750	225
Standard deviation	35.70	112.91	112.91	61.84
Standard deviation/mean cost (percent)	47.6	15.1	15.1	27.5
Premium (percent of mean cost)	23.8	7.5	7.5	13.9
Discretionary budget per member after five periods	0.14	0.05	0.45	0.25

Microinsurers A and C have the same membership but a different risk profile. Microinsurer A reinsures a rare event, whereas C reinsures a more frequent risk. Microinsurer A therefore pays a higher share of its expenditure as premium (47.6 percent versus 15.1 percent), but as this premium is lower than C's in nominal terms, A can expect a lower discretionary budget.[16]

Finally, a comparison of microinsurers A and D reveals another interesting aspect. Both microinsurers have the same group size, but A has one benefit whereas D has three. This risk diversification causes a threefold increase in claim load, a decrease in D's relative premium, and an increase in the discretionary budget. Once again, we conclude that D has a higher perceived utility than A from reinsurance.

This analysis suggests that the higher the microinsurer's claim load, the lower is the share of the premium *relative* to the microinsurer's total expenditure. Also, the higher the claim load, the higher is the discretionary budget because it is linked to the *nominal* value of the premium, which is higher. Furthermore, it seems that subscribing to reinsurance would be an optimal policy choice for microinsurers that offer a package with many benefits, including some that are not rare.

If the reinsurer is not solvent at all times, however, reinsurance would be impossible. This will be explored next.

Question 4: What is the reinsurer's balance and risk of insolvency?

The premium calculation has been based on the assumption that, in the long run, the reinsurer's risk of insolvency should not exceed 5 percent. For this purpose, it is not enough for the reinsurer's mean balance to be positive; the worst-case scenario has to be positive as well. If the reinsurer's business results in any one period were negative, reinsurance could, however, still work as long as enough resources were available to cover any operational deficit. In accounting terms, this translates into a requirement that the reinsurer's business results should be measured on the basis of accrued accounts, with surpluses and deficits transferred across accounting periods.

The reinsurer's balance has been simulated on the accrual basis, with the same specifications as those used for figure 7.4, but with only two pool sizes: 5 and 20 microinsurers. The new simulations show the reinsurer's business results during the first five periods. Figure 7.9 illustrates the balance in relation to the ceded risk. The ceded risk has been defined here as one-and-a-half times the sum of the standard deviation of the total cost of affiliated microinsurers. Figure 7.9A depicts the situation for a pool size of five microinsurers, and at two premium levels: 0.5*SD and 0.6*SD. Although the mean simulated balance is positive at both premium levels, the lower end of the variance of the results (that is, the worst-case scenario) at 0.5*SD clearly exposes the reinsurer to a negative balance in all years. The only business result that overcomes this limitation is achieved, in Period 5, when the premium is set at 0.6*SD. Figure 7.9B shows the reinsurer's balance at a pool size of 20 microinsurers. Here, the mean is identical to that of the smaller

FIGURE 7.9A   **Reinsurer's Balance, Pool of Five Microinsurers**

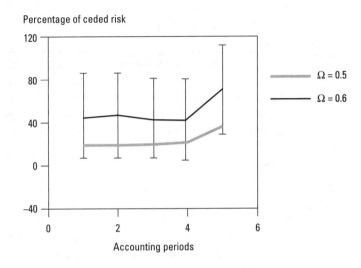

Percentage of ceded risk

$\Omega = 0.5$

$\Omega = 0.6$

Accounting periods

FIGURE 7.9B   **Reinsurer's Balance, Pool of 20 Microinsurers**

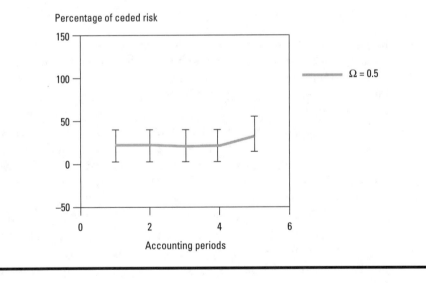

Percentage of ceded risk

$\Omega = 0.5$

Accounting periods

pool, but because the larger pool size greatly reduces the variance, the reinsurer's viability can be secured even with a premium of 0.5*SD. This result should be treated with some caution, however, as it may be different when the risk profile of the participating microinsurers is heterogeneous.

The variance discussed above implies that the reinsurer's solvency rate may be below the required level of 95 percent. The same simulation results were therefore used to derive the solvency rate. The results are presented in figure 7.10.

FIGURE 7.10   Reinsurer's Solvency

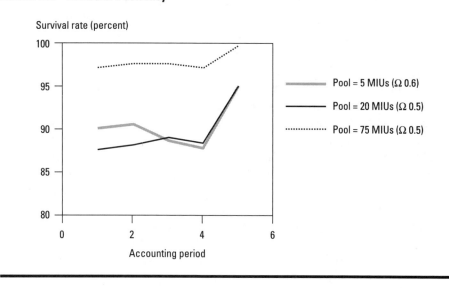

Here, the solvency rate does not reach the required 95 percent before the end of Period 5, when the pool is composed of 5 or 20 microinsurers. For the sake of comparison, the pool of 75 microinsurers is also shown. This large pool can secure the required solvency rate from the first period with a premium of 0.5*SD (but not with a lower premium—as already shown in figure 7.4).

In conclusion, the condition of 95 percent solvency is not met during the first four periods when the pool is no larger than 20 microinsurers and the lowest possible premium is set (discussed under Question 2). When the pool includes 75 microinsurers, this problem is eliminated, and the reinsurer can reach solvency of 95 percent or more from the first period.

As a pool that large at start-up of reinsurance seems unlikely, an alternative solution to secure the reinsurer's required solvency rate might be to begin operations with sufficient funds to provide the necessary financing for worst-case scenarios during the first four periods. The impact of external funding on the reinsurance operation is discussed in the next section.

Question 5: What impact does external funding have on reinsurance?

As we have seen, small microinsurers joining small reinsurance pools are exposed to a dual vulnerability. First, their variance is likely to be high, which translates into higher premiums, because these are calculated on the basis of variance. Second, small pools also cause an increase in the premium to secure the reinsurer's solvency at 95 percent from start-up. Since reinsurance for community-based schemes is likely to start with a small pool, quantifying the small-size surcharge and finding ways to release microinsurers from it would be desirable. Such an approach would be in line with the purpose of reinsurance as a mechanism offering financial sustainability to microinsurers at an affordable cost.

The question thus is: What size subsidy will both allow each microinsurer to pay only the minimum premium (0.5 of its SD) and also secure the reinsurer's solvency at 95 percent from the first period on? This quantity was obtained by comparing the full premium needed to the reduced premium over the first five periods. The results are shown in figure 7.11. As can be seen, the subsidy would be 26 percent of the premium for the stereotypic microinsurer[17] when the pool includes only 5 microinsurers. The subsidy would drop to 3 percent when the pool increases to 40 microinsurers. It stands to reason that this level of subsidy would be different, probably higher, when the pool is composed of microinsurers with a heterogeneous risk profile. Also, after five years, the subsidy would no longer be necessary because the reinsurer would be financially self-sufficient at the same premium for any pool larger than 20 microinsurers.

This insight points to the important impact of external resources on the way to achieve equity among microinsurers buying reinsurance. Once such resources are available, the reinsurer can negotiate the same premium level with each microinsurer regardless of the pool it affiliates to.

Besides the premium subsidy, the reinsurer needs to secure resources to pay for risk-management services (discussed in Feeley, Gasparro, and Snowden chapter 22, this volume).

FIGURE 7.11   Subsidy Needed to Limit the Premium to $\Omega = 0.5$

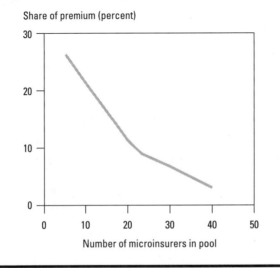

CONCLUSIONS

This model offers a way to quantify microinsurers' vulnerability and to examine the effectiveness of reinsurance as a remedy to it. The discussion has been limited to considerations that can be predicted by the application of statistical laws, and the focus has been on the effect of fluctuations in the microinsurers' and the reinsurer's total benefit expenditures.

The model assumes that microinsurers can fund their mean cost of benefit expenditure.[18] This assumption allows comparison of microinsurers and large health schemes, where it is often assumed that revenues should equal cost recovery. The simulations have shown that, even if this condition is satisfied, only 20 percent of the microinsurers will avoid insolvency within a time frame of five accounting periods. This longer-term view of community-based schemes is relatively rare in the literature, where operations are more often described for short or unspecified time frames, when accidental clustering of cost-generating events may cause insolvency. It has been shown that claim load is the critical predictor of the microinsurer's financial situation. When the claim load is relatively low or when the variance in total cost is relatively large, microinsurers cannot stabilize their financing autonomously, and reinsurance can provide financial stabilization.

Variance in total cost can stem from a small claim load or from a great variation in unit cost. A small claim load is likely to occur either when the group is very small or when the event is very rare. The model described here is suited to all these circumstances.

The reinsurance model can be applied when the SD of each affiliated microinsurer's total benefit cost is known. The reinsurer's success is highly sensitive to the accuracy of this SD; a 20 percent error in SD value can signify the difference between the reinsurer's long-term solvency or bankruptcy. The SD can be calculated only when the risk probability is known. In reality, the estimate of risk is often unreliable, and methods for improving it (discussed in Auray and Fonteneau, chapter 8), are likely to be introduced only when support for risk-management techniques is available.

Even when risk probability is known, the reinsurer is still affected by affiliated microinsurers' pool size and the heterogeneity of risk profiles. The larger the pool, the better the reinsurer can spread risk and thus reduce the variance of its business outcome. When the pool is small, the effect of heterogeneous risk profiles requires a higher premium for stabilization.

Therefore, reinsurance may be very vulnerable in its initial years of operation, even if the pool is large. To remain financially stable during these years, the reinsurer must secure sufficient reserves to cover unpredictable error in risk estimates and the possibility that developing an optimal pool size might take several years.

In any event, reinsurance premiums cannot be set lower than half the SD of each microinsurer's total cost, and several circumstances require higher premiums.

If every microinsurer paid the same minimal rate, subsidies would have to cover the difference in the reinsurer's income for the first four years.

Reinsurance is useful for two main reasons: It helps improve the microinsurer's solvency and gives the microinsurer access to resources from accumulated surpluses that can be spent instead of held as reserves. While both components are important and interrelated, enhanced access to resources would likely appeal more to the reinsurer's potential clients, since discretionary budgets seem more tangible than protection against a risk that is hard to visualize. On the other hand, policymakers and donors may be more interested in securing micro-insurers' long-term viability, and a subsidy to support this development may prove more attractive to microinsurers than ongoing financial support for their continued operations.

Some of the proposed model's limitations should also be recalled. First, the model does not deal with catastrophic risk.[19] Second, some statistical assumptions about real-life situations may be weak, for instance, the assumption that events are independent or that all unit costs are distributed according to a single law. These assumptions, necessary at the conceptualization phase, should be verified during piloting for each microinsurer. Third, the model assumes a distinction between insurable and uninsurable events and deals only with the former. This taxonomy (discussed in Vaté and Dror, chapter 6, this volume) does not always offer a clear-cut distinction between the two types of event. Finally, the administrative costs of operating reinsurance have been ignored in the simulations described here. In the long run, however, these costs would have to be covered by premium income or through other resources and would have to be affordable.

ANNEX 7A A MATHEMATICAL MODEL

Let us consider n microinsurers and T periods. We observe that:
$X(i, t, .)$ represents the aggregate benefits that microinsurance unit (microinsurer) i must pay at the end of period t. The dot indicates that at the beginning of the period this amount is unknown. We assume that $X(i, t, .)$ is a random variable for which the distribution function $F(i, t, x)$ is known. $\overline{X}(i,t)$ designates the mean of $X(i, t,.)$.

$m[\overline{X}(i,t)]$ is the amount set up as reserves by the microinsurer at the beginning of period t to pay its aggregate benefits for period t. This sum shall be expressed in relation to $\overline{X}(i,t)$.

$h[\overline{X}(i,t)]$ is the sum the microinsurer must pay before it can claim from the reinsurance. This amount has been called the *reinsurance threshold*.

We assume that $m[\overline{X}(i,t)] \geq h[\overline{X}(i,t)]$.

$\Delta(i, t)$ is the premium paid by microinsurer i to the reinsurer for period t. Microinsurers may reaffiliate for t periods, $t = 1, ..., T$.

Case A1—Microinsurers n sign a reinsurance contract for one period.

If microinsurer i did not sign a reinsurance contract, its probability of survival α_{i1} is equal to:

$$\alpha_{i1} = P[m[\ \overline{X\ (i,1)}\ ] - X(i, 1, .) \geq 0] = P[X(i, 1, .) \leq [m[\ \overline{X\ (i,1)}\ ]].$$

Let us calculate the probability of survival β_{1i} in the case where the microinsurer decides to sign a reinsurance contract. For this, we define random variable $Z(i, t, .)$ as follows:

$$Z(i, 1, .) = \begin{cases} m[\overline{X\ (i,t)}] - X(i, t, .) - \Delta(i, t) & \text{if} \quad X(i, t, .) \leq h[\overline{X(i, t)}] \\ m[\overline{X\ (i,t)}] - h[\overline{X\ (i,t)}] - \Delta(i, t) & \text{if} \quad X(i, t, .) > h[\overline{X(i, t)}] \end{cases}$$

$$\beta_{1i} = P[Z(i, 1, .) \geq 0]$$

And:

$$P[X(i,1,.) \leq Min\{[m[\ \overline{X\ (i,1)}\ ]- \Delta(i,1), h[\ \overline{X\ (i,1)}\ ]\}]+P[\{m[\ \overline{X\ (i,1)}\ ]-h[\ \overline{X\ (i,1)}\ ] - \Delta(i,1) \geq 0\} \cap \{X(i,1,.) > h[\ \overline{X\ (i,1)}\ ]\}]$$

Yet if:

$$\Delta(i,1) > m[\ \overline{X\ (i,1)}\ ] - h[\ \overline{X\ (i,1)}\ ]\ \text{then:}$$

$$P[\{m[\ \overline{X\ (i,1)}\ ]-h[\ \overline{X\ (i,1)}\ ] - \Delta(i,1)0\} \cap \{X(i,1,.) > h[\ \overline{X\ (i,1)}\ ]\}] = 0$$

if

$$\Delta(i,1) \leq m[\ \overline{X\ (i,1)}\ ] - h[\ \overline{X\ (i,1)}\ ]\ \text{then:}$$

$$P[\{m[\ \overline{X\ (i,1)}\ ] - h[\ \overline{X\ (i,1)}\ ] - \Delta(i,1)0\} \cap \{X(i,1,.) > h[\ \overline{X\ (i,1)}\ ]\}] = P\ [X(i,1,.) > h[\ \overline{X\ (i,1)}\ ]]$$

Where:

If $\Delta(i,1) > m[\ \overline{X\ (i,1)}\ ] - h[\ \overline{X\ (i,1)}\ ]$ then $\beta_{1i} = P[X(i,1,.)\ m[\ \overline{X\ (i,1)}\ ]] - \Delta(i,1)]$

If $\Delta(i,1) \leq m[\ \overline{X\ (i,1)}\ ] - h[\ \overline{X\ (i,1)}\ ]$ then $\beta_{1i} = 1$

Thus:

If $\Delta(i,1) > m[\ \overline{X\ (i,1)}\ ] - h[\ \overline{X\ (i,1)}\ ]$ and $\alpha_{i1} \geq \beta_{1i}$, then microinsurer i has no interest in reinsuring itself.

If $\Delta(i,1) \leq m[\ \overline{X\ (i,1)}\ ] - h[\ \overline{X\ (i,1)}\ ]$ and $\beta_{1i} = 1$, then microinsurer i has every interest in reinsuring itself as this will guarantee its survival.

Let us now look at the problem of the reinsurer.

Benefits paid to microinsurer i at the end of period t is a random variable that we designate by $W(i, t, .)$ and which is equal to:

$$W(i, t, .) = \begin{cases} 0 & \text{if} \quad X(i, t, .) \leq h[\overline{X(i, t)}] \\ X(i, t, .) - h[\overline{X(i,t)}] & \text{if} \quad X(i, t, .) > h[\overline{X(i, t)}] \end{cases}$$

It can be proven that the distribution function of variable $W(i, t, .)$, noted as $G(i, t, w)$ is equal to:

$$\begin{cases} 0 & \text{if} \quad w < 0 \\ G(i, t, w) = F(i, t, h[\overline{X(i,t)}] & \text{if} \quad w = 0 \\ F(i, t, w + h[\overline{X(i, t)}] & \text{if} \quad w > 0 \end{cases}$$

Consequently, if $\overline{W(i,t)}$ is the mean of $W(i, t, .)$ and σ^2_{Wit} its variance, then:

$$\overline{W(i,t)} = \int_{-\infty}^{+\infty} wdG(i, t, .) = \int_{0}^{+\infty} wdF(i, t, .) \text{ and } \sigma2Wit = \int_{-\infty}^{+\infty} w^2dG(i, t, .) - \overline{W(i,t)}^2$$

Let B_0 designate the funds the reinsurer has on hand at the onset of its activity, and $s(n, t)$ its administrative costs for the period t when it reinsures n microinsurance units.

We note that $A(n, t)$ equals $B_0 - \sum_{j=1}^{t} s(n, j)$,

The insurer's probability of survival at the end of the first period, γ_1 is equal to:

$$\gamma_1 = P[A(n, 1) + \sum_{i=1}^{n} \Delta(i, 1) - \sum_{i=1}^{n} W(i, 1, .) \geq 0] = P[\sum_{i=1}^{n} W(i, 1, .) \leq A(n, 1) + \sum_{i=1}^{n} \Delta(i, 1)]$$

The analytical expression of the convolution product law for random variables $W(i, 1, .)$ is obtainable only in specific cases.

Example

Here we assume, regardless of microinsurer i, that $X(i, t, .) = X(t, .)$ and random variables $X(i, t, .)$ are independent pairwise. We know (Bass 1974) that if n is greater than or equal to 30, a normal law containing mean $\overline{W(i,t)}$ and variance σ^2_{Wit}/n can approximate the law of random variable Z_{nt} defined by $1/n \sum_{i=1}^{n} W(i, t, .)$

In this case:

$$\gamma_1 = P[Z_{n1} \leq 1/n [A(n, 1) + \sum_{i=1}^{n} \Delta(i, 1,)]]$$

As the distribution of financial risk is the same for each microinsurer, we can reasonably put forth the hypothesis that they will all obtain the same contract in terms of premiums and reinsurance thresholds. Thus, regardless of whether $i = 1, ..., n$, we have $\Delta(i,1) = \Delta(1)$ and $h[\overline{X(i,1)}] = h[\overline{X(1)}]$, whereby:

$$\gamma_1 = P[Z_{n1} \leq \frac{A(n, 1)}{n} + \Delta(1)] = P[\mathbf{Z}_{n1} \leq [\frac{A(n, 1)}{n} + \Delta(1) - \overline{W(1)}] \sqrt{n} / \sigma_{W1}]]$$

where $\mathbf{Z}_{n1}$ is the random standard variable associated to Z_{n1} and $\overline{W(1)} = \overline{W(i,t)}$, $\sigma_{W1} = \sigma^2_{Wi1}$ regardless if $i = 1, ..., n$.

If the reinsurer is willing to accept a bankruptcy risk of $0.05 = 1 - \gamma_1$ then we have:

$$[\frac{A(n, 1)}{n} + \Delta(1) - \overline{W(1)}] \sqrt{n} / \sigma_{W1} = 1.65$$

Where:

$$\Delta(1) = \overline{W(1)} - \frac{A(n, 1)}{n} + 1.65\sigma_{W1} / \sqrt{n}$$

and, as the microinsurer is interested in reinsurance only when $\Delta(1) < m[\overline{X(1)}] - h[\overline{X(1)}]$, this reinsurance model can be considered only if:

$$0 < \overline{W(1)} - \frac{A(n, 1)}{n} + 1.65\sigma_{W1} / \sqrt{n} < m[\overline{X(1)}] - h[\overline{X(1)}]$$

Case A2—Microinsurers n sign a reinsurance contract for T periods, T > 1.

Let us calculate the survival probability β_{Ti} for microinsurer i in the case where it signs a reinsurance contract for T periods.

$$\beta_{Ti} = P[Z(i, 1, .) \geq 0, Z(i, 2, .) \geq 0, ..., Z(i, T, .) \geq 0] = \prod_{t=1}^{t=T} P[Z(i, t, .) \geq 0]$$

Consequently, regardless if $t = 1, ..., T$, $\Delta(i,t) \leq m[\overline{X(i,t)}] - h[\overline{X(i,t)}]$ the survival of the microinsurer i is certain throughout the entire period T.

To calculate the reinsurer's survival probability, we will suppose that the reinsurance contract binds each microinsurer to the reinsurer for T periods; that the amount of the premium for each period was determined when the contract was signed: and, to simplify matters, that the reinsurer's survival is calculated only at the end of period T. This last hypothesis implies, for example, that, in case of losses over one or more periods, the reinsurer can obtain interest-free financing of the deficit, repayable from profits in the future.

Within the context of these hypotheses, the reinsurer's survival probability at the end of period T is equal to:

$$\gamma_T = P[A(n,T) + \sum_{t=1}^{t=T} \sum_{i=1}^{n} \Delta(i, t) - \sum_{t=1}^{t=T} \sum_{i=1}^{i=n} W(i, t, .) \geq 0] = P[\sum_{t=1}^{t=T} \sum_{i=1}^{i=n} W(i, t, .) \leq A(n,T) + \sum_{t=1}^{t=T} \sum_{i=1}^{i=n} \Delta(i, t)]$$

Example

If we look again at the example above, where we suppose that microinsurers n are similar, even if $i = 1, ..., n$, $X(i, t, .) = X(t, .)$, and if we suppose that time frame T is short enough for the microinsurers' benefit distributions to remain constant, that is $X(t, .) = X(.)$, then:

W(i, t, .) = W(.) for all $i = 1, ..., n$ and all $t = 1, ..., T$

If product nT is greater than 30, we know that random variable Z_{nT}, defined as

$\frac{1}{nT} \sum_{t=1}^{t=T} \sum_{i=1}^{n} W(i, t, .)$, can be approximated with a normal law containing mean

and variance σ^2_W/nT, where $\overline{W}$ and σ^2_W are, respectively, the mean and variance of W(.).

We then have:

$$\gamma_T = P[Z_{nT} \le \frac{1}{nT} [A(n, T) + \sum_{t=1}^{t=T} \sum_{i=1}^{i=n} \Delta(i, t)]]$$

and if $\Delta(i, t) = \Delta$ for all $i = 1, ..., n$, $t = 1, ..., T$, which seems reasonable in this case as the microinsurers are similar, we obtain, with a 95 percent survival probability for the reinsurer:

$$[\frac{A(n, T)}{nT} + \Delta - \overline{W}]\sqrt{nT}/\sigma_W = 1.65$$

Where:

$$\Delta = \overline{W} - \frac{A(n, T)}{nT} + 1.65\sigma_W/\sqrt{nT}$$

and the condition that guarantees the interest of the reinsurance process:

$$0 \le \overline{W} - \frac{A(n, T)}{nT} + 1.65\sigma_W / \le m[\overline{X}] - h[\overline{X}]$$

ANNEX 7B CALCULATING THE REINSURANCE PREMIUM

In the following simple example, the reinsurance premium can be calculated analytically.[20]

Let us consider a case where more than 30 identical microinsurers sign identical reinsurance contracts for one time period. The law of large numbers allows us to state the following: the reinsurer operates under the condition that its risk of bankruptcy will not exceed 5 percent. The reinsurance premium Δ payable by each microinsurer must satisfy the following equation:

$$\Delta = \overline{W(1)} - \frac{A(n, 1)}{n} + 1.65\sigma_{W1}/\sqrt{n}$$

Where:

$\overline{W(1)}$ is the mean of a random variable W(1) equal to benefits paid by the reinsurer during Period 1,

σ_{W1} is the SD of the random variable W(1),

n is the number of microinsurers pooled by the reinsurance contract,

A(n,1) is the reinsurer's initial capital, minus administrative costs for the first period.

The equation indicates that, when the number of reinsured microinsurance units increases and the reinsurer's initial capital increases more slowly, the reinsurance premium will lean toward $\overline{W(1)}$. In this case, reinsurance will be attractive for microinsurers only when the premium $\overline{W(1)}$ is lower than the safety margin (that is, proportional to the microinsurer's own benefit expenditure variance) and when the reinsurance threshold is equal to the mean cost of the microinsurer's benefits.

The next example illustrates a case where the distribution probability of each microinsurer's business results is available. A uniform distribution of benefits payable by the microinsurer to its members is assumed, on an interval of [0, 10] ₪. In this case, without reinsurance, the microinsurer needs 10 ₪ at the beginning of each period to ensure its solvency. With reinsurance, the microinsurer would need to secure only the mean cost, 5 ₪, (the reinsurance threshold), because the reinsurer bears all costs above it, plus the premium. The mean value of benefits the reinsurer must pay a microinsurer i is 1.25 ₪ with an SD of 1.61. This has been calculated using the following algorithm[21]:

$$G_{i1}(w) = \begin{cases} 0 & \text{if } w < 0 \\ 0,5 & \text{if } w = 0 \\ \dfrac{2w + 10}{20} & \text{if } 0 < w \le 5 \\ 1 & \text{if } 5 < w \end{cases}$$

which leads us to $\overline{W(1)} = \dfrac{10}{8} = 1.25$ and $\sigma_{i1}^2 = \dfrac{5*10^2}{192} = 1.61^2$

The information obtained from the above calculation can now be placed in the equation above, with mean benefit $\overline{W(1)} = 1.25$, and $\sigma_{W1} = 1.61$, to obtain the reinsurance premium. The results are shown in table 7.1.

ANNEX 7C CALCULATING THE MEAN BENEFIT EXPENDITURE AND ITS VARIANCE

To calculate each microinsurer's mean benefit expenditure and its variance, payable at the end of period T, we note:

a(i, t) is the number of individuals covered by microinsurance i at period t.

b(i, t) is the number of benefit types included in the package of microinsurance i during period t.

D(i, j, k, t, .) is the number of occurrences of claims k during the period t for individual j covered by microinsurance i. We assume that D(i, j, k, t, .) is a discrete random variable (whose distribution follows the Poisson law, for example).

E[D(i, j, k, t, .)] is the mean of D(i, j, k, t, .).

Var[D(i, j, k, t, .)] is the variance of D(i, j, k, t, .).

C(i, j, k, t, .) is the amount paid by microinsurance i to individual j each time a claim k is submitted during period t for this individual. We assume that C(i, j, k, t, .) is a random variable.

E[C(i, j, k, t, .)] is the mean of C(i, j, k, t, .).

Var[C(i, j, k, t, .)] is the variance of C(i, j, k, t, .).

T(i, j, k, t, .) is the random variable defined by :

$$T(i, j, k, t, .) = \begin{cases} 0 & \text{if } D(i, j, k, t, .) = 0 \\ C_1(i, j, k, t, .) & \text{if } D(i, j, k, t, .) = 1 \\ C_1(i, j, k, t, .) + C_2(i, j, k, t, .) & \text{if } D(i, j, k, t, .) = 2 \\ \quad\cdots & \quad\cdots \\ C_1(i, j, k, t, .) + \ldots + C_s(i, j, k, t, .) & \text{if } D(i, j, k, t, .) = s \\ \quad\cdots & \quad\cdots \end{cases}$$

where:

$C_s(i, j, k, t, .) = C(i, j, k, t, .)$ for all s.

It follows that:

$X(i, t, .) = \sum_j \sum_k T(i, j, k, t, .)$ (NOTE: this variable is defined in annex 7A.)

$\overline{X}(i, t) = \sum_j \sum_k \overline{T}(i, j, k, t)$

Where $\overline{T}(i, j, k, t)$ is the mean of T(i, j, k, t, .)
And if the variable T(i, j, k, t, .) is independent, then:

$Var[X(i, t, .)] = \sum_j \sum_k var[T(i, j, k, t, .)]$

Expression of $\overline{T}(i, j, k, t)$:

$\overline{T}(i, j, k, t) = E[0]Prob[D(i,j,k,t,.)=0]+\ldots+E[C_1(i,j,k,t, .) + \ldots + C_s(i,j,k,t,.)]$
$Prob[D(i,j,k,t,.) = s]+ \ldots$

$$\overline{T}\,(i,\,j,\,k,\,t) = E[C(i,j,k,t,\,.)]Prob[D(i,j,k,t,.) = 1] + \dots + sE[C(i,j,k,t,\,.)]$$
$$Prob[D(i,j,k,t,.) = s] + \dots$$

$$\overline{T}\,(i,\,j,\,k,\,t) = E[C(i,\,j,\,k,\,t,\,.)]\,E[C(i,\,j,\,k,\,t,\,.)]\sum_{s=0}^{s=\infty} sProb[D(i,\,j,\,k,\,t,\,.) = s] =$$

$$E[C(i,\,j,\,k,\,t,\,.)]E[D(i,\,j,\,k,\,t,\,.)]$$

$$\overline{T}\,(i,\,j,\,k,\,t) = E[C(i,\,j,\,k,\,t,\,.)]E[D(i,\,j,\,k,\,t,\,.)]$$

Thus:

The mean cost paid by microinsurer i to individual j at the end of period t for claim(s) k is equal to the mean cost of claim(s) k paid by microinsurer i during period t multiplied by the mean number of occurrences of claim k during the period t for individual j.

Expression of Var[T(i, j, k, t, .)] :

$$Var[T(i,\,j,\,k,\,t,\,.)] = E[T(i,\,j,\,k,\,t,\,.)^2] - \overline{T}\,(i,\,j,\,k,\,t)$$

$$E[T(i,j,k,t,.)^2]=E[0^2]Prob[D(i,j,k,t,.)=0]+ \dots + E\{[C_1(i,j,k,t,\,.) + \dots + C_s(i,j,k,t,.)]^2\}$$
$$Prob[D(i,j,k,t,.) = s] + \dots$$

$$E[T(i,j,k,t,.)^2] = E(C(i,\,j,\,k,\,t,\,.)^2)\sum_{s=0}^{\infty} sProb\,[D(i,\,j,\,k,\,t,\,.) = s] + 2\,[E(C(i,\,j,\,k,\,t,\,.)^2]$$

$$\sum_{s=2}^{\infty} C_s^2 Prob[D(i,\,j,\,k,\,t,\,.) = s]$$

$$E[T(i,j,k,t,.)^2] = E(C(i,\,j,\,k,\,t,\,.)^2)\,E(D(i,\,j,\,k,\,t,\,.) + 2\,[E(C(i,\,j,\,k,\,t,\,.)^2]\sum_{s=2}^{\infty} C_s^2$$

$$Prob[D(i,\,j,\,k,\,t,\,.) = s]$$

$$Var[T(i,j,k,t,.)]= E(C(i,\,j,\,k,\,t,\,.)^2)\,E(D(i,\,j,\,k,\,t,\,.) + 2\,[E(C(i,\,j,\,k,\,t,\,.)]^2\sum_{s=2}^{\infty} C_s^2$$

$$Prob[D(i,\,j,\,k,\,t,\,.) = s] - E[C(i,j,k,t,.)]^2 E[D(i,j,k,t,.)]^2$$

$$Var[T(i,j,k,t,.)] = E(C(i,\,j,\,k,\,t,\,.)^2)\,E(D(i,\,j,\,k,\,t,\,.) + E[C(i,j,k,t,.)]^2\{2\sum_{s=2}^{\infty} C_s^2$$

$$Prob[D(i,\,j,\,k,\,t,\,.) = s] - E(D(i,\,j,\,k,\,t,\,.)^2\}$$

$$Var[T(i,j,k,t,.)]= E(C(i,\,j,\,k,\,t,\,.)^2)\,E(D(i,\,j,\,k,\,t,\,.) + E[C(i,j,k,t,.)]^2\{\sum_{s=2}^{\infty} s(s-1)$$

$$Prob[D(i,\,j,\,k,\,t,\,.) = s] - E(D(i,\,j,\,k,\,t,\,.)^2\}$$

But:

$$\sum_{s=2}^{\infty} s(s-1) \, \text{Prob}[D(i, j, k, t, .) = s] = \sum_{s=2}^{\infty} s^2 \, \text{Prob}[D(i, j, k, t, .) = s] - \sum_{s=2}^{\infty} s$$

$$\text{Prob}[D(i, j, k, t, .) = s]$$

$$\sum_{s=2}^{\infty} s^2 \, \text{Prob}[D(i, j, k, t, .) = s] = E(D(i, j, k, t, .)^2) - \text{Prob}[D(i, j, k, t, .) = 1]$$

$$\sum_{s=2}^{\infty} s\text{Prob}[D(i, j, k, t, .) = s] = E(D(i, j, k, t, .)) - \text{Prob}[D(i, j, k, t, .) = 1]$$

Therefore:

$$\sum_{s=2}^{\infty} s(s-1)\text{Prob}[D(i, j, k, t, .) = s] = E(D(i, j, k, t, .)^2) - E(D(i, j, k, t, .))$$

And:

$$Var[T(i,j,k,t,.)] = E[D(i,j,k,t,.)]E[C(i,j,k,t,.)^2] + E[C(i,j,k,t,.)]^2\{E[D(i,j,k,t,.)^2] - E[D(i,j,k,t,.)^2] - E[D(i,j,k,t,.)]\}$$

$$Var[T(i,j,k,t,.)] = E[D(i,j,k,t,.)]E[C(i,j,k,t,.)^2] + E[C(i,j,k,t,.)]^2\{Var[D(i,j,k,t,.)] - E[D(i,j,k,t,.)]\}$$

$$Var[T(i,j,k,t,.)] = E[D(i,j,k,t,.)]Var[C(i,j,k,t,.)] + E[C(i,j,k,t,.)]^2Var[D(i,j,k,t,.)]$$

Thus:

The variance of the cost paid by microinsurer i to individual j at the end of period t for claim k is equal to the sum of the variance of the cost of claim k paid by microinsurance i during period t multiplied by the mean number of occurrences of claim k during period t for individual j belonging microinsurer i, plus the square root of the mean cost of claim k paid by microinsurer i during period t multiplied by the variance of the number of occurrences of claim k during the period t for individual j.

Example:

If distributions of D(i, j, k, t, .) and C(i, j, k, t, .) are given by these tables :

D(i, j, k, t, .)	0	1	2	3	4
Probability	0.2	0;2	0.2	0.2	0.2

C(i, j, k, t, .)	1	2
Probability	0.25	0.75

Then:

$E[D(i,j,k,t,.)] = 2$ and $Var[D(i,j,k,t,.)] = 2$

E[C(i,j,k,t,.)] = 1.75 and Var[C(i,j,k,t,.)] = 0.1875

Thus:

E[T(i,j,k,t,.)] = 2.1.75 = 3.5 and Var[T(i,j,k,t,.)] = 2.0.1875 + 1.75^2.2 = 6.5

In this case it easy to compute the distribution of T(i,j,k,t,.):

T(i,j,k,t,.)	0	1	2	3	4	5	6	7	8
Probability	256/ 1280 = 20%	64/ 1280 = 5%	208/ 1280 = 16.25%	100/ 1280 = 7.81%	181/ 1280 = 14.14%	120/ 1280 = 9.38%	162/ 1280 = 12.66%	108/ 1280 = 8.44%	81/ 1280 = 6.32%

And it is easy also to compute the mean and the variance of T(i,j,k,t,.):

E[T(i,j,k,t,.)] = 3.5 and Var[T(i,j,k,t,.)] = 6.5

Therefore:

$$\overline{X}(i, t) = \sum_{j=1}^{a(i, t,)} \sum_{k=1}^{b(i, t,)} E[D(i, j, k, t, .)] \, E[C(i, j, k, t, .)]$$

and

$$Var[x(I, t, .)] = \sum_{j=1}^{a(i, t,)} \sum_{k=1}^{b(i, t,)} \{E[D(i,j,k,t,.)]Var[C(i,j,k,t,.)] + E[C(i,j,k,t,.)]^2 Var[D(i,j,k,t,.)]\}$$

Particular case:

If we assume that occurrences of each claim are independent of individuals and that costs are also independent of individuals, we have:

D(i, j, k, t, .) = D(i, k, t, .) and C(i, j, k, t, .) = C(i, k, t, .) or all j and k.

In this case we have:

$$\overline{X}(i, t) = a(i, t) \sum_{k=1}^{b(i, t,)} E[D(i, t, .) \, E[C(i, t, .)]$$

and

$$Var[X(i, t, .)] = a(i,t) \sum_{k=1}^{b(i, t)} \{E[D(i,j,k,t,.)]Var[C(i,j,k,t,.)] + E[C(i,j,k,t,.)]^2 Var[D(i,j,k,t,.)]\}$$

ANNEX 7D CALCULATING THE EFFECTS OF REINSURANCE

Using the previous example as the basis for an analysis of the impact of reinsurance over time, and assuming that all parameters remain unchanged (distribution probability of microinsurers' balance sheets, the number of reinsured microinsurers, and 5 percent limit on the reinsurer's insolvency risk), the central limit theorem can now be applied. Thus, if the reinsurance contract extends over a number of periods T, the premium Δ paid by each microinsurer for each period must equal:

$$\Delta = \overline{W} - \frac{A(n, T)}{nT} + 1.65\sigma_w / \sqrt{nT}$$

Where:

$\overline{W}$ is the mean of random variable W equal to benefits paid by the reinsurer each period,

σ_w is the SD of random variable W,

n is the number of microinsurers,

T is the duration of the reinsurance contract,

A(n,T) is the reinsurer's initial capital, decreased by its managing costs for periods T.

This example can be extended to a more general case, where

$$A(n, T) = B_0 - Ts(n)$$

where B_0 is the reinsurer's initial capital and we assume that, for each period, administrative costs s(n) depend only upon the number of reinsured units and that initial seed capital will be depleted over time. As this capital is depleted, the reinsurance premium will increase. By the same token, when the reinsurer accumulates surpluses during the same period, it can decrease the required premium. The general mathematical expression of the condition when the premium is likely to decrease over time is that this situation will occur when the derivative of Δ as a function of time is negative. The results of this derivation are the following:

For any given n, if $T \geq \dfrac{1.47B_0^2}{n\sigma_w^2}$, then premium Δ decreases as the duration T of the contract increases.

This relationship implies that the larger the number of microinsurers in the pool (n), and the greater the variance of the reinsurer's benefit expenditure (σ_w), the shorter the time from the initiation of the contract to the point when the premium will start to decrease.[22]

Simulated results, corroborating that a larger number of pooled microinsurers can reduce the premium, and that the impact of a larger pool tapers off at a certain size, are provided in figure 7.4.

NOTES

1. A review of the actuarial literature reveals the existence of numerous reinsurance models, which differ in the content and complexity of the benefit package (Outreville, chapter 3, this volume). Various simulation software packages have been developed

to assess the impact of these benefit packages in specific settings (Geneva Association 1982; Brown and Galitz 1983, 1984). However, these models and software were designed for use in the economic context of industrial countries and have not been effective when used in the context of microinsurance units in developing countries.

2. This variance is a function of group size; the ratio between the variance and the expected mean decreases as group size increases (Dror 2001).

3. The large number of microinsurance units is needed to apply the law of large numbers.

4. The assumption of uniform distribution is valid when there is no reliable information on the risk probability and on the variance of benefit cost. Any alternative assumption about distribution would probably have given a lower premium.

5. To avoid confusion between the acronyms MU (monetary unit) and MIU (microinsurance unit), the symbol ⋒ (stylized MU) is used here, without designating any specific currency.

6. Under this distribution law, the variance is equal to the mean.

7. Under this distribution law, the variance is equal to twice the mean.

8. The *Social Re Data Template* is described in appendix A, this volume. The data needs are discussed in detail in chapter 16, this volume.

9. This is a result of the complexity of the probability laws for microinsurers' business results and of the complex analytical expression predicting the probability of the reinsurer's bankruptcy (a convolution product of truncated laws).

10. A Poisson law was used, as is usual in such a case; the parameter used is the mean of each cost-generating event within the population.

11. CHI2 law was used for simplicity, but any other law would do.

12. The business result is a function of the distribution of cost-generating events it has to pay and the distribution of unit costs that apply to these events.

13. Monte Carlo simulation consists of generating pseudo random numbers following a given probability distribution with a view to obtaining empirically the probable distributions of random variables (see also glossary entry for this term at end of this volume).

14. This assumes that the microinsurer's members pay all their contributions in full and on time.

15. $(0.5*35.70)/75 = 23.8$.

16. In relative terms, all microinsurers can expect the discretionary budget to be around 80 percent of premiums paid.

17. $n = 500$, $P = 1$ percent, unit cost $= 15$, average total cost $= 75$, SD $= 35.70$.

18. The role of subsidies in achieving full recovery rate is discussed in Busse, chapter 13, this volume.

19. In this context, *catastrophic risks* generate higher expenses than the worst-case scenario predictable by the applicable statistical laws. Such cases can occur through such events as epidemics affecting the whole community, acts of nature, and the like.

20. The analytical calculation of the reinsurance premium is often impossible because of the complexity of the probability laws for microinsurers' business results and the complex analytical expression predicting the probability of the reinsurer's bankruptcy (a convolution product of truncated laws).

21. Annex 7A explains the principles underlying the algorithm.

22. For any given T, if $0{,}825\ \sigma_w\sqrt{nT} - T[ns'(n) - s(n)] \geq B_0$, then premium Δ decreases as the number of reinsured microinsurers n increases ($s'(n)$ designates the first derivative of s).

REFERENCES

Bass, J. 1974. *Elément de calcul des probabilités*. 3d ed. Paris: Masson.

Brown, Z.M., and L. Galitz. 1983. *The ASIR System*. Working Paper No. 66. Geneva: Geneva Association.

_____. 1984. *The ASIR System*. Working Paper No. 76. Geneva: Geneva Association.

Dror, D.M. 2001. "Reinsurance of Health Insurance for the Informal Sector." *World Health Organization Bulletin* 79(7):672–78.

Geneva Association. 1982. "The ASIR Model." *The Geneva Papers on Risk and Insurance* 7 (October 25):279–392.

Lesage, J.J. 1999. *Modélisation des systèmes réactifs*. Paris: Hermès Ed.

Monsef, Y. 1997. "Modeling and Simulation of Complex Systems Concepts." In E. Kerckhoffs, H. Pierreval, R.N. Zobel, and A. Lehmann, eds., *Frontiers in Simulation*. Society for Computer Simulation. Manchester: Department of Computer Science, University of Manchester.

CHAPTER 8

Local Consensus and Estimates of Medical Risk

Jean P. Auray and Robert Fonteneau

Reinsurance, as described in this book, seeks to stabilize microinsurance units (MIUs) by protecting them from both the risk of fluctuations in costs and the expense of paying for uninsurable costs (such as routine vaccinations or preventive care, including HIV/AIDS), which should be paid from other sources. Reinsurance does not attempt to replace or integrate all health-related activities.[1] The issue here is developing the methodology to separate the areas where reinsurance should intervene from those where other structures should assume the financial responsibility. In the industrial countries' national systems, where such separation is nonexistent, competition over resources can be observed between medical care and education, infrastructure, or social assistance. This competition should not be replicated at the level of small and poor communities.

Reinsurance of microinsurers must offer predictable solutions while recognizing the diversity of situations in which these units function. Demand for care reflects a 2:3 gap between actual and desirable spending for health care considered essential (UNICEF 1998, UNDP 1998).[2] But demand elasticity varies according to household income and the perception of cost/benefit (or quality) of the care received. In other words, elasticity is not entirely rigid (Jack 2000).

LOCAL CONSENSUS AT THE COMMUNITY LEVEL

Local consensus is a strong indicator of perceptions of the cost-benefit ratio of care or its quality. This assertion is based on the primordial role of direct local participation, through MIUs, in four out of eight domains of care in developing countries (WHO 1988): basic health information and education, maternal and child health, treatment of prevalent diseases and traumas, and access to essential drugs at affordable prices (Monekosso n.d.).

Within each of these four categories, access to care varies greatly, depending on the local resources available. Recent studies (Berman 2000) suggest that

The authors acknowledge, with thanks, helpful comments on a draft of this chapter made by Daniel Tounissoux, Professor of Mathematics and Informatics at University Claude-Bernard, Lyon, and by Nicolas Nicoloyannis, Professor of Mathematics and Informatics, University Lumière, Lyon.

ambulatory personal health care has the potential for providing the largest immediate health status gains in low-income countries, particularly for the poor (Good 1953). However, this care, a huge financial burden for individual (poor) households, represents the major part of health expenditure in low-income countries (compared with less than 30 percent in industrial countries). Consequently, these people often cannot deal with their complex health problems, a situation aggravated by unhealthy competition between private (often unqualified) providers and the public sector in markets lacking in cost and quality control. This systemic shortcoming in many developing countries is not resolved by traditional medical planning, which pays insufficient attention to the interactions among health, individual, and social factors and the health care system at large (Fonteneau and Beresniak 2002). Thus, it is commonly recognized that individual health status is largely influenced by an individual's ability and propensity to choose a healthy environment and way of life.

FROM CONSENSUS TO METHODICAL ESTIMATES

Microinsurers could exercise a natural role in defending the all-important healthy environment by representing the group vis-à-vis local actors in the health care system. If microinsurers are to do so, they must win the confidence of consumers and providers alike by fashioning a reliable compromise between true and perceived assessments of cost/benefit and quality of care. But when resources are tight and the prevailing rationale seeks to increase resources instead of rationing them effectively, funds are unlikely to be allocated to obtaining reliable information on costs and on utilization. Reinsurers need this information to estimate risk probability, morbidity patterns, and local health costs. This indispensable information is usually missing (WHO 2000).

Lacking adequate data at the local level and recognizing that local needs and priorities may be poorly reflected in global or national data, what alternative methods can be used to obtain the data needed to improve microinsurers' operations and stabilize their finance through reinsurance? Some qualitative "consensual methods" (for example, role play and oral autopsies) are known but rarely used at the village level. In Bangladesh, for example, only 7 percent of village health promoters engaged in such exercises (Taha 1997; Berwick and Nolan 1998). Some alternative methods must therefore be found to estimate the data reinsurers need to do business with microinsurers.

Repeated observations of the number of occurrences (k) of an event in a group numbering n individuals can provide an estimate of its risk. This method, known in probability theory under the term *balloting scheme*, is explained below.

A microinsurer might view participation in a balloting scheme first and foremost as a means of improving its operating efficiency, but not as an objective in itself. Therefore, its commitment to persevere in multiple repetitions of such an exercise over time may be limited. This exercise should allow the reinsurer to distinguish, as objectively as possible, the kinds of risks that reinsurance would cover, as distinct from the uninsurable risks that would be financed through other sources (Vaté and Dror, chapter 6, this volume).

ESTIMATING THE PROBABILITY P OF AN UNKNOWN EVENT

Suppose we have an urn full of balls, including a proportion p of white balls. Because there are so many balls, we cannot see them all, count the white balls, or know the precise value of p. We can only hope to find an approximate value for p. To do this, we perform the following experiment. In a series of withdrawals, we remove n balls from the urn and count the number of white balls each time.

We then know that the probability of counting exactly k white balls is equal to: $\binom{n}{p} p^k (1-p)^{n-k}$. The number of white balls observed at the end of the experiment is a random variable in a binomial distribution B(n,p) of parameters n and p. The proportion of white balls removed from the urn at the end of this experiment is therefore (k/n). We can perform many similar, independent trials the same way, noting the proportion of white balls observed each time.

In this way, we construct an estimator P(.) for the unknown proportion p of white balls in the urn. We know the distribution of this estimator. The different values of P(.) are those in set {0, 1/n, 2/n, 3/n, ... , k/n, ... , (n-1)/n, 1}, and the probability of P(.) is k/n (for all k ∈ {0, 1, ..., n-1, n} is $\binom{n}{p} p^k (1-p)^{n-k}$. This type of distribution is sometimes called a *binomial frequency*.

At the end of the experiment, we are able to obtain two items: a point estimation of p and a confidence interval for p. As we do not know p, the distribution of P(.) remains entirely theoretical. If, at the end of the experiment, we observe exactly k white balls out of n withdrawals, then k/n will be a point estimation for the unknown proportion p. This information is interesting, but it is only an "approximate value" of p. It would be useful to know how to assess the quality of this approximation, for that will enable us to determine a confidence interval. Taking into account the distribution of P(.) we deduce that the confidence interval at level α (in general, we choose α = 0.05 or α = 0.01) is the result of:

$$I_\alpha = [(k/n) - a_1, (k/n) + a_2]$$

where a_1 and a_2 are numbers

$$a_1 = (k_1/n) \text{ and}$$
$$a_2 = (k2/n)$$

where k_1 and k_2 are two whole numbers defined by:

$$k_1 = \text{Max}\{j \in Nn; p0 + p1 + \dots + pj \le \alpha/2\}$$

$$k_2 = \text{Min}\{j \in Nn; p0 + p1 + \dots + pj \ge 1 - \alpha/2\}$$

Expressions in which:

$N_n = \{0, 1, 2, ..., n-1, n\}$

and

$P_h = \binom{n}{p} p^k (1-p)^{n-k}$, for all $h \in N_n$

As the value of p is unknown in the expression of p_k, we replace p by the approximate value (k/n) of p, which is none other than the point estimation obtained in our experiment.

The direct calculation of values a_1 and a_2 is not easy, but it can be simplified in certain situations.

The Case of Normal Distribution

In the first situation, n is large enough and p is neither too close to 0 nor to 1. In practice, this indicates the simultaneous occurrence of two conditions: np>5 and n(1−p)>5. As p is unknown, in verifying this condition, we replace p by the point estimation (n/k). Thus, distribution B(n,p) is a normal distribution N(np,) $\sqrt{np(1-p)}$.

In these conditions, we can prove that random variable P(.) − p is part of distribution N(0, $\sqrt{\frac{p(1-p)}{n}}$). From this, we deduce a confidence interval at risk level

a for p: $I_\alpha = [\frac{k}{n} - u_{\alpha/2} \sqrt{\frac{p(1-p)}{n}}, \frac{k}{n} + u_{\alpha/2} \sqrt{\frac{p(1-p)}{n}}]$.

The Case of Poisson Distribution

In a second setting, p is small enough (that is, $p < 10^{-2}$) and n is large enough (this condition is linked to the preceding by np > 50). Thus, distribution B(n, p) is a

Poisson distribution P(np). In other words, in this case: $\binom{n}{p} p^k (1-p)^{n-k} \approx e^{-np} \frac{(np)^k}{k!}$.

In these conditions, variable P(.) is a discrete variable with values {0, 1/n, 2/n, ...,

k/n, ... (n−1)/n, 1}, where the value for k/n is part of probability $e^{-np} \frac{(np)^k}{k!}$. This

practically defines a distribution, insofar as the sum $\sum_{k=0}^{n} \binom{n}{p} p^k (1-p)^{n-k}$ barely

differs from 1 in the conditions we have posited. This can be verified. We verify that the expected value of P(.) is equal to p and that its standard deviation is equal

to $\sqrt{\frac{p}{n}}$.

This gives us a confidence interval I_α at risk level α for the value of p, as follows:

$I_a = [(k/n) - a_1, (k/n) + a_2]$

where a_1 and a_2 are two numbers defined by:

$a_1 = (k_1/n)$ and
$a_2 = (k2/n)$

where k_1 and k_2 are two integers defined as:

$k_1 = \text{Max}\{j \in Nn; p0 + p1 + \ldots + pj \leq \alpha/2\}$

$k_2 = \text{Min}\{j \in Nn; p0 + p1 + \ldots + pj \geq 1 - \alpha/2\}$

expressions in which we have:

$N_n = \{0, 1, 2, \ldots, n - 1, n\}$

and

$$p^h = e^{-np} \frac{(np)^h}{h}, \text{ for all } h \in Nn.$$

Conditions ($p < 0.01$ and $np > 50$) ensure that k_2 is well within N_n. Thus, if we suppose that $n = 5000$, $\alpha = 0.05$, and $p = 0.01$, then $k_1 = 36$ and $k_2 = 64$. In practice, however, p is unknown and we are replacing it by its point estimation k/n. If, for example, $n = 5000$ and $k = 45$, then we find a confidence interval at risk level $\alpha = 0.05$, $k_1 = 31$, and $k_2 = 58$, where $a_1 = 0.0062$ and $a_2 = 0.0116$, which gives us interval $I_\alpha = [0.0028, 0.0206]$.

The Monte Carlo Simulation Method

These different examples correspond to situations in which the probability p of an event's occurring is estimated through observations. Such situations are obviously of interest, for they enable us to determine, in addition to the point estimation of p, a confidence interval and information concerning the distribution of the estimator P(.) of p as well. Having information on both the point estimation and the distribution is particularly useful in the context of Monte Carlo simulations.

Indeed, if p is a parameter that must figure in a model (as is the case for the reinsurance model described in chapter 7, this volume), it is in our every interest to perform not a single calculation using the point estimation of parameter p, but diverse calculations where, for each new calculation, the value of p is drawn at random according to the distribution of the estimator P(.) of p. In this case, we do not obtain an outcome for the model (to which a confidence interval can generally not be associated), but an empirical distribution of the results, which is much closer to reality. This is the interest of the Monte Carlo model. Today, with high-performance computers, the Monte Carlo model has become easily operational, even in the field.

Nevertheless, in one situation this method fails: when the point estimation of p is zero. If p were truly nil, this would not pose a problem because the event considered would never arise. But this situation can easily arise when the real (unknown) value of p is very close to zero, without actually being zero. Although rare, this event is not impossible so that estimating its probability as zero would be a mistake.

The problem is not too serious if we are working with simulations and have a confidence interval. But if the point estimation is nil, a confidence interval cannot be determined or, more exactly, this confidence interval is reduced to a zero value, which is incompatible with a situation in which p differs from zero.

This problem can be approached in several ways, particularly in the realm of linguistics dealing with the frequency of verbal phrases. This type of situation falls into the category of "zero-frequency problems" where the "Leaving-One-Out" method is applied. This method is based upon the works of Good (Ney, Essen, and Kneser 1995; Good 1953; Katz 1992), which will not be examined here.

The general design of a methodology to build a confidence interval in the above situation, for which a confidence interval is not easy to establish, is given in box 8.1.

ESTIMATES BASED ON CONSENSUAL EXPERT OPINIONS: NGT OR DELPHI METHODS

Nonetheless, under some circumstances observations that can be modeled in the forms discussed so far cannot be obtained. In those cases, "expert opinion," based on experience or intuition, would be the only source of information (that is, the experts "estimate" or "think" that the probability of a given event's occurring is p). If there is only one opinion—or several identical opinions—we have only a single value for estimating the probability p. Later we shall see how

---

BOX 8.1   GETTING A CONFIDENCE INTERVAL WHEN K = 0

Since our context requires the use of simulations, we suggest a simple solution to construct a confidence interval in which the diverse values to be applied in the simulations can be extracted. For this, we return to our first illustration, the urn full of balls.

Taking the random variable $X(.)$, which represents the number of white balls removed from an urn containing a proportion p of white balls after n withdrawals, we can determine the probability of event $X(.) == 0$, knowing that p is different from 0, where

$P[X(.) = 0 / p \neq 0]$. Thus: $P[X(.) = 0 / p \neq 0] = (1 - p)^n$.

This number is the probability of not observing any white balls in n nonexhaustive withdrawals from an urn containing white balls in a proportion p (not equal to zero). Regardless of the integer n (greater than 1), this number naturally decreases if p increases; just as for a given p, it decreases as n increases.

The points plotted on the graph represent the functions that associate p with $(1 - p)^n$ for values of n ranging from n = 1 to n = 100.

(Box continues on the following page.)

BOX 8.1 (continued)

Values of exp(n ln(1 − p)

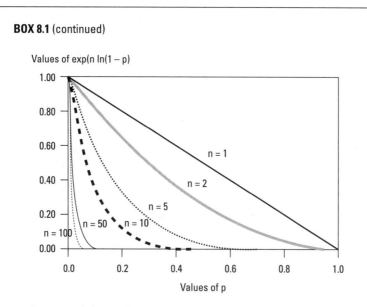

Since we did not obtain a single white ball in n independent withdrawals, we can now see whether the values of p other than zero are nonetheless plausible. For example, from the graph, we observe that for n = 5 and an urn containing 10 percent of white balls (p = 0.1), the probability of not finding any white balls is 0.60, which is obviously far from negligible. On the other hand if n = 10, this probability is only 0.37.

Under these conditions, we can construct an interval containing values of p, which, considering that no white balls were found, would be likely, and thus reject unlikely alternatives.

We construct a test as follows.

Let $\pi \in [0, 1]$. We will examine the following hypothesis H_0 where p designates the real unknown proportion of white balls:

$$H_0: p \geq \pi$$

which we will test against the alternative hypothesis:

$$H_1: p < \tilde{\pi}$$

We consider a risk a of type 1 error rate and calculate the probability of the event "X(.) = 0 knowing H_0". Thus:

$$P[X(.) = 0 \,/\, H_0] < (1 - \pi)^n$$

Consequently, if $(1-\pi)^n \leq \alpha$, we would reject hypothesis H_0 at a risk α of type 1 error rate.

The critical values of π in relation to α and n, that is, values $\pi(\alpha,n)$ which, for a given α and n, are such that we reject H_0 if $\pi > \pi(\alpha,n)$. We find $\pi(\alpha, n) = 1 - \sqrt[n]{\alpha}$ are provided in annex 8A, for $\alpha = 0.05$ and $\alpha = 0.01$.

(Box continues on the following page.)

BOX 8.1 (continued)

We now consider that, under the observed conditions, an interval in which the values of p could reasonably be extracted during the simulation is, for a given risk α interval $[0, \pi(\alpha, n)] = [0, 1 - \sqrt[n]{\alpha}]$.

For example, if $n = 100$ and $\alpha = 0.05$, all values of p greater than 0.0295 will be considered unlikely from the observations made. We shall therefore consider the "5 percent confidence interval" as $[0, 0.0295]$.

WHAT DISTRIBUTION ON THE CONFIDENCE INTERVAL?

We still need to determine the distribution on this interval from which the values of p must be extracted for a Monte Carlo simulation.

Different ways can be considered. A first approach consists of thoroughly exploiting the logic that led to the construction of interval $[0, \pi(\alpha, n)]$, and extracting values for p from a distribution where the density $f_1(.)$ is defined on $[0, \pi(\alpha, n)]$ by $f_1(x) = K(1 - x)$ n, K being a coefficient for which the value is:

$$K = \frac{n + 1}{1 - (1 - \pi(\alpha, n))^{n+1}}$$

A second approach consists of extracting values for p on $[0, (\alpha, n)]$ according to a density distribution $f_2(.)$ defined by $f_2(x) = \frac{2}{\pi(\alpha, n)} \left(1 - \frac{x}{\pi(\alpha, n)}\right)$. In this approach, the probability that P(.) will have a value p decreases as p increases. In a certain manner, this approach considers that the probability of a value p decreases as it moves away from 0, without taking the number of withdrawals n into consideration.

A third approach consists of making tosses in a uniform distribution on $[0, \pi(\alpha, n)]$.

The last two approaches would probably tend to inflate probabilities for the largest values of p, thus artificially enlarging the confidence interval. These two approaches would be worth considering in a context where the objective of the simulation is to estimate outcomes in the most unfavorable situation possible (for example, the case of an insurer trying to estimate the worst-case number of cost-generating events it might have to compensate (that is, a probability that is most certainly exaggerated).

to exploit a single value. However, if there are several conflicting opinions, we must try to draw up a synthesis (preferably a single one) of the information extracted from these opinions.

There are several well-known techniques to do so. Box 8.2 describes the most widely used methods: nominal group techniques (NGT) or Delphi.

BOX 8.2   NGT OR DELPHI METHODS

One way to synthesize expert opinions before gathering complementary information is by applying a group technique such as NGT or the Delphi method. Here, we simply mention these processes. For more information on this subject, see Delbecq, van de Ven, and Gustafson (1986).

The NGT method enables us to obtain a consensus by assembling the experts for a meeting at the same time and in the same place. At the outset, each expert states his or her opinion in writing. The opinions are then compiled, commented upon, and discussed. At the end of the debate, a synthesis is elaborated, either by a vote or a preference-aggregation process. The major drawback to the NGT procedure is that, like a classical play, it demands unified action, time, and place. This convention is not always compatible with the schedules of contemporary experts.

The Delphi method is somewhat easier, in that it requires unity of action. Its operation allows simultaneous collection, validation, discussion, and synthesis of experts' opinions. Theoretically, it forestalls domination by a few public opinion leaders, preserves each participant's anonymity, and allows measurement of dissenting or hostile voices. However, it takes a good bit of time (at least 45 days) and requires strong and continuous motivation of participants, who have to be available and skillful in answering questionnaires.

In the end, regardless of the method used, the result is the same: a single, synthesized version of the experts' opinions is elaborated as an estimate of probability.

ESTIMATES BASED ON NONCONSENSUAL EXPERT OPINIONS: "MAXIMUM LIKELIHOOD" AND BAYESIAN METHODS

Consensus methods are not always desirable or easy to implement, and a single opinion is sometimes preferred. Other methods may be preferable. For example, the information provided by the experts could be exploited directly by a random drawing of the expert opinion that will be retained. Yet, we still need to establish the probability distribution. In the absence of any specific information, uniform distribution could be assumed.

But perhaps one expert's opinion is more credible than those of the others. To make that decision, we need some minimal amount of information about the occurrence of the event for which we are studying the probability of p.

These two approaches are summarized in box 8.3.

Regardless of which of these methods is applied (or any other process, for that matter), the value retained for p is, at least initially, only approximate. It would therefore be wise to consider in the simulation not only the value proposed for p but also a margin of error.

BOX 8.3   NONCONSENSUAL METHODS

Maximum Likelihood Estimator

If we know, through a first experiment with a number of cases n (where n is not too big), that the event occurs k times, we could apply the ratio (k/n) as the base value for p. We could then assign weights to the experts reflecting the proximity of their opinions to k/n, the observed ratio [a method known as the maximum likelihood estimator (MLE)]. We could do this in several ways. The closer an expert's opinion to the observed (k/n), the higher would be the value of the weight assigned to that opinion. If an expert's opinion exactly matches the observation, that would be the only opinion retained. However, since that result could be partially coincidental, it may be desirable to draw upon the other experts' opinions as well.

In this case, we could rank the expert opinions, giving first place to the one closest to the observation, second place to the next closest, and so on. In this way, the opinions are assigned weighted values reflecting this ranking.

Bayesian Method

The Bayesian method determines the "most credible expert," knowing that in the experiments observed, event n occurred k times. If we assign each expert a number from 1 to N_e, and designate k_i as the number of times that expert i, i ∈ {1, ..., N_e} predicts the occurrence of the event if the experiment is carried out n times, and if we consider the following random variables:

X(.): number of times event p was observed in n independent experiments
E(.): number of the expert who is "right" (that is, the predicted value k_i is the value k effectively observed)

then we can calculate the probability that the expert who is right is expert i, knowing that we observed result k. This probability, designated as P[E(.) = i / k], is as follows:

$$P[E(.) = i / k] = \frac{P[k/E(.) = i] \ P[E(.) = i]}{P[k]},$$

an expression in which $P[k] = \sum_{k=0}^{n} P[k/E(.) = 1]$.

We would trust the expert who is "the most probable, in light of the outcomes observed." The following example illustrates this method.

Suppose we have three experts (Ne = 3) and their opinions concerning the probability of the event are:

Expert 1: $p_1 = 0.3$
Expert 2: $p_2 = 0.5$
Expert 3: $p_3 = 0.6$.

(Box continues on the following page.)

BOX 8.3 (continued)

We then perform 100 experiments, and the event is produced 40 times (k = 40). We have

P[E(.) = 1/k = 40] = 0.4386
P[E(.) = 2/k = 40] = 0.5602
P[E(.) = 3/k = 40] = 0.0013

In this case, Expert No. 2 is slightly more credible than Expert 1 (note that the result obtained with the MLE method would be different).

In most real-life situations, even if one expert's opinion on the value of p seems more reliable, it would be unwise to completely disregard all other opinions. It would be particularly interesting to seek expert opinion for an interval I_α in which p has a "very high chance" of occurring. For example, "95 chances out of 100" (which would define an interval $I_{0.05}$), or "99 chances out of 100" (which would define an interval $I_{0.01}$). The reasonable approach to a simulation here would be to extract the values of p in this interval I_α, according to an agreed distribution. The mean $\overline{p}$ of this distribution could easily be determined by an MLE or the Bayesian process. But which distribution law should be used? Of course, the normal distribution law $N(\overline{p}, \sigma)$ could apply, where σ would be determined by the value α and the limits of interval I_α (based on the experts' opinions). However, this process, which is acceptable for values of p close to 0.5, becomes less acceptable as $\overline{p}$ moves closer to 0 or 1. In these cases, the real distribution is less and less likely to be symmetrical. Furthermore, there is a risk that the normal distribution could provide increasingly absurd values (less than 0 or greater than 1, depending on whether $\overline{p}$ is close to 0 or 1). It is therefore reasonable to search for another distribution law. In this case, a Beta distribution would be particularly suitable. Box 8.4 briefly describes the general design of such a distribution.

CONCLUSIONS

Applying risk-management techniques at the level of microinsurance units requires information that is often unavailable, at least initially. This information includes estimates of the probability that cost-generating events will occur, their mean cost, and the variance. When data are unavailable, other methods of estimation need to be used.

The microinsurers themselves may agree that they need to improve data recording, but until they do, in the short term, data gaps will have to be bridged by opinions of people the community considers best informed, and who can

BOX 8.4   BETA DISTRIBUTION

Here we are interested only in the Type I Beta distribution, but to simplify matters, we will just call it a Beta distribution.[3] A Beta distribution is one where the density is a function $\beta(.)$ defined by:

$$\forall\, x \in [0, 1]\ \beta(x) = \frac{x^{n-1}(1-x)^{p-1}}{B(n,\,q)}$$

$$\forall\, x \notin [0, 1]\ \beta(x) = 0$$

where n and q are two strictly positive real numbers, and where B(n, q) is defined by:

$$B(n,\,q) = \frac{\Gamma(n+q)}{\Gamma(n)\,\Gamma(q)}\,,$$

function $\Gamma(.)$ being defined, for all $x > 0$ by:

$$\Gamma(x) = \int_0^\infty t^{x-1}\, e^{-t}\, dt.$$

Numbers n and q are the parameters of the Beta distribution.

We show that, for a Beta distribution containing parameters n and q, the mean is $m = \dfrac{n}{n+q}$ and the variance is $\sigma^2 = \dfrac{nq}{(n+q+1)(n+q)^2}\,.$

If the mean m is known (according to an expert opinion), then we can express mean m and variance σ^2 in relation to the two parameters m (known) and n (to be determined), q being deduced from m and n by the ratio:

$$q = \frac{(m-1)}{m}\, n.$$

In addition, if we consider that there is only one probability $\alpha/2$ that the real value of p will be less than the value s (provided by the experts), then we can determine a value $n(\alpha, s)$ in such a way that the probability of the Beta distribution of parameters $(n(\alpha, s), q)$ being less than s with a mean m is $\alpha/2$.

Thus, the values of p will be extracted from distribution $B(n(\alpha, s))$, $(n(\alpha, s))$.

Example: suppose we estimate that the distribution of p must be a Beta distribution, with a mean of 0.78 (expert opinion) and that only 2.5 percent of the values of p are less than 0.15 (expert opinion).

Then m = 0.78.

We then apply an inverse Beta function to search for the corresponding value of $(n(\alpha, s)$; where $\alpha/2 = 0.025$, for a mean Beta distribution of 0.78 and a value s = 0.15. We find $n(\alpha, s) = 1.393$. Consequently q = 0.3928. For this Beta distribution (1.393; 0.3928), the mean is in fact 0.78, and the withdrawals will be carried out in this distribution.

influence communal consensus on the cost/benefit and the quality of health care benefits.

The role of local residents and local consensus should not be minimized in the search for objective markers. Consumers may provide important leads on what they consider acceptable and practical. Hence, expert opinion is an acceptable basis for risk estimates when local data are unavailable.

The methods discussed here can be operated in the context of the tools developed for the operation of reinsurance for microinsurance units such as simulations run with the *Social Re Toolkit*. These methods provide a practical guideline for planners and for those who implement the insurance plan, but need not be operated at the microinsurers' level.

ANNEX 8A

TABLE 8A.1   Table of Critical Values $\pi(\alpha, n)$

Extremity $\pi(\alpha, n)$ of the confidence interval $[0, \pi(\alpha, n)]$, at a 5 percent threshold, for a given a and n.

n	$\alpha = 0.05$	$\alpha = 0.01$
1	0.9500	0.9900
2	0.7764	0.9000
3	0.6316	0.7846
4	0.5271	0.6838
5	0.4507	0.6019
6	0.3930	0.5358
7	0.3482	0.4821
8	0.3123	0.4377
9	0.2831	0.4005
10	0.2589	0.3690
11	0.2384	0.3421
12	0.2209	0.3187
13	0.2058	0.2983
14	0.1926	0.2803
15	0.1810	0.2644
16	0.1707	0.2501
17	0.1616	0.2373
18	0.1533	0.2257
19	0.1459	0.2152
20	0.1391	0.2057
21	0.1329	0.1969
22	0.1273	0.1889
23	0.1221	0.1815
24	0.1173	0.1746
25	0.1129	0.1682
26	0.1088	0.1623

(Table continues on the following page.)

TABLE 8A.1 (continued)

n	$\alpha = 0.05$	$\alpha = 0.01$
27	0.1050	0.1568
28	0.1015	0.1517
29	0.0981	0.1468
30	0.0950	0.1423
50	0.0582	0.0880
100	0.0295	0.0450
200	0.0149	0.0228
300	0.0099	0.0152
400	0.0075	0.0114
500	0.0060	0.0092
1,000	0.0030	0.0046

NOTES

1. These include multidisciplinary problems governed by multiple criteria whose solutions are largely unknown and deserve further research (Vissade and others 2001).

2. This gap could be closed by an increase of international development aid, but it is unlikely to be closed by poor people themselves given their limited ability to pay.

3. Various developments concerning this distribution can be found in Ledermann (1985) and Saporta (1990).

REFERENCES

Berman, P. 2000. "Organization of Ambulatory Care Provision: A Critical Determinant of Health Performance in Developing Countries." *Bulletin of the WHO* 78(6):791–800.

Berwick, D., and T.W. Nolan. 1998. "Physicians as Leaders in Improving Health Care." *Annals of Internal Medicine* 28128–36.

Delbecq, A., A. van de Ven, and D. Gustafson 1986. *Group Techniques for Program Planning: A Guide to Nominal Group and Delphi Processes.* Middleton, Wis.: Green Briar Press.

Fonteneau, R., and A. Beresniak. 2002. *Les limites de la planification sanitaire en Afrique.* Hermès Scientific Publications—Santé et systématique. Paris: Hermès.

Good, I.J. 1953. "The Population Frequencies of Species and the Estimation of Population Parameters." *Biometrika* 40(December):237–64.

Jack, W. 2000. *Principles of Health Economics for Developing Countries.* WBI Development Studies. Washington, D.C.: World Bank.

Katz, S.M. 1992. "Estimation of Probabilities from Sparse Data for the Language Model Component of a Speech Recogniser." *IEE Transactions, Acoustics, Speech and Signal Processing* 35(3):400–401.

Ledermann, W., ed. 1985. "Statistics." *Handbooks of Applicable Mathematics*. Vol. 6 A and B. New York: Wiley.

Monekosso, G.L. n.d. *Health Minimum Package for All at the District Level*. Maseru, Lesotho: Bähr Mapping and Printing.

Ney, H., U. Essen, and R. Kneser. 1995. "On the Estimation of 'Small' Probabilities by Leaving-One-Out." *IEE Transactions on Pattern Analysis and Machine Intelligence* 17(12):1202–12.

Saporta, G. 1990. *Probabilités, analyse des données et statistiques*. Paris: Editions Technip.

Taha, A. 1997. "How to Make the Most of Village Health Promoters." *World Health Forum* 18(3/4):278–81.

UNDP (United Nations Devlopment Programme). 1998. *Cambodia Human Development Report*. New York: UNDP.

UNICEF (United Nations Children's Fund). 1998. *Implementing the 20/20 Initiative: Achieving Universal Effect to Basic Social Services*. New York: UNICEF, Division of Communication, with UNDP, UNESCO, UNFPA, UNICEF, WHO. September.

Vissade, L., and others. 2001. "Impact socio-économique de l'épidémie du SIDA en Afrique sub-saharienne sur les femmes et les enfants." *Journal d'économie médicale* 3:215–29.

WHO (World Health Organization). 1988."The Challenge of Implementation: District Health Systems for Primary Health Care." *Bulletin of the WHO* 78(6):791–800.

_____. 2000. "Health Services: Well Chosen, Well Organized." Chapter 3 in *The World Health Report 2000: Health Systems: Improving Performance*. Geneva: WHO.

CHAPTER 9

Insurance and Market Failure at the Microinsurance Level

Axel Weber

C ommunity-based health insurance schemes in developing countries and insurance schemes in wealthy countries operate under different conditions, but basic principles of insurance apply in both situations. In developing countries, conditions for a complicated system such as insurance require specific solutions. Any reinsurance activity will require intimate knowledge of these special environmental constraints.

In this chapter, we examine the challenges that typically confront community-based health insurance schemes, the microinsurers. Drawing on experience of how microinsurers have dealt with such challenges, we attempt to provide a "treasury" of best practices (annex 9A). The solutions described were gathered from various microinsurers around the world, but especially from Sub-Saharan Africa and South Asia.

TYPICAL CHALLENGES OF MICROINSURERS

Microinsurers must deal with multiple failures at every point in the health care system, starting with the market itself, the insurance and reinsurance systems, as well as systemic corruption and fraud.

Health Market Failure

The health market in which microinsurers operate is hampered by supply shortages, low client income, and lack of information about care possibilities and prices. In addition, the market is frequently split into a deteriorating public health system and an expensive private system.

Lack of supply. Microinsurers' first and most basic challenge is the lack of health care supply, the foundation of any insurance activity. Most target groups' health care

For their helpful comments on a draft of this chapter, the author thanks Volker Leienbach, Director, GVG (Gesellschaft für Versicherungswissenschaft und gestaltung), Cologne, Germany; and Jürgen Hohmann, Head of Health Insurance Sector Project, GTZ, Bonn, Germany.

environment is poor. In most developing countries, the majority of people live in the countryside, where there are no health care providers at all, or they are too far away or provide only rudimentary care. Some rural residents may have access to health posts or satellite clinics, but the closest hospital for complicated treatment is usually located in large and faraway cities. Often the hospital, too, provides only basic services. Qualified staff, drugs, materials, and equipment are often lacking.

Health insurance, unlike pension schemes, has a triangular structure. Besides clients and an insurance structure, health insurance needs health care providers. Without health care providers, health insurance makes no sense. However, health insurance can help develop the supply infrastructure.

In urban environments, the supply of health care providers is often better than in rural environments. Insurance that covers both urban and rural target groups under the same plan can pose problems of equity. In this case, depending on where they live, some people can easily obtain health care, while others have to travel long distances. This situation is difficult to handle for the insurer because it is hard to differentiate contributions to reflect relative access to care.

Health care providers are frequently public employees, which poses a special problem for health insurance schemes. In many developing countries, there is no official copayment for public providers, but they ask for under-the-table payments. In these cases, it is difficult for the insurer to cover costs. Demand for health care leads to direct spending by private households. Health insurance, however, should not encourage under-the-table payments. But even if insurers did try to cover these provider payments, on what could insurers base them? Without any official fee schedule, it would be difficult for the insurers to manage risk.

Lack of purchasing power. The main problem limiting the supply of good-quality health care is the lack of purchasing power. Most people in the target areas are very poor. The better-off drive to the nearest city for care at better-equipped private hospitals instead of using local providers. Thus, local providers are left with clients with weak resources, which leads to low standards of care. Public providers were established in many developing countries to provide health care in disadvantaged localities with low purchasing power. But because of deteriorating public budgets in most developing countries, the quality of public institutions is declining. Rural communities are therefore caught in a vicious circle: Lack of infrastructure discourages insurance activities, but infrastructure does not develop for lack of purchasing power. Lack of access to health care deepens poverty. In Cambodia, for example, more than half of the poorest people are poor because of an illness or health-impairing accident. Only improved health care financing methods can break this vicious circle.

Lack of information about care possibilities. Lack of resources not only inhibits demand but also people's knowledge about the possibilities for professional health care. When sick, they look to traditional healers and traditional recipes, not modern, professional health care institutions. People seek modern health care only as a last resort. By then, the disease is severe, and treatment costs are high.

Lack of information about prices. Many people are afraid to seek health care at modern institutions for lack of information about prices. Often, there is no general policy on tariffs and fees, either from the provider or from the government and, even if there is, patients nearly always have to make under-the-table payments. Prices are not transparent but arbitrary. The gap in education and the lack of fee schedules or price lists discourage people from seeking professional help for fear of the unforeseeable financial consequences.

Split-care markets. Frequently, the health care market is split between a public network and a private market. The public network is often deteriorating, because of lack of funds and poorly paid and motivated practitioners who lack materials and drugs for treatment.

The private market includes doctors who are employed and paid by public institutions, but who run a private practice on the side, earning additional income. These doctors refer patients to their private consultations in the afternoon. This practice is not surprising, as the salaries of many doctors in public facilities are low, sometimes below the subsistence level for a family. However, insurers cannot encourage this practice by funding these doctors' private activities.

Insurance Market Failure

The development of insurance in many developing countries is inhibited by distrust and scanty knowledge of insurance practices, as well as lack of know-how, high transaction costs, lack of cash and financial intermediaries, high dropout rates, lack of competition, and unsustainability.

Distrust of insurance. People in many countries have had bad experiences with financial institutions or health insurers. The microinsurers' target groups are poor and afraid to turn over their resources to an institution they do not know. For this reason, microinsurance schemes have to overcome strong suspicions and reluctance. Events such as the crash of the Cooperative Bank in Uganda in 1999, resulting from fraud, reinforce peoples' fears.

Lack of information about insurance protection. Many people simply do not understand the concept of insurance. It takes time to explain insurance and risk sharing. The idea of handing over money that will be used to pay for other peoples' health care is hard to explain—and to absorb. Their main fears are about paying money "for nothing" (i.e., when they are not ill) and paying for others, especially the very poor who are sick more frequently than the better-off. Support is therefore weak at the outset among microinsurers' target populations.

Lack of know-how. It takes initiative, know-how, and qualified staff to set up and run an insurance scheme; these are often unavailable. The target group does not normally take the initiative or provide administrators. Know-how usually comes from external promoters, which raises a problem of sustainability. Expertise is expensive. Qualified insurance managers, and even clerks, expect salaries much higher than the target groups' household income. Insurers often lack the financial wherewithal to afford professional staff. The typical microinsurer, with between 1,000 and 5,000 members, would spend more than 50 percent of its contribution income to maintain professional administration. The microinsurer thus often remains dependent on external aid to cover know-how and administrative expenses. This is especially true for schemes that insure against the costs of small and frequent risks.

High transaction costs. Given the lack of infrastructure, communication and transport networks are minimal in most target areas. There are no banks, no post offices or mail services, no roads, and no telecommunication equipment. As a result, transaction costs are high, for example, to collect contributions, file and process claims, register and renew membership, keep members informed, and recruit new members.

Lack of money. The target groups in many countries lack cash—they either have none at all or do not regularly have cash. They do their usual transaction in kind. Although some schemes accept contributions in kind, most insurers need cash to function.

Lack of financial intermediaries. For lack of financial infrastructure, cash must be used for most financial transactions. Without banks to accept deposits, insurers keep their financial reserves in cash to pay the costs of health care. Doing business only in cash raises transaction costs (for example, interest forgone) and invites theft and fraud.

High dropout rates. Membership in most microinsurance schemes is unstable, with high dropout rates. Many microinsurers have to replace half their membership every year. Awareness campaigns recruit new members, but many existing members do not renew. Such members usually reason that since they did not fall ill, they do not need insurance. High dropout rates have several adverse effects. They increase administrative costs because the microinsurer has to make extraordinary efforts to acquire enough new members to maintain a viable membership threshold. Only the unhealthy stick with the plan (adverse risk selection).

Lack of competition. Many microinsurers are local monopolies, with no competition from other schemes in the area, and no pressure to strive for excellence. This is the only explanation for the survival of schemes whose administrative costs eat up 70 percent of their budget.

Lack of sustainability. Balancing income and expenditure is a problem for most schemes from the outset. The reasons for this problem include lack of data that would allow the calculation of "sufficient" contribution; administrative costs that exceed financial capacity; and cutting benefits or raising contributions for fear of losing members. Funding by donors enables these schemes to survive, but at the cost of heavy dependence on the donors.

Many schemes do not even know what their real costs are. Some schemes, particularly those run by hospitals, commingle their finances with health care providers' funds. Others do not count costs borne by donors. Such overlooked costs include staff salaries paid by donors; the cost of staff employed by a hospital that works for the insurer; overhead for project or hospital rooms and infrastructure; and public providers' services given to insurance members without adequate remuneration. The income from contributions is used to raise hospital staff salaries. The public budget bears the cost of care. Many schemes also try to provide more services than their members' financial capacity can support.

Administrative costs present a special problem. The schemes' small size and their members' financial limitations do not allow hiring qualified staff and purchasing necessary equipment. Under these circumstances, it is difficult to make the schemes sustainable. This problem decreases as membership grows and the frequency and size of insured risk decreases.

Adverse Selection

A special problem many schemes have to deal with is adverse risk selection. Members try to join the scheme when they see an advantage in it—when they are sick or pregnant. They often drop out when they recover or when they see that they have paid contributions without getting any benefit from the scheme. Adverse selection can put a scheme out of business if it does not take protective measures.

Moral Hazard

Moral hazard can come from the insured as well as from providers.

From insureds. Early in their membership, many members "try out" benefits to see if the insurance scheme works. For this reason, a cost bulge typically occurs with new members. Apart from this, the amount of moral hazard from members depends on the benefit package. The risk of moral hazard is high if low-cost benefits such as consultations and drugs are paid and no copayment is required. On the other hand, if more expensive benefits such as surgery and hospital treatment are covered, the exposure to moral hazard is lower. No one would want to undergo abdominal surgery, for example, just to collect insurance benefits.

From providers. Some providers deliver unnecessary services. The risk largely depends on the type of payment they receive. Fee-for-service payments invite moral hazard problems, whereas capitation payments give no incentive to overtreat patients.

Reinsurance Failure

Reinsurance makes sense only if the basic insurance premium is calculated to cover average costs. Reinsurance can deal with risks, but it cannot solve a chronic deficit on client insurance. To reinsure microinsurance schemes, a group of microinsurers must be gathered to enable risk sharing. Finally, reinsurance needs a sound basis for risk calculation. Many microinsurers have anecdotal evidence about most of the data needed, but no reliable statistics or accounting.

Corruption and Fraud

Corruption, so common in developing countries, may seriously hamper an insurance scheme's chances of success. Fraud may originate with the insured, who claim fictitious health care costs or with administrators, who divert monies collected by the insurer.

Failure of Risk Coverage

Sound risk analysis is the basis of useful insurance so that plans can provide only the services clients need. The main benefit of health insurance, especially for the poor, would be coverage of *catastrophe risks* (illnesses or accidents with devastatingly expensive treatment in terms of the average household budget). However, experience shows that people who agree to pay contributions expect to obtain more than coverage for rare catastrophe risks. Insurance against catastrophes alone is harder to sell than comprehensive coverage.

Objective and subjective needs have to be separated. *Objective needs* can be *medical* (prevention, diagnostics, injuries, and available treatments) and they can be *financial* (coverage against the risk of treatment costs too large for an individual). *Subjective needs* are based on individual preferences, not objective criteria.

Theoretically, any medical condition requiring diagnosis and treatment can be covered by health insurance. However, because of financial and other restrictions, microinsurer benefit packages are very limited. From the medical point of view, first priority should be given to preventive, life-saving, and disability diagnostics and treatments, especially those proven most cost-effective. That is why most microinsurance schemes concentrate on such services.

However, financial needs (risks) may differ from medical needs significantly. Some costs of health services may be affordable for most households. Examples of these services include outpatient consultations, most ordinary drugs, and the like. Although these services may be important from a medical point of view, their coverage may be a low priority from an individual's financial point of view. Individuals or families may assign highest priority to coverage for services that could bankrupt them. These services involve mainly catastrophe risks, for example, hospitalization for surgery, a complicated delivery, treatment of serious malaria, or a ruinous accident. Contrary to the common wisdom, preventive measures save health insurance costs only for a few conditions, such as contagious diseases.

From the insurer's point of view, risk is defined by the expected value of the costs (the costs of benefits covered times the respective probability) and by the variance of the expected costs, especially its relation to total turnover. The probability of an insurance case (or an accumulation of cases in an epidemic) can be low, but the costs can be high and the occurrence sporadic. Thus, in technical terms, not only are the probability and the amount of the possible damage important, but also the standard deviation of the expected value of the damage, the maximum loss, and its size relative to the insurer's turnover. This is one reason insurance companies maintain reserves or reinsure their portfolio.

The individual household views risk slightly differently. The first consideration is similar to the insurer's, the cost of illness. However, household income as well as health care costs have to be considered. Unlike insurers, individual private households cannot link revenue to the number of members. The health risk increases with the number of family members—but not necessarily with a corresponding increase of revenue. However, the variance will be much larger because the sample is smaller, a common effect without risk sharing. This effect is also heavier and less unpredictable, the higher the individual damage from each occurrence and the lower the probability. This means more frequent but less costly events are much easier for households to handle than less frequent but more costly events, even if the expected value of both is equal. Potential costs cannot simply be multiplied by the probability. The variation also means that the financial impact on the household's budget has to be taken into account. Mathematically, the expected value may be the same. But the maximum value of an event's damage must be compared with an indicator expressing its impact on the household's economic situation—which may be the income of the household or, in some environments, the family or the village. For example, the probability of needing bypass surgery in the next year may be 0.001. If the operation costs 1,000,000 pesos, the expected value is 1,000 pesos, which is not very high. However, if the risk occurs, an average family cannot pay, or pays but goes into bankruptcy.

Other risk aspects aggravate the situation of most individual households. If a household has to pay for a bypass on credit, interest charges have to be added to the costs. For example, if the interest rate is 15 percent a year, the household's expected average costs will double. This is one of the reasons people lose their property bit by bit in many poor countries.

A household has little choice about health care. If an accident damages a bicycle, motorcycle, or car, repairs can be postponed, at least temporarily. But if a family member falls seriously ill, treatment is the only acceptable option. Not treating the sick or injured person at all is not a true option or choice but the result of a desperate economic situation. When the family's breadwinner falls ill or has an accident, its income is cut off. This is a different kind of risk, not similar to that of health insurance.

Finally, apart from the effect of risk sharing, which is the main difference between individual households and insurers, the risk itself is intrinsically different. The benefits of insurance really come into play in the event of catastrophes. Not many microinsurance schemes take this into account, but one exception is the Groupe de recherche et d'échanges (GRET) scheme in Cambodia. (See box 4.5 in Balkenhol and Churchill, chapter 4 of this volume.)

Insurance can demonstrate all its benefits, especially in events that put an insurmountable burden on individuals. First-line, cheap health care services are not a classical insurance benefit, however, despite their importance from medical and social points of view.

Nevertheless, good health insurance may mitigate risk by improving primary care services and controlling its costs. For people who cannot afford cheap basic health care services, some kind of coverage may be necessary. Even if insurance does not pay for it, everyone would benefit from improvements in primary care. The insurers would also benefit because broad primary care would help reduce costs in other fields that are covered.

Many microinsurance schemes pay for health care services (even if they are cheap) until they run out of money. If the budget is exhausted or very small, expensive treatments, not the cheap ones, are cut out first.

SOLUTIONS TO TYPICAL CHALLENGES OF MICROINSURERS

The following sections provide some common solutions to the most typical forms of problems related to insurance and microinsurance.

Health Market Failure

Insurmountable though these problems may seem, some microinsurers are solving them. In doing so, they have learned lessons that may help others, new to the community health insurance business (annex 9A and box 9.1).

Lack of supply and lack of purchasing power. Insurers should start in areas that have a supply of health care. Insurance cannot be created without a health care market, but it can help build that market. Insurance concentrates and increases purchasing power. Thus, with the establishment of health insurance, the market may develop, expanding both the supply of care and equality of access. An efficient insurance mechanism has an impact not only on the number of providers but also on the price, quality, and availability of care. The effect of insurance thus extends beyond risk sharing. These side effects help even the uninsured population.

BOX 9.1   HOW DO MICROINSURERS DEAL WITH CLASSICAL INSURANCE PROBLEMS?

Like private and social health insurance, microinsurers are vulnerable to some market failures from moral hazard, free riding, adverse selection, information asymmetry, cost escalation, risk pooling, and catastrophes.

Moral hazard. Moral hazard denotes price sensitivity of elastic demand and price indifference of inelastic demand. Moral hazard originates mainly from three phenomena: demand-induced overutilization, supply-induced overutilization, and system-induced mechanisms linked to insurer behavior (including premium calculations) that encourages the first two causes. Here, two features must be kept in mind: the risk covered and the information available to the insurer about the insured. If health insurers could respond only to risk aversion, they could be expected to limit the benefit package to a few random, inelastic, high-impact, low-frequency risks. However, health insurance schemes operate under imperfect conditions, and insurers do not limit their activity only to random catastrophic risks. Microinsurers, for the time being, are exposed neither to a competitive market nor to regulations constraining the definition of insurable risks. Benefits are determined in light of the community's ability to pay. Furthermore, sometimes overutilization is preempted by qualifying conditions (such as a benefit cap), set to emphasize multilateral over unilateral utility. Bearing in mind that small communities can establish a consensus on what constitutes inelastic utilization, and that utilization information circulates within the community, microinsurers seem to be less exposed than large insurers to demand-induced moral hazard, at least for high-cost events. Nor are these schemes exposed to system-induced moral hazard as long as they do not operate complex provider payment systems. As for supply-induced moral hazard, since supply is often the limiting factor in the operation of microinsurers, lack of competition may encourage supplier-induced moral hazard. Any shielding may be temporary in nature, and this risk may increase as curative care grows.

Free riding. A free rider obtains a benefit but does not contribute to the cost. The free-riding issue is inherently linked to imperfect information on user behavior. Private health insurers have tried to forestall this situation by excluding some risks from the benefit package. This exclusion may provide safety against free riding, but it has been viewed as one of private insurance's main market failures, one that gave rise to government provision of social insurance (Stiglitz 1988, p. 344). Nonetheless, free riding can exist as long as free riders can hide their advantage, particularly from the insurer. Considering the quick spread of information within small communities and the ease with which microinsurers can adjust decisions to take account of such information, the options for free riding are considerably reduced in this context. Free riding has occurred, however, where members' identity was poorly controlled.

(Box continues on the following page.)

BOX 9.1 (continued)

Adverse selection. When people with a high probability of health-loss predominate in the membership and the healthy do not join, adverse selection occurs. Some types of occupations entail higher exposure to risk than do others, and some persons' living conditions expose them to specific types of risks. In large and heterogeneous groups, the cheapest way to minimize insurer exposure to adverse selection is to randomize the health risk by insuring groups selected for characteristics other than health status. Other solutions employed by commercial insurers include individual risk rating or personalizing deductibles according to "experience rating." Microinsurers cannot tap into large population groups, nor can they apply risk rating, which would be too expensive and contrary to the principles of community solidarity. Microinsurers may be exposed to some risk of adverse selection, mainly at start-up, particularly if the most vulnerable individuals within the community are also the most risk averse (which may be a weak assumption). Enlarging membership might provide some shielding from this problem, for example, by requiring whole families to join together or requiring at least 60 percent of a village to join (as is practiced in parts of Uganda).

Information asymmetry. Information asymmetry can occur on the demand and the supply side. *Demand-side* asymmetrical information occurs when the client cannot exercise informed choice on the optimal care needed. Provider choices are assumed to respond to practicing good medicine, retaining patient satisfaction, and perpetuating high income. All three elements are usually linked to increased use. Microinsurers are shielded only by limiting their benefit package. *Supply-side* asymmetrical information means that the provider has insufficient information on the outcome of treatment and engages in defensive or trial-and-error treatment, which increases the cost of care. It can also occur when a patient withholds vital information from the provider.

Microinsurers can reduce their exposure to information asymmetry mainly through control over the benefit package and through negotiations with providers.

Cost escalation. When either the demand side or the supply side seeks more (or more technologically sophisticated) treatment than required, cost escalation occurs. In some developing countries, insurance schemes add "loading costs" to the regular medical expenses in order to pass on to the customers extra costs for premium collection or high bank or credit costs. Such schemes may also factor in the difficulty of obtaining reinsurance, or its high cost. Microinsurance can reduce the risk of cost escalation by holding overhead costs of collection and administration to the bare minimum. Microinsurers can also reduce this risk by negotiating fees with providers and by structuring the benefit package around items that are less sensitive to individual choice (Vaté and Dror, chapter 6, this volume).

(Box continues on the following page.)

BOX 9.1 (continued)

Risk pooling. In risk pooling, the insurer gathers similar but unrelated risks, in effect spreading risk over a larger number of cases. Classical insurance sorts people across multiple heterogeneous communities representing a similar though un-related risk and not otherwise connected by intrinsic characteristics. Micro-insurance clusters persons who are bound together first and foremost by be-longing to the same homogeneous community, and also by sharing a willingness to bear together some health contingencies. In the absence of risk pooling, indi-vidual microinsurers may be exposed to more frequent high-severity claims.[1] Additionally, a microinsurance unit struck by a pandemic-like occurrence would experience a very serious financial risk except in the unlikely event it could pool risks with other communities. The more realistic option would be ceding risk through reinsurance.

Catastrophes. A single rare event (for example, an earthquake) or a few huge claims could wipe out a microinsurer's financial resources, leaving the insurer unable to meet its obligations to the other insured. Microinsurers are not neces-sarily any more exposed to catastrophes than other insurers, but initial evidence from Uganda suggests that they could be more exposed to high-severity claims.[2]

Source: Adapted from Dror and Jacquier 1999 and from Dror and Duru 2000.

Lack of information about care possibilities. Some schemes cooperate with commu-nity health workers or village chiefs, who receive training concerning health care possibilities. Other schemes, which do not rely on "multipliers," run information campaigns. However, insurers may have an interest in not initiating large de-mand—which could overwhelm the system.

Lack of information about prices. Some schemes try to allay patients' fear of being surprised by high prices by emphasizing negotiated fixed prices and posting them at the entrance to the facility. This practice has diverted demand from providers with opaque prices to providers with transparent prices, even if insurance does not cover them entirely. Consumer protection of this kind costs insurers nothing but it does help patients financially.

Split-care markets. One way of dealing with the split-care market is to sign con-tracts with providers, excluding this option. Doctors get contracts that allow them to earn their living in the hospital, but in exchange they must commit themselves to working exclusively in the hospital that employs them. A codex is agreed between health insurer and hospital, ensuring this exclusivity and stipulating sanctions for fraudulent behavior. This arrangement could help many public hospitals improve their services by attracting and keeping qualified staff if they also pay them competitive salaries. This will be possible only through (official) user charges and copayments.

Insurance Market Failure

One of the main reasons microinsurers collapse is for lack of sufficient clients. The main sources of market failure are distrust, lack of information, lack of know-how, high transaction costs, lack of cash, lack of financial intermediaries, high dropout rates, lack of competition, and lack of sustainability.

Distrust of insurance. Many microinsurers receive support from donors and use this support, together with the donor's name, as a selling point. The insurance idea can also be promoted by cooperating with local stakeholders such as village chiefs, public administrations, hospitals, and other local providers, or by teaming up with well-known health care providers or organizations such as cooperatives or microcredit institutions.

Lack of information about possibilities. The concept of microinsurance has to be explained. Many target groups have no idea what insurance is about and need some basic information to understand it. That is why well-run microinsurers invest in social marketing, for example by promoting tours tailored to local customs and the target groups' educational background, involving local multipliers, circulating folders using texts in local dialects or explanatory drawings instead of written texts, or cooperating with radio and television. Insurance could be a way to correct the negative impact of the introduction of user fees.

Lack of know-how. Most microinsurers get technical advice from international organizations and donors, both on start-up and later on operations. In a few instances, scheme initiators or administrative staff come from the target groups, but these are exceptions. First, people have to learn to think and behave like entrepreneurs, using entrepreneurial techniques and logic.

High transaction costs. Cooperating with local stakeholders (for example, village chiefs or heads of associations and cooperatives) in the areas of information, contribution collection, registration, and claims processing can cut high transaction costs. Costs can be cut by reducing the number of contacts, for example, by collecting contributions only once or twice a year on set dates or cooperating with banks, if there are any. Providers could be made responsible for collecting contributions, or insurers could establish local offices in the main hospitals, which are already staffed with clerks. Coverage could be limited to high-cost risks such as complicated deliveries or surgeries instead of including small risks such as primary care services.

Lack of cash. To circumvent the problem of lack of cash, some insurers have experimented with contributions in kind instead of cash payments. This is a possibility if the goods traded are homogeneous, easy to store and transport, and if the insurer can easily sell the goods. Another possibility is cooperating with other risk-related projects (such as rice banks).

Lack of financial intermediaries. Many microinsurers have bank accounts but, because their clients and providers do not, they continue to deal mainly in cash. Insurers can try to work closely with banks when setting up the schemes, for example, by negotiating good service conditions and investing in information. Nevertheless, most of their transactions will still be in cash.

High dropout rates. Few microinsurers have solved the high dropout rate problem. The best strategy is to involve local stakeholders, which reduces anonymity in the insurance transaction, thereby raising the social costs of canceling membership. For the same reasons, members should be involved in governance and control of the insurance scheme. As an incentive to renew, members could be offered a discount on contributions or premiums. Microinsurers should also invest in systems to store information, including records on dropouts (to be excluded from membership) and reinstatement during a specified penalty period.

Lack of competition. Competition between health insurers is a way of exercising social control over management. Where there is no such control via competition, other ways must be found to link demand and supply, for example, involving members in designing benefit packages and contributions and involving stakeholders in scheme administration.

Lack of sustainability. To overcome lack of sustainability, strategies should include reducing administrative costs. A good way to do this is by making the insurance and benefit package as simple as possible, working with volunteers instead of professional staff, and tapping all available community support. To improve the likelihood of prompt payment of contributions, for example, microinsurers should look to village chiefs, community members, and stakeholders for help in collecting contributions. Other means include containing claim costs through contracts with providers and analyzing members' needs and their ability to pay. Finally, microinsurers should consider reinsuring the scheme, especially if it covers high risks. There is a tradeoff between administrative costs and elements such as compliance and reduction of moral hazard. The less schemes invest in administration, the less capable they are of making the scheme sustainable. For this reason, most schemes depend heavily on knowhow and other support from donors. Broad strategy and practical guidelines in general would help microinsurers become sustainable.

Adverse Selection

To reduce adverse selection, many microinsurers have found practical solutions such as waiting periods; compulsory membership (for example, in the case of marriage or affiliation with a cooperative); and group coverage (for example, whole families or a minimum percentage of a community or a cooperative).

Moral Hazard

Proven tools for reducing moral hazard include setting claim limits for insureds and careful choice of provider-payment mechanisms.

From insureds. To reduce moral hazard from their members, many schemes set limits for claims. Such limits have proved especially useful in fields where members can easily influence demand, for example, primary consultations. Moral hazard from the insured is less problematic if the insurance covers mainly catastrophe risks (nobody elects surgery just to collect benefits, but many people consult a doctor if it is free). Microinsurers can also influence moral hazard from the insured by introducing copayments.

From providers. The main tools for reducing moral hazard from providers are through the choice of an appropriate provider-payment mechanism (for example, capitation instead of fee for service) and use of effective quality-control and patient-referral systems. Implementing these measures, however, requires know-how and compliance on the part of the providers.

Corruption and Fraud

One proven method for reducing the risk of corruption and fraud is community involvement and social control. In communities where people know each other, the risk of corruption is lower than in large, anonymous communities. The design of the benefit package and the administrative procedures can also help overcome this risk. To head off the risk of cheating on benefits, many community-based schemes have introduced membership cards with photos of the family covered.

Failure of Risk Coverage

Sound risk analysis is a cornerstone of insurance. This means providing only services that clients really need. To find out what those services are requires inquiries and sound studies on the risks involved in illness and accidents. Often, those are not the risks covered by existing schemes. For example, catastrophe risks are frequently not covered but they are one of the main causes of poverty. Faced with a catastrophic health event, families borrow money or sell land and cattle to pay for treatment, but these goods are the basis of their subsistence.

Insurance of catastrophe risk is the only way to help the target groups out of this dilemma. Catastrophic diseases might be defined by cost, diagnosis, or definition of a threshold. A cost definition might say, for example, that costs exceeding two months' income of the target group will be covered up to a maximum amount. A diagnosis definition might name the most frequent causes of surgery and clinical treatments that would be covered by fixed-case payments. A threshold definition might state that members pay treatment costs up to set ceiling, beyond which insurance picks up the bill. In this case, "catastrophe" means accumulated costs of treatment, not the cost of only one intervention.

The coverage of catastrophe risks is also a challenge for reinsurance, but it can have an impact on coverage and administration of these cases. Catastrophic risks are easier to administer than many small risks because they occur less frequently.

CONCLUSIONS

This overview of microinsurers' challenges and solutions has shown that the existing schemes have grown up in a difficult environment. Three elements have impelled their creation:

- Withdrawal of public funds from health care financing in many developing countries

- Providers' difficulties in collecting their fees from patients

- External initiatives, mainly from nongovernmental organizations and other stakeholders

The involvement of local stakeholders, the adaptation to local customs, and the development of special techniques to overcome microinsurers' typical problems have incubated a series of schemes still operating today in many developing countries. Nevertheless, most of these schemes are still struggling with problems, including high dropout rates, large deficits (often covered by donors or by local government units), and fraud. Reinsurance schemes that plug into these experiences can improve the survival chances of those microinsurance schemes' by improving supervision, technical assistance, and financial sustainability. This counts especially for schemes handling catastrophic diseases.

ANNEX 9A Insurance Problem Solving, Selected Countries

Problem	Solution	Guimaras (Philippines)	OHPS (Philippines)	Kiziisi (Uganda)	Ishaka (Uganda)	GRET (Cambodia)
HEALTH MARKET FAILURE						
Lack of supply and lack of purchasing power	Start in areas where there is supply of health care.	●	●	●	●	●
Lack of information about care possibilities	Cooperate with community health workers or village chiefs.	n.a.	n.a.	●	●	n.a.
Lack of information about prices	Negotiate fixed prices and advertise them.	●	●	●	●	●
Split market for care	Sign contract with providers.	●	●	●	●	●
INSURANCE MARKET FAILURE						
Bad experience with insurance, lack of trust	Team up with well-established organizations such as cooperatives or microcredit institutions.	●	●	n.a.	n.a.	n.a.
	Team up with well-known health care providers.	n.a.	n.a.	●	●	●
Lack of information about possibilities	Do social marketing.	n.a.	●	n.a.	n.a.	n.a.
Lack of know-how	Seek technical advice from international organizations and donors.	●	●	●	●	●
High transaction costs	Cooperate with local stakeholders (for example, village chiefs or heads of associations and cooperatives).	●	●	●	●	●
	Collect contributions only once or twice a year on a fixed date.	●	●	●	●	●
	Cooperate with banks.	n.a.	●	n.a.	●	n.a.
	Cooperate with health care providers and make them responsible for collecting contributions.	n.a.	n.a.	●	●	n.a.

Problem / Solution						
High transaction costs (continued)						
Open local offices in main hospitals, staffed by clerks.	n.a.	n.a.	n.a.	n.a.	•	n.a.
Cover high-cost risks (for example, complicated deliveries, appendectomy) instead of small risks.	n.a.	n.a.	n.a.	n.a.	n.a.	•
Lack of money, transactions in kind						
Accept contributions in kind in lieu of cash payments.[a]	n.a.	n.a.	n.a.	n.a.	n.a.	n.a.
Difficulty investing and banking money						
Cooperate as much as possible with banks.	n.a.	n.a.	n.a.	n.a.	•	n.a.
Invest through reinsurer.	n.a.	n.a.	n.a.	n.a.	n.a.	n.a.
High dropout rates						
Involve local stakeholders as much as possible.	•	•	•	•	•	•
Keep record of the dropped out members.	•	•	n.a.	•	n.a.	n.a.
Invest in information.	•	•	•	•	•	•
Involve members in scheme governance and control.	•	n.a.	n.a.	n.a.	•	n.a.
Offer discount on contributions for contract renewal.[b]	n.a.	n.a.	n.a.	n.a.	n.a.	n.a.
Lack of competition						
Involve members in design of benefit packages and contributions.	•	n.a.	n.a.	•	•	n.a.
Lack of sustainability						
Reduce administrative costs.	•	n.a.	n.a.	•	n.a.	n.a.
Maximize compliance in contribution collection.	•	•	•	•	•	•
Do realistic analysis of members' needs and their ability to pay.	•	•	•	•	•	•
Reinsure, especially if scheme covers higher risks.[c]	n.a.	n.a.	n.a.	n.a.	•	n.a.

(Table continues on the following page.)

ANNEX 9A (continued)

Problem	Solution	Guimaras (Philippines)	OHPS (Philippines)	Kiziisi (Uganda)	Ishaka (Uganda)	GRET (Cambodia)
Adverse selection	Institute waiting periods.	•	•	•	•	•
	Introduce group coverage.	•	n.a.	n.a.	n.a	n.a.
	Introduce compulsory membership.	•	n.a.	n.a.	n.a.	n.a.
MORAL HAZARD						
Insureds	Set limits for claims.	•	•	•	•	•
	Cover catastrophe risks.	n.a.	n.a.	n.a.	n.a.	•
	Collect copayments at first contact with providers.	n.a.	n.a.	n.a.	•	•
Providers	Institute payment through capitation.	n.a.	•	n.a.	n.a.	•
	Introduce quality control activities.	•	•	n.a.	n.a.	n.a.
	Create effective referral system.	n.a.	•	n.a.	n.a.	n.a.
Corruption, abuse, and free-riding	Involve community and social control.	•	n.a.	n.a.	n.a.	n.a.
	Introduce membership cards with photos of insured family.	•	•	•	•	•
Failure of risk coverage	Initiate inquiries and sound studies about risks.	•	n.a.	n.a.	n.a.	•
	Insure against catastrophe risk.	n.a.	n.a.	n.a.	n.a.	•

n.a. Not applicable.
GRET Groupe de recherche et d'échanges.
OHPS ORT Health Plus Scheme.
a. This option has been tested in some rural environments in China and in Peso for Health, Negros Oriental Province, Philippines.
b. This option is being discussed by several schemes in the Philippines.
c. In the context of an association of all schemes in Uganda, this option is being discussed.

NOTES

1. Conditions are imperfect, given difficulties in identifying risks across a large and heterogeneous population, public regulation of the insurance industry, or imperfect competition between different benefit packages. Because commercial insurers know they offer benefits that are likely to be used and that they cannot change the benefit package during the life of the contract, they buy stop-loss reinsurance to lower their exposure to the insured risk.

2. According to data from the Kisiizi (Uganda) relating to four trimesters in 1999, the probability of surgery was very low (0.02 cases per insured household)—but the members considered hospitalization and surgery their highest priorities for coverage since, if they had to pay for it themselves, they would be unlikely to afford it. In one case, the cost of such surgery accounted for more than 70 percent of the total benefit cost for that period. Although the event was not subject to moral hazard, the microinsurance unit could not cover this benefit without a mechanism to shield it from insolvency, resulting from a high-cost claim for a low-probability event. A single event with such a small probability should not normally put the entire group at risk of bankruptcy.

BIBLIOGRAPHY

Arube-Wani, John. 1997. *Exploring the Potential for Community Health Insurance and Pre-Payment Schemes. Towards the Development of Alternative Health Financing Options in Uganda* Consultant Report. Ministry of Health. Kampala, Uganda.

Atim, Chris. 1998. *Contribution of Mutual Health Organizations to Financing, Delivery and Access to Health Care. Synthesis of Research in Nine West and Central African Countries.* Technical Report 18. Bethesda, Md.: Abt Associates Inc., Partnerships for Health Reform Project.

Basaza, Robert. 1998. "Voluntary Health Insurance: The Impact of and Prospects for Voluntary Health Insurance in Sub-Saharan Africa." Discussion Paper.

Cassels, Andrew. 1997. *A Guide to Sector Wide Approaches for Health Development.* Geneva: World Health Organization.

CIDR/EZE. 1999. *Community Based Health Insurance in Luweero Area, Uganda.* Feasibility Study Report. Luweero.

Dror, David, and Christian Jacquier. 1999. "Micro-Insurance: Extending Health Insurance to the Excluded." *International Social Security Review* 52(1):71–97.

Dror, D.M., and G. Duru. 2000. "Financing Micro-Insurance: Perspectives and Prospectives." Proceedings. Seventh International Conference on System Science, Budapest.

Hutchinson, Paul. 1998. *Equity and Access to Medical Services in Uganda. The Effects of Income, Gender and Proximity.* Social Protection Series. Washington, D.C.: World Bank.

Jitta, J. 1996. *Evaluation of Health Financing Reforms in Uganda. A Document Review of User Fees.* Discussion Paper.

McGaugh, Jhan. 1999. "Community Based Health Insurance: Experiences and Lessons Learned from East Africa." Proceedings of a Study Design Workshop, Mombasa.

Stiglitz, J.E. 1988. *Economics of the Public Sector*. New York: Norton. Quoted in A.B. Atkinson, *Income and the Welfare State: Essays on Britain and Europe*. Cambridge: Cambridge University Press, 1995.

UNDP (United Nations Development Programme). 1998. *Cambodia Human Development Report*. New York: UNDP.

PART 3

Implementation Issues

CHAPTER 10

Building Capacity and Strengthening Implementation at the Community Level

Sara Bennett and George Gotsadze

Experience in implementing microinsurance schemes for health care has been growing. With increased interest in protecting the poor against health care costs (WHO 2000), several reviews of microinsurance schemes have recently been conducted (Atim 1998; Bennett, Creese, and Monasch 1998).

In this chapter, we consider what can be learned from experience with microinsurance regarding implementation processes, particularly regarding financial stabilization and risk management. We build upon reviews and more recently published papers and reports to address three main questions:

- What capacity constraints have microinsurance schemes encountered in developing countries?

- What are the critical features for designing and implementing monitoring and evaluation frameworks for microinsurance schemes?

- What should be done to build capacity for microinsurance schemes in developing countries, particularly to enhance financial stability?

Microinsurance seems to be one of the few (or only) ways of protecting population groups outside the formal sector against health care costs while raising adequate revenue to deliver services. Because of poor design and management, however, these schemes often fail, or their coverage dwindles (Bennett, Creese, and Monasch 1998). A huge variety of schemes could be labeled "microinsurance." These schemes often serve different types of communities, with different objectives and different health care contexts. For example, microinsurance schemes have been implemented to provide health insurance for farmers in the Republic of Korea (Peabody, Lee, and Bickel 1995), to expand coverage of basic primary health care services in Guinea-Bissau (Chabot, Boal, and Da Silva 1991), or to provide insurance coverage to self-employed women workers in India (Vyas and Chatterjee 1995). The variety of scheme circumstances and objectives means that no "blueprint" for scheme design and implementation can be offered. The key to success, therefore, lies in strengthening the planning, implementation,

The authors would like to acknowledge the insightful comments provided by Chris Atim on an earlier draft of the chapter.

and monitoring processes so that scheme managers and designers understand their operating context, and how best to adapt scheme design to respond to objectives, context, and monitoring information.

CAPACITY CONCEPTS

Several alternative ways of conceptualizing capacity have been presented (Batley 1997; Grindle and Hildebrand 1995). To keep a relatively simple conceptual framework, we distinguish between only two types of capacity: individual skills and organizational capacity. Organizational capacity encompasses appropriate systems (for example, information and management), and adequate resources (for example, computers, and transportation).

Capacity Is Task Specific

Many different types of tasks go into design and implementation of a microinsurance scheme (figure 10.1). The capacity required to conduct each of these tasks varies both in terms of skills and organizational capacity. For example, conducting a legal situational analysis requires some understanding of the legal system, computing

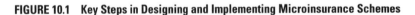

FIGURE 10.1   Key Steps in Designing and Implementing Microinsurance Schemes

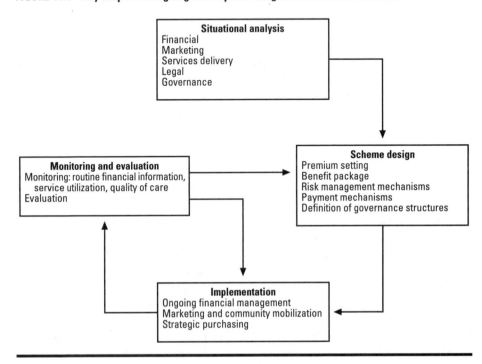

premium rates requires actuarial skills, and monitoring certain aspects of quality of care may require a functional health information system.

Capacity Is Actor Specific

The actors who design a scheme are usually different from the ones that implement it day-to-day. Frequently, external actors are involved in design, and local actors take on most routine management. Providers offering services under the scheme may also need particular capacities to participate (for example, the ability to follow set treatment protocols or bill for care). We therefore consider capacity constraints and approaches to capacity building for different groups of actors (namely technical advisers, scheme managers, and providers). Technical advisers could be local or international.

We do not consider the role of government agencies and governmental policy, often viewed as an integral part of capacity and sometimes critical in terms of building individual schemes' capacity. Issues regarding the relationship of the scheme to government are described elsewhere in this book (chapters 11, 12, 13, and 15, in particular).

EXPERIENCE DESIGNING AND IMPLEMENTING MICROINSURANCE

This section explains the boxes identified in figure 10.1. Monitoring and evaluation are considered in the next section.

Situational Analysis

Not many papers on microinsurance schemes describe the analyses conducted prior to start-up, probably because few are done. Situational analyses are usually more comprehensive when an external donor is involved in start-up and can support the costs of baseline household surveys and costing analyses. For example, the establishment of pilot microinsurance schemes in Rwanda, supported by the U.S. Agency for International Development (USAID), included a review of existing data on health care financing, health service utilization and costs, further analysis of routine ministry of health (MOH) data as well as assessment of existing local prepayment schemes, and provider and population interest in participating (Schneider, Diop, and Bucayana 2000). Box 10.1 catalogs analyses conducted in preparation for launching such schemes in Georgia.

A series of papers, supported by the International Labour Organization (ILO), investigated the feasibility of pilot microinsurance projects in four countries. They mainly focused on the broad economic context and extensive organizational analyses and gave less emphasis to the financial viability of schemes (van Ginnekan 1997). This seems to be a general trend: situational analyses conducted prior to scheme design focus on assessing different groups' interest in participating in the

---

BOX 10.1   GEORGIA: SITUATIONAL ANALYSES FOR RURAL SCHEMES

- Review of household survey data on morbidity, utilization of alternative services, and out-of-pocket payments

- Interviews with providers to assess interest in participating in scheme

- Focus group discussions with community to assess interest in participating

- Review of services currently delivered and community preferences for services to be included in benefit package

- Cost analysis of existing services and proposed benefit package

- Analysis of existing revenue sources for providers

- Legal analysis, especially relating to the legal status of microinsurance funds

The preparation was concluded with a three-day workshop with all key stakeholders, communities, local government representatives, providers, regional health authorities, and technical advisers, who discussed the findings of the preparatory analyses and their implications for scheme design.

Source: Bennett, Gotsadze, and Gzirishvili 2000.

---

scheme and on the appropriateness of existing organizational structures for managing and administering the scheme (Akanzinge 1997).

Experience in Scheme Design

As was the case for situational analyses, few documents describe in any detail how schemes were designed. Conclusions about capacity to design schemes must therefore be drawn from the design adopted. Many insurance schemes have run into difficulties that could have been avoided through improved scheme design (table 10.1).

Many of the scheme design failures noted in table 10.1 lead to increased financial risk. For example, a poorly defined or undefined benefit package means that it is impossible to cost the services likely to be delivered under the scheme and hence to set premiums on an actuarial basis. Problems of adverse selection and inappropriate design of the referral network will lead to higher costs than those initially envisaged.

In terms of scheme sustainability, a critical design aspect is premium setting. From what can be gleaned from the literature, premium setting is often an ad hoc process:

> When the insurance scheme was launched the premium was calculated by dividing the double of total IP [inpatient] bills by the district population; because it was expected that

TABLE 10.1   Common Design Shortcomings and Their Results

Design shortcoming	Result	Source
Failure to include mechanisms to prevent adverse selection such as compulsory enrollment of the whole family or village, restricted enrollment period, or waiting period for entitlement to benefits	Adverse selection: enrollment of higher risk cases, escalating premiums and costs, and decreasing membership	Bennett, Creese, and Monasch 1998
Poorly defined or undefined benefit package	Inability to cost services likely to be used and therefore to set realistic premiums	Bennett, Creese, and Monasch 1998; Musau 1999; Jutting 2000; Atim 1998; Somkang and others 1994; Kiwara 1997; Chabot, Boal, and Da Silva 1991
Inappropriate design of referral network	Failure to make best use of primary care and develop effective gatekeeper mechanisms for hospital care, and therefore higher costs	Bennett, Creese, and Monasch 1998
Ineffective exemption mechanisms	Exclusion of poor	Creese and Kutzin 1995
Failure to factor inflation rates into premium calculation	Underestimation of premiums damages financial sustainability	Musau 1999
Failure to negotiate in advance price of services with providers	Higher than anticipated prices leads to higher expenditures by microinsurance fund, damaging financial sustainability	Bennett, Creese, and Monasch 1998; Mills, Bennett, and Russell 2000
Failure to adopt measures to improve quality of care	Poor quality of provided medical services to the scheme members	Bennett, Creese, and Monasch 1998; Musau 1999
Absence of limited drug list, little attention to incentives created for overprescription	No attention to drug supply	Mwabu, Ainsworth, and Nyamete 1993; Litvack and Bodart 1993; McPake, Hanson, and Mills 1993

the admission rate would double. On top a security margin has been added (Somkang and others 1994).

The [premium] amounts were based on current estimates that the country's per capita expenditure on health is US$10, i.e., 6,000 Tshs [Tanzanian shillings]. This is about 500 Tshs per month or Tshs 20 per day (Kiwara 1997).

The premium-setting process in Guinea-Bissau, described by Chabot, Boal, and Da Silva (1991), is even more interesting. When, in one village, project staff suggested how much villagers should pay into the fund, most villagers declined to contribute. Subsequently, project staff elsewhere simply suggested that villagers should "pay whatever they felt to be sufficient." The amount contributed was small, but most villagers contributed. With the small amount of money collected, drugs could be purchased for only a three-month period:

> As the responsibility for the decision on the amount of payment had been in their [the villagers] hands, the project staff declined any loans or an advance of drugs during the months that followed the depletion of the stock. Thus villagers had to wait until the next harvest, when they again discussed how much everybody should contribute to the Abota. This time they more than doubled the amount (Chabot, Boal, and Da Silva 1991).

In Bwamanda (one of the more successful schemes documented), a more sophisticated approach to rate setting was taken, based on operating costs and projected population coverage, with the goal of shifting the hospital toward full cost recovery (Moens 1990). However, the model seems to have made no allowance for increased operating costs resulting from increased demand.

Thailand is the only developing country example where a reinsurance function already exists, although such a function has been discussed in the Philippines (Bautista, Yap, and Soriano 1999). Although the available documentation on Thailand does not discuss capacity constraints faced in designing the reinsurance scheme, Thailand has a well-established and competent bureaucracy compared with many other developing countries and substantial experience with designing health insurance schemes. It is unclear why so few countries and schemes have adopted a reinsurance program but it is probably related to the limited coverage of microinsurance programs, the widespread prevalence of government subsidies to public sector health care providers, as well as limited understanding of the reinsurance issue, and insufficient skills to establish such a function.

A necessary complement to overall scheme design is the design of specific management systems. The presence of adequate financial management systems at scheme start-up appears particularly important for financial sustainability. In the ORT[1] project in the Philippines, several management systems were defined during the project's preparation, including systems for recording membership, contribution payments, utilization of specific services, drug orders, purchases, and sales, and for financial accounting (Ron and Kupferman 1996). Several of these systems entailed components both at the central project level and in provider facilities.

Table 10.2 lists the management tools and systems employed in the pilot risk-pooling scheme in Rwanda. For many schemes, however, system design prior to project implementation appears to have been partial, evolving during the initial years of the scheme in response to problems identified.

Experience in Scheme Implementation

Information on the process of scheme implementation is more complete than that on scheme design or situational analysis. Review of the available literature suggests great variety between schemes in terms of the effectiveness of implementation measures.

Marketing and community mobilization. Most schemes conduct some special marketing campaigns, often in the form of community meetings. Some schemes (for

TABLE 10.2   Rwanda: Use of Management Tools and Systems Employed

Accounting and administrative tools	User	Purpose
Member patient registry (in addtition to already existing register for nonmembers)	Provider	Tracks members' drug and service utilization pattern in detail. To be used for comparison with nonmembers.
Monthly summary of member patient registry (in addition to monthly report on nonmembers)	Provider	Summarizes members' care as reported in detailed register. To be used for comparison with nonmembers.
Prepayment journal of members' care	Provider	Compares capitation payment to health centers with fee-for-service charges per sick member that would have been paid if health centers were reimbursed by fee for services.
Cash and bank book	Insurance scheme	Tracks cash and bank activities.
Revenue and expenditure journals	Insurance scheme	Summarizes daily revenues and expenditures as tracked in cash book.
Monthly treasury book	Insurance scheme	Monthly summary financial report on insurance scheme revenue and expenditures.
Membership book	Insurance scheme	Lists members' demographic and premium information.
Membership cards for three categories (individual, family, group)	Insurance scheme	Identity card entitles members to receive insurance scheme benefit package.
Members' sociodemographic information sheet	Insurance scheme	Summary of sociodemographic information on each member/family filled in when members sign up and pay premium.
Membership book on indigent members	Insurance scheme	List of indigent members exempt from paying premium.
Monthly summary report on new members and premium amount collected	Insurance scheme	Summary of new members per membership category and total premium amount collected.
Book on members leaving insurance scheme	Insurance scheme	List of members leaving insurance scheme.

Source: Adapted from Schneider, Diop, and Bucayana 2000.

example, Rwanda) took more innovative approaches such as radio interviews with scheme managers, newspaper coverage, and educational activities during Sunday church services—although despite these efforts enrollment in the Rwanda schemes was still relatively low (Schneider, Diop, and Bucayana 2000).

Lack of local ownership of schemes appears to be a relatively widespread problem that adversely affects enrollment. Many schemes engaged in only minimal consultation with communities; consequently, it is unlikely that the microinsurance product responds to the perceived needs of community members. If this is the case, then not even extensive marketing is likely to produce good results. Enrollment rates in many schemes reviewed are low. About half of the schemes reviewed by Bennett, Creese, and Monasch (1998) covered 20 percent or less of the targeted beneficiaries.

Schemes frequently use community members to sell membership cards. This can also be problematic if the community members are unsure of their role or what they must do. The situation described by Donaldson (1982) in Nepal is not atypical: "[O]f the 300 cards initially distributed to Badegaon Committee members, only 33 cards were sold, 247 cards were returned unsold, and 20 cards were unaccounted for."

Financial management. Implementation of strong financial management procedures is the Achilles heel of many microinsurance schemes:

> Major problems were found in financial administration. Because of inadequate recording procedures, lapses in recording of transactions, incomplete accounting books, it was impossible for the team to conclude on the completeness as well as the accuracy of financial statements (Somkang and others 1994).

> Supervision of funds collected became a great problem, as the reporting was poor and follow-up lacking (Mogedal 1984).

Among weaknesses identified by a team evaluating the Chogoria microinsurance scheme in Kenya in 1994 were the following:

- "The number of beneficiaries is not known precisely because data is [sic] not kept on size of families enrolled...

- "The actual cost of services used by members is not known because costing of patient services is not done routinely...

- "The frequency of beneficiaries' encounters at the hospital is not recorded or analyzed however the data is [sic] accessible" (Enright and others 1994).

This haphazard management style resulted in a loss of US$110,000 over a four-year period, shared between the hospital and the insurance company (McFarlane 1996).

In Bwamanda, among six key factors influencing the success of the scheme, the first two involved financial management, namely the managerial capacity of the health zone (especially financial management) and the investment policy for offsetting inflation (Moens 1990).

Papers published and reviews conducted during the 1990s emphasized the problems microinsurance schemes commonly encountered with financial management (Bennett, Creese, and Monasch 1998; Atim 1998). As a consequence, perhaps more attention is being paid to this issue. For example in Rwanda, monthly data on finances, enrollment, utilization, and costs were collected and analyzed from the prepayment schemes, as well as from provider units, and presented at monthly meetings of the steering committee (Schneider, Diop, and Leighton 2001). This intensive focus on the schemes' sustainability may also reflect donor preoccupations and the involvement of external technical assistance in their development.

Strategic purchasing. The role of strategic purchasing in microinsurance schemes received little attention in the literature until quite recently. Many schemes were so intent on raising revenues and promoting service utilization that they paid little attention to how well their funds were spent. Schemes working with private providers (for example, Self-Employed Women's Association in India and ILO-supported schemes in Dar es Salaam have paid most attention to this factor (Vyas and Chatterjee 1995; Kiwara 1997). In both cases, fairly effective mechanisms for strategic purchasing appear to have been developed (such as establishing quality standards for providers and reviewing fees charged). For other schemes, evidence about this role is so limited that it is difficult to draw conclusions about the capacity to conduct strategic purchasing.

Drawing from other parts of the literature on health sector reform (such as that on contracting out of services), it seems likely that neither scheme managers nor public health officials are accustomed to the types of negotiation involved in establishing contracts between a microinsurance scheme and a provider (Mills, Bennett, and Russell 2000). Furthermore, strategic purchasing requires regular information on the number, type, and quality of services furnished under the scheme, and this basic information is frequently incomplete.

LEARNING FROM EXPERIENCE

Monitoring and evaluation (M&E) are a critical part of any microinsurance scheme design and implementation. They serve a number of different purposes:

- *Correction of course.* Routine monitoring by scheme managers and communities, with the support of advisers and consultants, should detect problems at an early stage and enable changes or corrections in the design and implementation of schemes so as to forestall further problems.

- *Quantifying impact.* M&E allows estimation of schemes' impact on objectives, for example, whether improved financial accessibility has increased utilization of health care services or whether increased financial inflows have resulted in better quality of health services.

- *Understanding the reasons for success or failure.* To draw lessons for other initiatives, the reasons a particular scheme worked or did not work also have to be understood.

Getting the initial architecture of the scheme right and ensuring effective implementation is part of the challenge, but also important are identifying problems in scheme performance before the scheme breaks down and adapting scheme design to a continuously changing environment. The dimensions of monitoring identified in figure 10.1 (routine financial information, service utilization, quality of care) have been discussed above in terms of experience with scheme implementation. If routine information systems are not put in place as part of the implementation process, effective routine monitoring is unlikely to occur and proper evaluation may also be jeopardized.

M&E cannot be conducted according to a blueprint. Microinsurance schemes are diverse, both in goals and design, and M&E efforts must be adapted to fit each of them. Because many schemes suffer from lack of clear definition of goals and objectives, it is difficult not only to design the scheme itself but also to design an effective monitoring framework. M&E normally involves both internal and external components. While external evaluations may bring objectivity and significant skills not available among the microinsurance management team, scheme managers may not have adequate ownership of findings and consequently may not fully implement evaluation results. Particularly for an activity such as microinsurance, which depends so critically on the commitment and interest of not only scheme managers but also a broader group of stakeholders (for example, community members), an inclusive approach to designing and implementing M&E activities is desirable.

As for other dimensions of schemes considered above, the available documentation on M&E in microinsurance schemes is weak and incomplete. Published papers usually report specific evaluation findings or monitoring results on one or two issues, but they rarely report on the entire M&E framework. An exception to this is the series of reports on Rwanda (box 10.2). Again, this general lack of documentation probably reflects the schemes' lack of an appropriate M&E plan. Such a plan should be developed at start-up and amended as necessary. For lack of documentation, much of the discussion here is theoretical in nature.

Monitoring

Most schemes appear to do some monitoring (it would be difficult not to), particularly financial monitoring. Atim (2000) provides a comprehensive approach to monitoring mutual health organizations in Ghana (table 10.3). He defines four broad types of indicators (institutional development, effectiveness in service delivery, efficiency, and financial performance).

Reports on existing schemes use some of the indicators suggested in table 10.3, but to the authors' knowledge no scheme has comprehensive data over a period of time on the indicators identified above. Some of these indicators may have to be adapted to reflect different schemes' assorted management approaches. For example, many schemes would simply drop a member for failing to pay dues, so "percentage of members in arrears" would be irrelevant.

In addition to the dimensions identified above, organizational monitoring helps managers understand the context. For example, possible indicators include:

- Staff adherence to the policies defined by the organization

- Provider adherence to the contractual terms between scheme and health facility

- Completeness of an organization's records

- Completeness of the data collected

BOX 10.2   RWANDA: MONITORING AND EVALUATION IN A PILOT MICROINSURANCE SCHEME

The scheme in Rwanda was a pilot, externally supported activity and, as such, had greater inputs into M&E than many other schemes.

Some indicators were assessed monthly, others quarterly:

- *Monthly.* Membership numbers, routine financial indicators, and reenrollment rate.

- *Quarterly.* Provider utilization rates, selected quality indicators, and financial performance.

Planned evaluation covered:

- Patient satisfaction through patient interviews

- Stakeholder (beneficiaries, providers, managers) perceptions of scheme—focus group discussions

- Organizational performance

- Impact on household financial status and accessibility of care, particularly for vulnerable households (household survey)

- Cost of implementing pilot schemes.

Of all the M&E activities listed, the household survey is the only one likely to have significant associated costs. Schemes elsewhere could (and arguably should) easily implement other M&E activities.

Source: Schneider, Diop, and Bucayana 2000.

- Communication flow between providers and the scheme and between the scheme members and the organization

- Extent to which the scheme follows recording and reporting requirements.

Evaluation

Few published papers have attempted to conduct full evaluations of several microinsurance schemes using the same evaluation methodology, but there are two partial exceptions: Dave and Berman (1990) and Atim (1998). These case studies involved visits to all of the schemes evaluated, but they suffered from the usual problems of data quality that beset other reviews of microinsurance schemes. The lack of comparative evaluations is very problematic—and critical to the further development of this field.

The evaluations available for individual schemes usually focus on concerns expressed by their managers. Table 10.4 presents objectives, methods, and sources of information for three "typical" scheme evaluations. These evaluations are typical

TABLE 10.3   Ghana: Proposed Indicators for Monitoring Mutual Health Organizations

Indicator	Definition/examples
Institutional development	
Number of members/beneficiaries	Self-explanatory
Growth rate of membership/beneficiaries	Self explanatory
Participation rate, meetings	Number of attendees/expected number
Participation rate, elections	Number of members voting/number eligible to vote
Dues payment	Amount of dues collected/total amount expected
Percentage of members in arrears	Number of members with dues paid/total number of members
Coverage rate, target population	Number of members/total number in target population
Effectiveness in service delivery	
Utilization rate of health services by scheme beneficiaries	Number of consultations under scheme/number of beneficiaries
Coverage rate provided by scheme	Percentage of beneficiaries' total health care costs paid by scheme
Morbidity rate among members	Number of cases of illness among members/number of members
Mortality rate among members	Number of deaths among members/number of members
Quality of health care	Various (for example, waiting time, drug availability, cleanliness)
Efficiency	
Trends in health care expenditure per beneficiary	Total health expenditure by scheme/number of members
Trends in health care expenditure per category of service	Percentage of expenditure by type of service (for example, consultations, admissions, drugs)
Risk-management indicators	Various—corresponding to risk-management mechanisms adopted
Financial performance	
Current ratio	Current assets/current liabilities
Liquidity ratio	Liquid assets/current liabilities
Long-term solvency ratio	Total external liabilities/members' contributions
Ratio of dues to expenses or charges	Dues/annual expenses
Ratio of coverage of expenditure	Reserves/monthly expenses ratio
Ratio of operating costs to income	Operating cost/total annual receipts

Source: Adapted from Atim 2000.

only in that they reflect diverse concerns particular to the scheme evaluated. All three schemes identified in the table have undergone a number of evaluations over time that have focused on different aspects of the scheme.

Most of the longer-lived and more successful schemes have done frequent evaluations. For example, several evaluations of different aspects of the Bwamanda

TABLE 10.4   Objectives and Methods Employed by Three "Typical" Evaluations

	Bwamanda, Democratic Republic of Congo (1990)	Nkoranza, Ghana (1994)	Thai Health Card Scheme (1997)
Objectives	• Identify impact of scheme on accessibility of health care • Identify impact of scheme on financial accessibility of hospital	• Idenitfy impact of scheme on accessibility of inpatient care • Identify administrative strengths and weaknesses • Assess trends in average costs and income • Assess possibility of fixing fees • Make recommendations for improvements	• Compare utilization patterns of holders of different types of health cards • Assess allocative efficiency in terms of resources allocated to different levels of care • Assess financial sustainability • Assess efficiency of overall fund management • Assess reinsurance policy • Predict expansion of scheme
Methods/sources of information	• Review of administrative records • In-depth and structured interviews • Household survey • Community meetings	• Document review • Review of administrative records • Household survey • Interviews with stakeholders	• Postal questionnaire collecting existing administrative data on number of cards, service utilization, cost of providing services, fund allocation. • Interviews with key informants (fund managers)

Sources: Somkang and others 1994; Moens 1990; Pannurunothai and others 1997.

scheme in the Democratic Republic of Congo have been conducted (Moens 1990; Criel and van Lerberghe 1996; Criel 1992). Similarly, the Thai health card scheme has been evaluated many times. These evaluations have contributed to some fundamental refocusing of the Thai scheme, for example, a shift from limited benefits for enrollees (for example, a maximum of three outpatient visits a year) toward much greater coverage for catastrophes. In the Bwamanda case, a group of expatriate or external technical advisers led all the evaluations. In Thailand, Thais involved at the central level in scheme management or located in Thai universities conducted all evaluations (except the very first, conducted in the 1970s). Despite the lack of any hard supporting evidence, it seems likely that financial and skill capacity to conduct evaluations as needed, instead of depending on external resources and evaluators, is likely to contribute toward the success and sustainability of microinsurance schemes.

BUILDING CAPACITY FOR MICROINSURANCE SCHEMES—THE ROLE OF REINSURANCE

Chapter 5 of this volume presents a number of different causes of financial instability in microinsurance schemes, most of them directly linked to weak implementation processes and limited capacity (table 10.5). Catastrophes (such as epidemics or macroeconomic shocks) are the only source of financial instability unrelated to capacity issues. The other capacity problems listed in table 10.5, column two, stress lack of data prior to scheme start-up, poor scheme design (in terms of both administrative structures and systems and technical design), weak social marketing, and lack of attention to developing the skills of the individuals who are responsible for day-to-day management.

As chapter 5 points out, reinsurance schemes need to be complemented by other services for financial stability of microinsurance schemes. The third component of the reinsurance approach is "knowledge transfer and consulting services." This chapter has demonstrated the types of needs for knowledge transfer and consulting. Reinsurers could contribute to the financial stability of microinsurance schemes in many ways, including by training managers and community members, standardizing system development and implementation, providing standardized management and research tools, supporting schemes with consultancy services, and monitoring and evaluating performance.

Training Fund Managers and Community Members

More or less standardized country-specific training courses and training materials can be developed on such issues as basic principles of insurance; management

TABLE 10.5   Financial Instability and Capacity Constraints

Source of financial instability	Causes of financial instability—related to weak capacity
Inaccurate calculation of contributions	• Lack of reliable cost and utilization data • Inability of scheme organizers to interpret data and estimate premiums
Unsatisfactory compliance rate with premium payment	• Weak administrative structures, allowing money to leak from scheme • Members' failure to pay premiums, because scheme inadequately marketed or not designed to be adequately attractive to them
Random statistical fluctuations in claims	• Weak scheme marketing, leading to low enrollment and small group size
Fluctuations in unit cost of benefits	• Failure by scheme managers to negotiate set prices with care providers
Instability resulting from underestimation of risk probability	• Weak data on utilization and morbidity profiles, preventing accurate estimates of risk probability • Adverse selection and higher than expected risk (partly from poor scheme design, and perhaps also from poor marketing)
Catastrophes	• Unrelated to capacity issues
Administrative costs	• Unpredictably high administrative costs related to inefficient management structures

Source: Adapted from Dror, chapter 5, this volume.

system operation (especially financial management systems); health service delivery topics such as the use of treatment guidelines and protocols; rational drug use; and skills in negotiations, enabling scheme managers to obtain cost-effective service packages.

Standardized Management System Development and Implementation

Stable microinsurance schemes are dependent upon effective management systems within the scheme and strong management and information systems among providers. Reinsurers can develop standardized management information systems (and complementary manuals) for schemes in a particular country. They can also work with government and private sector providers to strengthen information systems among providers.

Generic Tools for Microinsurance Schemes

Many different materials are needed to satisfactorily complete all the key steps in designing and implementing microinsurance schemes (figure 10.1). Much effort could be saved, and higher quality results ensured, if there were standard country-specific instruments and tools, for example:

- Standardized contracts to formalize relations between the scheme and health care providers, the scheme and enrolled persons, and the scheme and the government

- Standardized spreadsheets to aid cost analysis, risk assessment, and premium setting

- Social marketing materials

- Research tools to explore local willingness to pay for alternative benefit packages and establish user satisfaction with schemes.

Consultancy Services

Even if prospective schemes receive extensive supporting materials, they are likely to need specialist advice. A reinsurer should facilitate access by local scheme managers and interested communities to well-qualified technical advisers who can assist with scheme design and implementation.

Ongoing M&E

Spotting and addressing problems of financial instability as early as possible is in the interest of the reinsurer-type agency. To this end, the agency must routinely monitor its schemes' key dimensions. In addition, the agency might evaluate schemes regularly to see how well they answer topical policy concerns.

Although microinsurance schemes' variety of objectives and structures make it difficult to promote global approaches, partners at the global level can play a big role in preparing the ground for reinsurers and supporting them in their work. Priorities for global-level action include:

- Improving understanding of the reasons for scheme success and failure through comparative analysis of scheme design, implementation, and management

- Supporting training courses for experts who might staff *Social Re*-type agencies or provide microinsurance schemes with consultancy services

- Developing generic tools for microinsurance schemes that could be adapted for use at the country level

- Disseminating—in easily accessible formats—emerging lessons of experience with microinsurance.

CONCLUSIONS

From schemes' experience with the processes involved in implementation, monitoring, and evaluation, we have attempted to draw lessons to strengthen these processes. Our effort has been considerably impeded by the lack of comprehensive information on scheme objectives, the design and implementation processes, and the tools used to monitor and evaluate their impact. We have had to rely exclusively on ad hoc reports by individual schemes.

A key conclusion must be that the international community should take a more proactive role to facilitate scheme documentation and evaluation in a way that allows comparison of different approaches. The establishment of reinsurers opens up a promising route for doing this.

Capacity problems commonly occur in relation to the many different tasks involved in preparing, designing, implementing, and monitoring microinsurance schemes. In some contexts, the observed capacity shortcomings occur in such basic procedures as maintaining adequate accounts, preventing theft of funds, or failing to define a benefit package. When confronted with these fundamental lacunae, a reinsurer would have to focus first on transferring basic knowledge and building capacity instead of on reinsurance proper.

Although financial sustainability is clearly a key property of a scheme, how it relates to other key properties is unclear, particularly to community involvement. In his evaluation of the Bwamanda scheme, Moens (1990) commented: "It is as crucial to realize the importance of community involvement as to recognize the limitations of the communities' financial management capacities to organize such type of risk coverage arrangements."

There is a potential conflict between setting up a microinsurance scheme in a way that preserves a strong sense of community ownership and establishing a solid financial and actuarial base. Acknowledging this tension raises further questions: How can technical advice best serve a community-initiated and -owned project? At what stages in the scheme and in what form should technical advice be given? How can technical decisionmaking skills best be transferred to community members? A stronger understanding of these process issues would facilitate the work of reinsurers.

In the past five years, focus has converged on microinsurance and its potential for protecting populations outside formal-sector employment from unpredictable and uneven health care expenditures. Scheme designers can now draw upon an emerging body of literature and lessons and an expanding pool of resources. Although the evidence is limited, these assets seem to be influencing scheme design and implementation in positive ways (Atim 2000).

We have come a long way during the past decade in understanding the factors that make a microinsurance scheme more or less successful, but we still have a long way to go. Considering the great diversity of objectives and design of microinsurance schemes, we cannot offer any universally applicable blueprint for success. The most promising strategy is to build capacity among scheme managers and advisers, and to simultaneously strengthen M&E activities so that problems can be rapidly identified and addressed as the scheme evolves. Reinsurance could play a key role in this process.

NOTE

1. ORT is an international nongovernmental organization that aims to improve the quality of life of the poor and the marginalized.

REFERENCES

Akanzinge, A.P.N. 1997. "The Characteristics, Achievements, Problems, Possible Solutions of the Community Financing Scheme for Hospital Admissions: Nkoranza District, Ghana, West Africa." Paper presented at the Interregional Meeting on Health Insurance for the Nonformal Sector, October 20–22, 1997. Geneva: World Health Organization.

Atim, C. 1998. *Contribution of Mutual Health Organizations to Financing, Delivery, and Access to Health Care: Synthesis of Research in Nine West and Central African Countries.* Technical Report No.18. Bethesda, Md.: Abt Associates Inc., Partnerships for Health Reform Project.

_____. 2000. *Training of Trainers Manual for Mutual Health Organizations in Ghana.* Bethesda, Md.: Abt Associates Inc., Partnerships for Health Reform Project.

Batley, R. 1997. "A Research Framework for Analysing Capacity to Undertake the "New" Roles of Government." *The Role of Government in Adjusting Economies.* Paper No. 23. Birmingham, U.K.: University of Birmingham.

Bautista, M.C.G, E.C. Yap, and E.S. Soriano. 1999. *Local Governments' Health Financing Initiatives: Evaluation, Synthesis, and Prospects for the National Health Insurance Program in the Philippines.* Bethesda, Md.: Abt Associates Inc., Partnerships for Health Reform Project.

Bennett, S., A. Creese, and R. Monasch. 1998. *Health Insurance Schemes for People Outside Formal Sector Employment.* Current Concerns, ARA Paper No. 16. WHO/ARA/CC/98.1 Geneva: World Health Organization.

Bennett, S., G. Gotsadze, and D. Gzirishvili. 2000. "Activities to Develop Health Financing Mechanisms in Western Georgia: Report to the International Medical Corps." International Medical Corps, Georgia. Unpublished.

Chabot, J., M. Boal, and A. Da Silva. 1991. "National Community Health Insurance at Village Level: The Case from Guinea-Bissau." *Health Policy and Planning* 61:46–54.

Creese, A., and J. Kutzin. 1995 "Lessons from Cost-Recovery in Health." Discussion Paper No.2. WHO/SHS/NHP/95.5 Geneva: World Health Organization.

Criel, B. 1992. "Community Financing Schemes: Give Them Time. Discussion of Two Prepayment Schemes Conducted at the District Level in Zaire." University of Antwerp, Belgium.

Criel, B., and W. van Lerberghe. 1996. "The Bwamanda Hospital Insurance Scheme: Effective for Whom? A Study of Its Impact on Hospital Utilization Patterns." Unpublished.

Dave, P., and P. Berman. 1990. *Costs and Financing of Health Care: Experiences in the Voluntary Sector.* New Delhi: Ford Foundation.

Donaldson, D. 1982. "An Analysis of Health Insurance Schemes in the Lalitpur District of Nepal." Thesis No 29712 (M. Pub. Health). University of Washington. Unpublished.

Enright, M., D. Kraushaar, D. Oatway, and G. Ikiara. 1994. *Developing Prepaid Health Programs in Kenya: A Private Insurance Assessment.* Arlington, Va.: PROFIT.

Grindle, M., and M. Hildebrand. 1995. "Building Sustainable Capacity in the Public Sector: What Can Be Done? *Public Administration and Development* 15:441–63.

Jutting, J., 2000. "Do Mutual Health Insurance Schemes Improve the Access to Health Care? Preliminary Results from Household Survey in Rural Senegal." Paper prepared for delivery at the conference on Health System Financing in Low Income Countries, November 30–December 1, 2000, CERDI, Clermont-Ferrand.

Kiwara, A.D. 1997. "Social Protection for the Informal Sector: Health Care Services Provision and Health Insurance Schemes." Paper presented at the Interregional Meeting on Health Insurance for the Nonformal sector, October 20–22, 1997. Geneva: World Health Organization.

Litvack, J.I., and C. Bodart. 1993. "User Fees and Improved Quality of Health Care Equals Improved Access: Results of a Field Experiment in Cameroon." *Social Science and Medicine* 37(3):369–83.

McFarlane, G.A. 1996. Personal correspondence to AFRO/WHO, November 1996.

McPake, B., K. Hanson, and A. Mills. 1993. "Community Financing of Health Care in Africa: An Evaluation of Bamako Initiative." *Social Science and Medicine* 36(11):1383–95.

Mills, A., S. Bennett, and S. Russell. 2000. "Government Purchase of Private Services." Chapter 6 in *The Challenge of Health Sector Reform: What Must Governments Do?* Basingstoke, U.K.: Macmillan.

Moens, F. 1990. "Design, Implementation and Evaluation of a Community Financing Scheme for Hospital Care in Developing Countries: A Prepaid Health Plan in the Bwamanda Health Zone, Zaire." *Social Science and Medicine* 30(12):1319–27.

Mogedal, S.M. 1984. "Local Health Insurance Supplementing National Efforts—Nepal." *Public Health Review* 12:286–90.

Musau, S.N. 1999. *Community-Based Health Insurance: Experiences and Lessons Learned from East and Southern Africa*. Technical Report No. 34. Bethesda, Md.: Abt Associates Inc., Partnerships for Health Reform Project.

Mwabu, G.M., M. Ainsworth, and A. Nyamete. 1993. *Quality of Medical Care and Choice of Medical Treatment in Kenya: An Empirical Analysis*. Technical Working Paper 9. Washington, D.C.: World Bank.

Pannurunothai, S., S. Srithamrongsawad, M. Kongapaen, and P. Thamwanna. 1997. *"Financing Reforms for the Health Card Scheme in Thailand: Utilization and Financing Study."* Unpublished.

Peabody, J.W., S.W. Lee, and S. Bickel. 1995. "Health for All in the Republic of Korea: One Country's Experience with Implementing Universal Health Care." *Health Policy* 31:29–42.

Ron, A., and A. Kupferman. 1996. *A Community Health Insurance Scheme in the Philippines: Extension of a Community-Based Integrated Project*. Geneva: World Health Organization.

Schneider, P., F.P. Diop, and S. Bucayana. 2000. *Development and Implementation of Prepayment Schemes in Rwanda*. Technical Report No. 45. Bethesda, Md.: Abt Associates Inc., Partnerships for Health Reform Project.

Schneider, P., F.P. Diop, and C. Leighton. 2001. *Pilot Testing Prepayment for Health Services in Rwanda: Results and Recommendations for Policy Directions and Implementation*. Technical Report No. 66. Bethesda, Md.: Abt Associates Inc., Partnerships for Health Reform Project.

Somkang, E., P. Akanzinge, T. Apau, and F. Moens. 1994. "Nkoranza Health Insurance Evaluation Report." Unpublished report. The Netherlands: Diocese of Sunyani, Ghana, and Memisa Medicus Mundi.

van Ginnekan, W., ed. 1997. *Social Security for the Informal Sector: Investigating the Feasibility of Pilot Projects in Benin, India, El Salvador and Tanzania*. Geneva: International Labour Organisation.

Vyas, J., and M. Chatterjee. 1995. "Organizing Health Insurance for Women Workers: The SEWA Experience." Paper presented at International Workshop on Health Insurance in India, September 20–22, 1995, IIM [Indian Institute of Management], Bangalore.

WHO (World Health Organization). 2000. *World Health Report 2000–Health Systems: Improving Performance*. Geneva.

CHAPTER 11

Role of Central Governments in Furthering Social Goals through Microinsurance Units

M. Kent Ranson and Sara Bennett

It must be realized that community financing is, at best, only a partial solution, that it may be more difficult and less effective than reallocation of current resources, and that governments have to encourage and facilitate—not impose—it.

—Wayne Stinson 1982, p. 42

In microinsurance, people prepay some health care costs and, through revenue pooling, the healthy cross-subsidize care for the sick.[1] Government is responsible for the overall performance of the health system. It has a responsibility to steer microinsurers so that they contribute to national health policy goals. Nonetheless, government involvement in microinsurance varies tremendously from one country to another.

Take as examples of the two extremes of government involvement the Health Card scheme in Thailand and the Bwamanda hospital insurance scheme in the Democratic Republic of Congo, both widely viewed as successful (annex 11A). Under the Thai Health Card scheme (between 1983 and 1994), financial management was conducted at the community level, but the design and implementation of the scheme (including setting of the premium and benefit package) were carefully laid out by the Ministry of Public Health (author's communication with Samrit Srithamrongsawats, 2000). In contrast, "the overall environment in which the [Bwamanda hospital insurance] initiative took place was characterized by the virtually total absence of the state, both in terms of resource allocation and in terms of planning, regulation, control, etc." (Criel 1998, p. 25). Based on the diverse experience of existing microinsurers, what can be concluded about the optimal nature and extent of government involvement?

This chapter explores the mechanisms that central governments can use to *facilitate* the development, sustainability, and impact of community-financed health insurance schemes (typically through ministries of health and social insurance schemes).[2] The first section establishes a theoretical framework for mechanisms

The authors acknowledge, with thanks, the useful comments on an earlier draft from Anne Mills, Head, Health Economics and Financing Programme, London School of Hygiene and Tropical Medicine, and from Cristian Baeza, Senior Health Economist, International Labour Office.

between government and community-financed health insurance (microinsurance) schemes. The second section reviews other authors' views on facilitating mechanisms and reviews and analyzes existing mechanisms. The last section summarizes the findings and makes suggestions regarding options available to policymakers. Throughout the chapter, the focus will be on developing countries.

CONCEPTUAL FRAMEWORK

A first step in considering how central government can further social goals through microinsurance is to assess whether or not such schemes are effective and sustainable. There is a real shortage of solid empirical evidence on this question; the studies and reviews that have been undertaken suggest that many schemes are shortlived and fail even to meet the goals they set for themselves (Stinson 1982; Bennett, Creese, and Monasch 1998). Despite this body of (less than positive) experience, several international agencies still seem to view such schemes as a possible means to improve access to cost-effective health care, particularly among the poor. The discussion below is based upon the *assumption* that microinsurance can, at a minimum, be a sustainable means to extend social protection in health, and therefore it is worthwhile for governments to consider how they can ensure that such schemes also serve broader social goals. Further research on the validity of this assumption—and under what conditions it holds—is critical to our understanding of the role that such schemes can play and consequently what government should (or should not do) to support them.

Figure 11.1 is a simple conceptual map of the associations between the government's health systems goals, obstacles to promoting these goals through microinsurance, and the categories of government mechanisms that can be used to overcome these obstacles. The two primary goals of microinsurance are to respond to the beneficiaries' health/financial needs (for example, improving access to care, preventing medical indebtedness, mobilizing health care resources, and empowering consumers) and to be financially viable and sustainable (including the ability to absorb financial shocks such as the costs of an infectious outbreak).[3] The government's broader health systems goals, to which microinsurance may be able to contribute, are better health in the target population, fair financing, and responsiveness (for example, "reducing the damage to one's dignity and autonomy, and the fear and shame that sickness often brings with it") (WHO 2000, chapter 2). Goals such as affordability, equity, accessibility, sustainability, and quality are proximal *(instrumental)* goals that are not intrinsically valuable but "are relevant rather as explanations of good or bad outcomes" (WHO 2000, p. 24). Similarly, democracy and participation are likely to be important determinants of the responsiveness of health systems but are generally not considered goals of the health care system. The goals of the microinsurer and government may not coincide. For example, a government mandate for community-financed health insurance schemes to include the poorest individuals or households—in the interest of

FIGURE 11.1   Government Goals for Microinsurers, Obstacles to Achieving Them, and Corrective Mechanisms

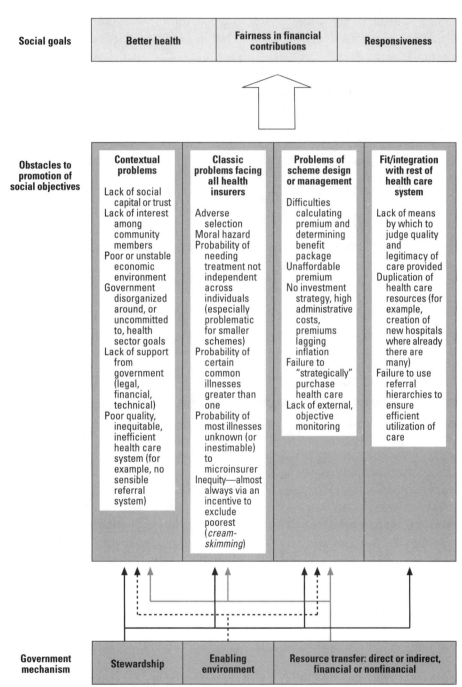

Source: Social Goals adapted from WHO 2000.

fairness of financing—might conflict with the schemes' goal of financial viability. Thus, when evaluating government mechanisms, it will be important to consider both sets of goals.

Another issue that requires further consideration, but which lies somewhat outside the scope of this chapter, is whether or not investing in microinsurance represents the most efficient means for government to achieve its social objectives. While microinsurance may represent one path to achieve improved equity, accessibility, and so on, other paths (such as greater government financing of health care) may, overall, be preferable. Ideally, governments should consider the range of strategies available to achieve goals before opting to support or work with microinsurers.

The extent of a government's commitment to its social objectives is also important in determining whether, and how, it should become involved in microinsurance. The following typology of government types is not fully developed but will allow us to explore potential negative impacts of government involvement in microinsurance and the best ways to avoid such impacts. Governments run the gamut of intentions and executive competence and are invariably a combination of these three types:

Type 1—Well-intentioned and well-executed government. Governments of this type offer the best prospects for developing an environment where microinsurers can serve social goals. However, despite the best intentions, government involvement can still change the nature of the scheme. Increased government regulation and control may change a community-financed scheme from bottom-up (participatory) to a top-down organization, where decisions are made centrally and handed down to scheme managers. Transparency, voice (or community participation), community ownership, and innovation may suffer. While some may consider community participation and ownership goals in and of themselves, there is also some evidence to suggest that community involvement can enhance the overall functioning of microinsurers. In India, for example, successes of the Mallur Milk Cooperative scheme (Dave Sen 1997) and the ACCORD scheme (Prasad 1998) were attributed in part to community organization, ownership, and participation. Lack of community participation, and isolation of the scheme from traditional and political leaders in the area, may have contributed to the downfall of the Barpali Village Scheme (Stinson 1982). In Nkoranza, Ghana, the lack of community involvement in scheme management was thought to be one of several problems that contributed to problems within the scheme (Atim 1999). Even the best of governments may find it difficult "to remain neutral in its approach of the (sometimes tense) relationship between an insurer and a provider (who may be a government facility)" (Criel 2000, p. 44).[4]

Type 2—Well-intentioned but poorly executed government. State action often has unintended consequences that create additional problems. For example, a government may enlarge or replicate microinsurance schemes, paying little attention to the traditional networks of social support that it is replacing. Likewise, government facilitation may prove harmful, if unstable or unreliable (for example, a scheme that comes to rely on government subsidies may be hard hit if the subsidies are withdrawn after a change in mandate or administration). This raises the critical question of government capacity to support such schemes.

Type 3—Poorly intentioned government. Government intervention may prove harmful in settings where government is corrupt or self-interested. Bureaucrats may prefer government-provided health insurance (social insurance) where they have direct control over resources. Alternatively, the government may see microinsurance as an easy source of income through extortion.

If government is corrupt, microinsurers should avoid government mechanisms. Under Type 2 government, capacity building may be needed, its nature and extent depending on the situation. Under a Type 1 government, experience in other settings may provide government with lessons on ways it should, or should not, intervene.

A variety of other factors may act as obstacles to microinsurers' operating successfully and contributing toward social objectives (figure 11.1). Contextual (environmental) problems relate to the economic, political, social, or cultural context in which the scheme operates. People in a poor or unstable economic setting, for example, may be unable or unwilling to participate in microinsurance. The classic problems facing all insurers include adverse selection, moral hazard, covariant risks (risks affecting groups of households, communities, regions, or nations), and unknown probability of illness (Barr 1998). Schemes may also fail to meet social objectives because of problems of design and management, for example, failing to increase premiums to keep pace with inflation and rising health care costs. Finally, microinsurers may fail to contribute to social goals if they are not well integrated with the rest of the health care system. For example, a hospital-based insurance scheme may adequately cover the risks of a high-cost hospital admission, but in the absence of a network of preventive, primary, and referral services, it may function inefficiently or fail to attract the people who need it most.

Certain government mechanisms may lessen or overcome obstacles to the success of microinsurers and their promotion of social objectives. The mechanisms used by government to facilitate microinsurance can be categorized as stewardship, creation of an enabling environment, and transfer of resources, both financial and nonfinancial. Stewardship covers developing a policy framework; implementing relevant legislation; mandating or obliging someone to perform certain activities; monitoring and regulating the quantity, quality, and price of insurance and health care; and generating and disseminating information on disease prevalence and treatment costs. The creation of an enabling environment is a broader concept that includes ensuring economic and political stability and preventing corruption in the legal, health care, and banking systems (these mechanisms are somewhat "soft" and generally fall outside the realm of the ministry of health). The transfer of resources to microinsurance may occur directly, from government to insurer, or indirectly, from government to health care provider (usually government-owned) or the insured. Resources (financial or otherwise) may be transferred regularly or routinely or only when the scheme faces bankruptcy. Non-financial transfers include targeted technical or managerial support or provision of a reinsurance function, wherein groups of microinsurers create a "solidarity" fund for protection against covariant risks.

As indicated by the arrows in figure 11.1, government stewardship mecha-nisms are usually directed toward controlling the price, quantity, and quality of insurance available on the market by regulating certain aspects of scheme design and management and ensuring that health insurers (and health care financing methods) are well integrated with the health care system. Government mecha-nisms that help provide an enabling environment for microinsurance may counter the contextual problems (for example, lack of interest or social capital in the target group) that hinder these schemes. Transfer of resources is most likely to tackle the "classic problems" of insurers (for example, the provision of reinsur-ance to counter covariant risk), or problems of scheme design and management (for example, targeted technical assistance, or financial bailout, when a scheme faces bankruptcy as a result of low premiums or overly generous benefits).

POTENTIAL AND ACTUAL MECHANISMS FOR INFLUENCING MICROINSURANCE SCHEMES

Here we describe more specifically each type of mechanism used by government to facilitate microinsurance (stewardship, creation of an enabling environment, and transfer of resources, both financial and nonfinancial). Then we discuss the goals (both microinsurance and health system) to which they might contribute and describe, where possible, scenarios in which the mechanism has been used in different places (table 11.1 and annex 11A).

Stewardship

In its stewardship role, government develops a policy framework and regulations, monitors microinsurer activities, and shares information.

Developing a policy framework. A policy framework should define the role microinsurers will play in the bigger picture of health care financing as well as the roles of other stakeholders in microinsurance (government, external donors, health care providers, and beneficiary groups). A framework should make clear which populations are best covered by microinsurance and which populations the government will cover. For example, the government of Thailand has clearly identified who should be covered by the Thai Health Card scheme (the nonpoor, largely farmers) and who falls under other schemes (the poor, elderly, children,

TABLE 11.1   Government Mechanisms in Use

Mechanism	Place used and nature of mechanism
STEWARDSHIP	
Developing policy framework	• GUINEA-BISSAU—Abota Health Insurance Schemes. Clear government guidelines exist. • INDONESIA—Dena Sehat. Government provides guidelines and training packages. • REPUBLIC OF KOREA—National Health Insurance (NHI) Class II scheme for self-employed and NHI Class IV scheme for rural populations. Government has played an important role in setting and implementing policy.
Mandating certain activities	• BANGLADESH—Gomoshathaya Kendra and Grameen Health Program (Pilot Scheme)/Grameen Health Centres. Government directive to provide preventive services, family planning, and health education, free for all, irrespective of family subscription to health insurance.
Monitoring and regulating insurance	• GUINEA-BISSAU—Abota Health Insurance Schemes. Scheme is subject to government accounting. • MADAGASCAR—Les Pharmacies Communautaires (PHACOM). Government establishes drug list (formulary) from which PHACOMs can order for their health centers. • NEPAL—Lalitpur Medical Insurance Scheme. Scheme is organized within regulations set by government. Government prepares essential drug list. • PAPUA NEW GUINEA—Pomio Government Health Centre. Scheme is subject to government accounting—officer in charge reports to Provincial Health Authority every six months. Government decides on categories of patients exempted from copayment (not premium). • PAPUA NEW GUINEA—Gaubin Health Centre. Financial reports, including both revenue and expenditure, are submitted at end of each quarter to provincial health office. • PAPUA NEW GUINEA—Tinsley Medical Insurance Scheme. Financial reports on both revenue and expenditure are submitted at end of each quarter to provincial health office. • PHILIPPINES—Federated Primary Health Care Mother's Club—Surigao City. It is registered with Securities and Exchange Commission and must maintain financial integrity. • TANZANIA—UMASIDA. Subject to government accounting procedures—Cooperatives Act controls fund reporting and accounting. Constitution of scheme has been approved by Ministry of Home Affairs. • UGANDA—Kisiizi Hospital Health Scheme. Ministry of Health evaluates scheme regularly and makes recommendations.
Monitoring and regulating health care	• PHILIPPINES—Tarlac Health Maintenance Program. Scheme follows hospital accreditation requirements issued by Philippine Medical Care Commission/Philippine Health Insurance Corporation. Department of Health provides essential drug list in National Drug Formulary, a list of reimbursable drugs and medicines. • TANZANIA—UMASIDA. Government plays implicit regulatory role by registering private providers and ensuring they deliver quality care.
ENABLING ENVIRONMENT	
Ensuring economic and political stability	• CHINA—Cooperative Medical System (CMS). Central government had key role in establishing economic and social system conducive to formation of CMS.
Social animation	• MADAGASCAR—Associations des Amis de la Santé (AAS). Government agency, l'Unité d'Appui Communautaire, sensitized and mobilized community to set up AAS.
TRANSFER OF RESOURCES	
Cash transfers	• REPUBLIC OF KOREA—National Health Insurance (NHI) Class II scheme for self-employed and NHI Class IV scheme for rural populations. Government pays 50 percent of premium.

(Table continues on the following page.)

TABLE 11.1 (continued)

Mechanism	Place used and nature of mechanism
Cash tranfers (continued)	• PHILIPPINES—Tarlac Health Maintenance Program. Channeled foreign assistance in preparation of management information system. • UGANDA—Kisiizi Hospital Health Scheme. Ministry of Health signed memorandum of understanding with hospital, undertaking to underwrite any scheme losses in first two years, up to a maximum of Ush 18,000,000 (US$13,300). Scheme would not be sustainable on membership fees alone (cost recovery 55 percent). Government has covered deficit. • CHINA—Cooperative Medical System. Central government paid staff salaries at higher level facilities. • CONGO, DEM. REP. OF—Bokoro. Government is responsible for "payment of some salaries." • CONGO, DEM. REP. OF—Kongolo Health Centre. Government pays salary of one nurse. • GUATEMALA— ASSABA, Community Health Financing Scheme. Primary care facilities are organized and financed by government. • INDIA—Voluntary Health Services, Medical AID Plan. Government finances 75 percent of community health project and 25 percent of hospital and ancillary services. • INDONESIA—Dena Sehat. Government continues to fund health care at health centers. • MADAGASCAR—Associations des Amis de la Santé (AAS). Government cofinances health posts. • MALI—Molodo (owned by government health center). Government pays two of three nurses' salaries. • PAPUA NEW GUINEA—Pomio Government Health Centre. Government pays salaries. • PAPUA NEW GUINEA—Palmalmal Health Centre. Government pays salaries. • PAPUA NEW GUINEA—Tinsley Medical Insurance Scheme. Government pays 80 percent of salaries and operating costs. • UGANDA—Tororo Hospital Treatment Cards. Government pays for all hospital operating costs, partially offset by user fees and premiums. • UGANDA—Pallisa Community Development Trust. Government pays for essential drug supplies, training and supportive supervision, and bicycles for immunization.
Nonfinancial transfers	• GUINEA-BISSAU—Abota Health Insurance Schemes. Government subsidizes cost of 12 essential drugs and also provides some "simple equipment." Village health workers (primary caregivers under scheme) are nonpaid volunteers. They do receive training and supervision from government workers. • INDIA—Self-Employed Women's Association. For scheme's first two years, government (through semiautonomous Government Insurance Corporation) was responsible for both pooling and reimbursement, but not for revenue collection. Otherwise, no transfer of resources. • KENYA—Chogoria Hospital Insurance Scheme. Ministry of Health has provided technical assistance through Kenya Health Care Financing Project, funded by U.S. Agency for International Development. • NEPAL—Lalitpur Medical Insurance Scheme. Government supplies every health post with annual stock of essential drugs. • PHILIPPINES—Tarlac Health Maintenance Program. Government provided technical assistance in preparation of program's benefit package and premium calculation. • UGANDA—Kisiizi Hospital Health Scheme. Ministry of Health provided technical assistance as well as computer equipment and peripherals.

Source: Unpublished database compiled to write *Health Insurance Schemes for People Outside Formal Sector Employment* (Bennett, Creese, and Monasch 1998).

and formal-sector workers (annex 11A). Government's policy must be well coordinated, and the state should avoid targeting safety-net programs to specific types of individuals or households (for example, children, the elderly) if doing so is likely to damage existing group schemes (World Bank 2001, p. 149).

The policy framework may further indicate the types of health care interventions best covered by microinsurance, a topic still being debated. Microinsurance might best complement the government system by covering high-cost, hospital-based care in countries where the government health system focuses on providing an "essential package" of primary health care interventions (World Bank 1993). In countries where government hospital services are of acceptable quality and accessibility, microinsurance might best fill in the gaps by covering primary-level curative care (at health centers, community hospitals).

In Guinea-Bissau, the Ministry of Public Health has outlined specific responsibilities for village leaders that are related to community-level prepayment schemes (box 11.1; Eklund and Stavem 1995, pp. 210–11). The primary goal of

---

BOX 11.1   GUINEA-BISSAU: PARTICIPANT RESPONSIBILITIES

The responsibilities defined by the Ministry of Public Health for participants in community health insurance prepayment schemes include:

- The village decides on the prepayment scheme fees (whether per capita, per adult, or per household) and on the timing of payments.

- The village must collect funds under the prepayment system to ensure that initial drug supplies are continually replenished. Drugs are sold to USBs (village health posts) with substantial subsidies, set at the central level and equal across regions.

- Some villages create special health subcommittees to oversee USB operations, but in the smaller villages the political committee executes those responsibilities.

- The village provides labor and most construction materials for building the health post. The Ministry of Public Health provides materials for windows, doors, and hinges.

- The government supplies simple equipment, including a metal cupboard for storing drugs, a bed, a stretcher, four chairs, one obstetrical stethoscope, one lantern, a kit of posters and other teaching aids, and an initial stock of drugs estimated to last for six months (for the population of each village).

- The village selects one or more residents to be trained as village health workers and midwives.

Source: Eklund and Stavem 1995, pp. 210–11.

the prepayment schemes in Guinea-Bissau is to improve the availability of drugs and first aid in "widely scattered" rural villages. The policy framework allows a high degree of autonomy in scheme management (the village decides who will manage the scheme, who will do the work, and what the premium will be) and holds the village accountable for such work as constructing a health post and replenishing initial drug stocks.

Regulating microinsurance. Government may regulate almost any function of microinsurance, including revenue collection (insurance price or premium), pooling, and purchasing of health care (contents of the benefit package, "quantity" of coverage for specific interventions, speed of reimbursement, nature of provider payment, quality of covered health care services). The World Health Organization (WHO), for example, argues that the pooling function of health insurers—which determines the extent of redistribution from healthy to ill, and wealthy to poor—can be maximized by regulations that enforce community rating (adjusting for the average risk of a group), portable employment-based pooling (insurance that a worker keeps when changing jobs), and equal minimum benefit packages (access to the same services in all pools) (WHO 2000, p. 103). Standard economic theory also sheds light on regulations that can be used to optimize the efficiency of microinsurance. For example, Barr (1998, pp. 287–88) writes about government interventions for dealing with adverse selection and moral hazard.

A mandated activity is one that *must* be performed, and mandates are usually specified in law (Musgrove 1996, p. 6).[5] The government of Bangladesh, for example, mandates that two large insurance schemes operating in the country (Gomoshathaya Kendra [GK] health care system and Grameen health program) provide "preventive services, family planning and health education, free for all, irrespective of family subscription to the health insurance scheme" (Desmet, Chowdhury, and Islam 1999, p. 928). The impact of this mandate—an attempt to improve equity of the health care system and provide priority preventive care—is not clear. The GK system insures roughly one-quarter of its target population, yet the uninsured account for a disproportionately small 1.5 percent of GK clinic attendees (Desmet, Chowdhury, and Islam 1999).

An alternative approach to mandating, which may be used to deal with adverse selection and moral hazard, is to require membership in a microinsurance scheme. Making insurance compulsory prevents low risks from opting out and the externalities caused by noninsurance. This approach could be implemented by starting coverage before birth to cope with the congenitally and chronically ill, preventing insurance companies from withholding coverage from high-risk individuals, and regulating the conditions under which microinsurers could increase premiums. Key questions here are, How feasible is community-level mandating in developing countries, where many unknowns (for example, income, population base) make social health insurance unfeasible? Does mandating membership in a scheme automatically change the scheme's nature, so that it is viewed as a government imposition instead of a community initiative? In the district of

Boboye, Niger, the Ministry of Public Health implemented a scheme in which people were required to pay an "annual tax" that was pooled at the district level, managed by a health committee (nongovernment), and used primarily to finance pharmaceutical products (Diop, Yazbeck, and Bitran 1995). Although not discussed by the study's authors, community participation in this pilot scheme seems to have been minimal.

Government regulation has occurred around many microinsurers, but the literature provides only limited information on the reasons for such regulation and its impact. Until recently in India (January 2000), only state agencies were permitted to sell insurance. In Georgia, only private health insurance companies may manage an insurance scheme. At least in the case of Georgia, this intervention would appear to be a case of poorly intentioned government (protecting the business of a few private insurers) instead of a government attempting to achieve social goals. Depending on the extent to which such restrictions are coupled with monitoring and enforcement, they can seriously hinder microinsurers.

The monitoring and enforcement implicit in many regulations is resource- and skill-intensive and might not be feasible for many developing-country governments. This situation applies particularly to risk adjustment, ensuring a basic minimum benefit package, and community rating (WHO 2000). Evidence on the effectiveness of health sector regulation in developing countries is limited, but the evidence that does exist points to major problems confronting government in implementing regulation (Mills 2000, chapter 7). Although regulating health insurance may be somewhat more straightforward than regulating health services, the difference is marginal, and lack of government capacity to regulate is a major constraint.

Several microinsurers are reportedly subject to government accounting regulations (table 11.1). These regulations are intended to catch any fiscal irregularities, and so protect the scheme's financial viability and its members. The UMASIDA scheme in Tanzania, like other health insurance organizations in the country, is registered with the Ministry of Home Affairs (van Ginneken 1997). Reporting and accounting of UMASIDA funds is controlled by the Cooperatives Act, but how these funds are "controlled" is not clear (Bennett, Creese, and Monasch 1998). It would probably be quite straightforward to figure out what kind of control is exerted—but again this "control" is probably of a very generic nature and does not help to achieve social goals in any broad way but just to prevent misuse of funds. In some cases, governments have prepared essential drug lists limiting insurance-covered drugs (for example, the PHACOM scheme in Madagascar, the Tarlac Health Maintenance Program in the Philippines, and the Lalitpur Medical Insurance Scheme in Nepal; Bennett, Creese, and Monasch 1998). This can encourage efficiency (and also safety) and, as a consequence, financial viability.

Monitoring and regulating health care. Governments can assist microinsurers by indicating which providers are eligible to enter into a contract with an insurer (typically based on some quality-of-care measure). Such action can help a microinsurer optimize the quality and efficiency of health care purchased. In selecting its providers, the Tarlac Health Maintenance Program in the Philippines uses the hospital accreditation requirements issued by the Philippine Medical Care Commission/Philippine Health Insurance Corporation (Bennett, Creese, and Monasch 1998). Failure of the government of India to regulate or accredit hospitals means that some health care, financed under the Self-Employed Women's Association (SEWA) Medical Insurance Fund, has been of poor, if not dangerous, quality (Ranson and John 2001).

Information sharing. Government can provide information that is useful to insurers in setting premiums and benefit packages. This might include information on disease prevalence, relative quality of facilities, and relative or recommended cost of different interventions. Governments can also ensure that the parties responsible for the schemes have the opportunity to share experiences and discuss strategies. An "umbrella" body may serve as a useful partnership forum (Bennett, Creese, and Monasch 1998). An example of such an umbrella body is the Uganda Community-Based Health Financing Association (Musau 1999).

Creating an Enabling Environment

The creation of an enabling environment, although clearly important, encompasses a broad range of activities. In fact virtually every government activity, from economic promotion to education, could be seen as contributing to an enabling environment. This vast range of activities cannot be covered here. We focus only upon activities directly linked to microinsurance, social animation, legal recognition, and control of corruption.

Social animation. Government may act as a catalyst for helping disparate parts of the community work together. In Madagascar, the government agency l'Unité d'Appui Communautaire sensitized the community to set up the community-financed insurer, Associations des Amis de la Santé (AAS) (Bennett, Creese, and Monasch 1998).

Legal recognition of businesses/ventures. To have legal status in many countries, schemes have to register as a club, cooperative, nongovernmental organization (NGO), or some other type of organization. Once registered, the scheme is formally bound by whatever regulations cover that type of organization. Normally, these regulations include some provision for presenting full accounts to members (and possibly to government). A legal framework should allow microinsurers to establish contracts with health care providers and to seek assistance or compensation if a provider fails to fulfill the contract. The organization's status may also affect whether or not it pays taxes; if so, how much; and what happens to any profit (for example, reinvested or distributed to members). These laws are part of government efforts to create an enabling environment for all types of businesses.

Control of corruption. Under-the-counter payments, if widespread, can present a significant barrier to the development of microinsurance. For a microinsurer to operate successfully, providers must depend upon formal payments alone for their pay (otherwise beneficiaries pay double). However, providers are often reluctant to refuse informal payments, a large and tax-free addition to their income. Although it is generally thought that governments can play an important role in aiding the removal of informal payments, there are few concrete suggestions on ways to do so.

Transfer of Resources

Government can transfer resources to microinsurers directly, indirectly, or through reinsurance.

Direct transfer. The government can make financial contributions directly to a microinsurer, either regularly or during financial crisis. In two cases, the National Health Insurance scheme in the Republic of Korea and the Thai Health Card scheme, government makes a matching contribution equal to the amount collected in premiums (annex 11A). Governments can also provide technical and managerial assistance to individual schemes. Technical skills may be required to assess ability and willingness to pay; analyze cost and expected income; calculate fees, premiums, and other charges; measure utilization; develop systems (financial, management, or health information) for recording routinely all income and expenditures, and conducting monitoring and evaluation. In the Philippines, the Tarlac Health Maintenance Program was provided technical assistance to prepare its benefit package and calculate premiums. Uganda's Ministry of Health provided the Kisiizi Hospital Scheme with technical assistance as well as computer equipment and peripherals. With financial support from the Department for International Development (DfID), Uganda's Ministry of Health acted as financial guarantor to the Kisiizi Hospital Health Scheme up to a loss equivalent to Ush 18 million (US$13,300) during its first two years of operation. In 1997/98, the government contributed Ush 10 million to the scheme in "compensation" for excess claims arising from a malaria epidemic (Musau 1999, p. 21). All these transfers would be likely to facilitate scheme financial viability. Some might also facilitate efficiency.

Indirect transfers. Indirect transfers through providers seem common, particularly when the providers are government owned. Schemes in which the government covers staff salaries at the health care provider include the Cooperative Medical System in China, the Bokoro and Kongolo schemes in the Democratic Republic of Congo, the ASSABA in Guatemala, the AAS in Madagascar, and the Tororo Hospital Treatment Cards scheme in Uganda. Government can make financial contributions to households (or communities) and recommend or require (for example, by providing vouchers) that they be put toward community-financed health insurance. Such transfers may be risk equalizing if they compensate for socioeconomic differences (and hence differences in risks) between households and regions.

"Tied transfers." Tied transfers (direct and indirect) are subsidies that encourage use of preventive care, primary care, and essential drugs (for example, bicycles provided specifically for use in offering immunizations). The government of Guinea-Bissau subsidizes the cost of the 12 essential drugs used by the Abota schemes. Similarly, the government of Nepal supplies the Lalitpur Medical Insurance scheme with its annual stock of essential drugs.

One important question concerns the best way for government to provide financial support—as direct subsidies to a scheme, as indirect subsidies through providers, or as tied subsidies. Economists usually prefer untied to tied subsidies. Assuming a rational and fully informed insurer and insured population and a competitive insurance market, insurers are theoretically more likely than government to use these funds efficiently, given competitive market forces. However, it may be argued that subsidies would be more efficiently used if channeled through government providers or tied to certain goods or activities, considering the many imperfections of the health care market (for example, information asymmetries, externalities, monopoly providers). Problems arise due to the government's intentions (poorly versus well intentioned) and effectiveness (poorly versus well executed). Tied subsidies from a poorly intentioned or poorly executed government could hinder a microinsurer's ability to achieve social goals. For example, government subsidies for immunizations and other preventive care may deter a microinsurer from fulfilling the goals set by scheme planners and members such as protection from the high costs of hospital care. Similarly, subsidies channeled indirectly through government providers may not promote efficiency, if the government facilities are undersupplied and understaffed, as they often are. At present, there are insufficient data to suggest that one type of subsidy is superior to others. Research may help to determine the impact of different types of subsidy on health insurance and health care consumption, and ultimately, on the distal health systems goals.

Reinsurance. Government may set up a reinsurance scheme (or solidarity fund). Participating microinsurers contribute to this pool, and the resources are used to finance unexpected expenditure (for example, epidemics and other covariant risks). Government may establish this fund but not contribute to the pooled resources or establish the fund and make some contribution to the pooled resources (a combination of reinsurance and subsidy). Among developing countries, a reinsurance fund has been established only in Thailand. The Thai government has established a pool at the central level to facilitate risk sharing among provincial and community funds. The individual schemes send 2.5 percent of premium revenues to this central fund. This fund appears to be used either when people need health care outside their province of residence or costly services (for example, referral to a university hospital). As a result of managerial problems rather than a lack of suitable cases, this fund has been underutilized (only 10 percent of the fund was used in 1995 and 1996), according to Pannarunothai and others (2000). Given the very limited experience, it is not clear what financial resources, managerial capacities, or broader institutional features a government would have to possess to successfully reinsure. It seems that while reinsurance may not place quite the same extensive demands upon government capacity as social health insurance, it still requires actuarial, financial, and regulatory skills, which are frequently lacking in developing countries. As an alternative to reinsurance—one for which the infrastructure is already in place in most developing countries—government could heavily subsidize the cost of what is perceived as necessary but high-cost care. Government ownership of public facilities where such services are provided obviates the need for reinsurance.

SUMMARY, DISCUSSION, AND CONCLUSIONS

Sadly, despite the intense interest in the role of microinsurance, empirical evidence is still lacking about the extent to which microinsurance can help serve broader social goals, and the circumstance under which it—rather than other tools at a government's disposal—is likely to be the most effective means to pursue such social goals. Prior to implementing mechanisms to work with micro-insurers, governments should seriously consider whether this is the best strategy to further its objectives.

Having made this decision, governments can facilitate the development, viability, and impact of microinsurance through a variety of mechanisms that have been used in developing countries. The objective in implementing the mechanism and the actual impact of the mechanism are rarely reported in the literature.

The most common type of mechanism is the indirect transfer of resources from government to microinsurer, usually in the form of free or reduced-cost health care services at government facilities. There are also many reports of scheme regulation by government, but the precise nature of the regulation is often not evident. Seldom-used mechanisms include reinsurance, legislation that confers official status on the schemes, mandates that would require schemes to perform certain activities or enroll certain populations, and mechanisms to share health-related information with schemes (for example, on disease prevalence or cost of care).

With some confidence we can conclude that:

- Broad policy statements by government are helpful, particularly in creating an environment conducive to building confidence in microinsurers (otherwise people may worry that schemes will be shut down).

- Regulation of microinsurers should be embarked upon only with caution in developing countries. Given capacity constraints and the fact that regulation is so often perverted to serve private interests, it should be used with a very light touch. Tighter government control over schemes may stifle innovation and limit their variety, another reason for not encouraging too much regulation. Any regulation used should be simple and easy to understand.

- Mandating scheme membership, for example at the level of local or village government, is an interesting idea, but we have limited evidence on how it works and how feasible it is to implement in the contexts where microinsurance can make the biggest contribution.

- Environment is important—but we have little understanding of the impact of government measures on environment (how frequently does government succeed at uniting disparate groups?). Nor do we fully understand the effects of the environment upon the scheme (for example, how important is trust among members, or between members and the insurer or provider, to the success of a scheme?).

- Technical assistance of adequate quality is desirable and not very controversial.

- Financial support is critical but it is not clear how this should be delivered. Is it best to provide regular and sustained financial support or only when schemes are financially strained (for example, resulting from poor investment strategy, a disproportionately old or sick enrolled population, or premiums set too low)? If governments provide support in the first two scenarios, they run the risk of fostering inefficiently managed schemes. However, this type of support may be required if governments do wish to encourage coverage of populations that are poorer and at higher risk of illness. Microinsurers may require reinsurance against covariant risks, but the question is whether, to what extent, and how reinsurance should be coupled with other forms of financial/technical support.

International donors can do much to facilitate beneficial mechanisms between government and microinsurers.

- They can recommend that poorly intentioned governments (Type 3) stay away from microinsurance.

- They can help build capacity among well-intentioned but poorly executed governments (Type 2).

- Among well-intentioned, well-executed governments (Type 1), they can recommend mechanisms discussed above, encourage research on the relative impact of mechanisms, and help disseminate the lessons learned.

Future research should examine the association between specific mechanisms and their impact on microinsurers' goals (for example, financial viability or consumer satisfaction) and health-system goals (equity, efficiency, and universal coverage).

The optimal package of mechanisms will vary from one country to another, and within one country as it moves through different stages of development, particularly as health insurance coverage increases. For example, in a developing country with a small formal sector (5 to 10 percent of the population), government might best limit its activities to establishing a receptive economic and policy environment, perhaps including broad policy statements relevant to different actors in the health care system. As the formal sector grows, and the health care and health financing system become more complex (encompassing some form of social insurance as well as for-profit and microinsurance), government might implement targeted financial and nonfinancial schemes to facilitate microinsurance development and foster efficiency and equity. Once microinsurers are well established, government might implement specific regulations to standardize the price, volume, and quality of insurance available in the country, with universal social security coverage the goal.[6]

ANNEX 11A FIVE CASE STUDIES

INDIA—SELF-EMPLOYED WOMEN'S ASSOCIATION

References: Ranson and John 2001; Chatterjee and Vyas 1997.

Location: Ahmedabad, Gujarat, India.

Members: The Medical Insurance Fund covers some 32,000 members in 10 districts. To join the Fund, one must be female, between the ages of 18 and 58, and a member of the SEWA, an organization of poor, self-employed women.

Scheme description: SEWA's Integrated Social Security Scheme was initiated in 1992. It provides life, medical, and asset insurance (against the loss of house or working capital in case of flood, fire, or communal riots). The Medical Insurance Fund is owned and managed by SEWA, an NGO. Women joining the Fund either pay a yearly premium or a fixed deposit. For *hospitalization* (outpatient care is not covered), the insured seeks care from the public or private provider of her choice and pays out-of-pocket for the hospitalization at the time of discharge. She must then submit doctors' certificates and receipts to SEWA. If the claim is approved, the insured receives reimbursement to a maximum of 1,200 rupees. Certain chronic ("preexisting") diseases are excluded from coverage. Women who join by paying the fixed deposit (instead of the annual premium) are entitled to certain special benefits (for example, reimbursement for cataract surgery, hearing aids, and dentures).

Government mechanisms: *Initially technical support, now nothing.* During the first two years of the scheme (1992–94), SEWA collected premiums and passed them on to the United India Insurance Company (UIIC), a semiautonomous government agency. The UIIC was responsible for reviewing claims, deciding the amount of reimbursement, and making the reimbursement. A number of problems were responsible for the discontinuation of this partnership: women often could not produce the documentation required; collecting the documentation involved high travel and photocopying costs; claims were often processed late; and the UIIC did not cover certain types of hospitalization (for example, occupational illnesses and gynecological diseases). Today, government plays a minimal role: no regulation of health care or (nonprofit) health insurance providers and no financial or technical transfers.

UGANDA—KISIIZI HOSPITAL HEALTH SOCIETY

Reference: Musau 1999.

Location: Rukungiri district of southwestern Uganda.

Members: 6,580 individuals (in 1,400 households in 32 Engozi (burial and ambulance) societies). The target population is the 100,000 people living in the catchment area of this 180-bed, Church of Uganda mission hospital.

Scheme description: the minister of health launched the Kisiizi Hospital Health Society in August 1996. The scheme is managed by the hospital (two full-time staff in the Community-Based Health Care Department) with inputs from chairmen of Engozi societies. Premiums are collected every three months by local Engozi societies. Premiums vary according to family size. Benefits include discounts on outpatient and inpatient care at Kisiizi Hospital and outreach clinics (including chronic diseases and delivery, if the patient goes for regularly scheduled checkups). Members pay only the copayment fee on a hospital admission; the scheme pays the hospital directly for the rest of their treatment.

Government mechanisms: *Stewardship, financial and nonfinancial transfers.* The scheme is recognized and supported by the Ministry of Health (MOH) and actively supervised through its Planning Department. How the commissioner of insurance views the schemes in Uganda is not yet clear. The Uganda Community-Based Health Financing Association is clarifying this and other legal issues on behalf of all the member schemes.

At the inception of the scheme, the MOH, through funding from the DfID, agreed to underwrite losses during the first two years up to a maximum of Ush 18 million (US$13,300). The MOH also implicitly accepted responsibility for losses arising from epidemics and reimbursed the scheme for a loss of Ush 8.5 million from a malaria epidemic in 1998. The MOH also provided computer equipment and peripherals, and under the DfID project, technical assistance.

RWANDA—PILOT SCHEMES IN THREE DISTRICTS

Reference: Schneider, Diop, and Sosthene 2000.

Location: Three of Rwanda's 40 health districts (Kabutare, Byumba, and Kabgayi).

Members: 88,000 members in first year of operation. The target population is the 1.1 million people living in the three districts.

Scheme description: Initiated in 1999, the schemes are managed within communities, usually in collaboration with health care providers. By paying an annual premium of FRw 2,500 per family, members are entitled, after a one-month waiting period, to a basic (government or church-owned) health center package, covering all services and drugs provided at their preferred health center; ambulance referral to the (government or church-owned) district hospital; and a limited package at the district hospital (C-section, overnight stay, physician consultation). Members pay a copayment of FRw 100 per episode of care at the health center. Prepayment schemes reimburse health centers by capitation payment and the hospital by a per-episode payment.

Government mechanisms: *Stewardship, financial and nonfinancial transfers.* Rwanda's National Health Policy of 1995 laid the groundwork for developing and implementing community-based health financing schemes. The MOH launched the prepayment schemes and conducted an awareness campaign (newspaper, radio, TV) in the three districts. A steering committee of government, donor, church, and community representatives from the central and regional levels plays the role of the strategic decisionmaker, overseeing the development and implementation process. At the district level, community representatives, meeting in workshops, discussed the health care services that they thought should be covered, and sent their findings to the steering committee. Based on these findings, the steering committee wrote the by-laws, the schemes' legal basis, and the contract between prepayment schemes and providers.

Funded by the USAID, the schemes receive extensive technical support and monitoring through the MOH, but no government money. Health facilities receive about 10 percent of their total revenue from the government in the form of salaries paid to government employees at the health center.

THAILAND—THAI HEALTH CARD SCHEME

References: Pannarunothai and others 2000; author's communication with Samrit Srithamrongsawats.

Location: Thailand, countrywide.

Note: The scheme was "community-based" between 1983 and 1994. Now it is "owned and managed" by the government of Thailand.

Members: 1.24 million members (25 percent of the target population). The target population is farmers and workers in the informal sector.

Scheme description: Established 1983 as a pilot study, the scheme, designed by the government of Thailand, was expanded to the whole country in 1987. From 1983 to 1994, the fund was managed at the community level; now it is managed at the provincial level. The scheme covers comprehensive basic health service packages, excluding some dental and cosmetic health services as well as services in the private wards. Cardholders have to go to designated public facilities for care.

Government mechanisms: A pre-health card entitles the bearer to health care. Thailand previously had a good deal of experience with village drug funds, nutrition funds, sanitation funds, and mother-child health funds.

Phase 1 (1983–87). Initially, the premiums, collected by health volunteers, were retained at the community level. The unit of membership (individual versus family), cost of the card, and benefits covered varied considerably from province to province and within provinces. The government did not provide direct subsidies to the scheme. However, because all health care purchased under the scheme was public, indirect transfers were likely through the government providers. The Ministry of Public Health (MOPH) was involved in monitoring and evaluation, with support from German Technical Corporation (GTZ), perhaps more so in project districts.

Phase 2 (1987–94). The health card scheme was incorporated into the structure of the Sixth National Health Development Plan in 1987. In 1991, a Health Insurance Office was established at the MOPH to execute the National Health Card Programme. A formal information system was introduced in project provinces. Schemes were managed at the provincial level, but provinces also "agreed" on card price, beneficiaries, benefit packages, referral requirements, and fund management and allocation.

Phase 3 (1994 to present). Now managed at the provincial level, the scheme receives a 50 percent ("matching") government subsidy. The original scheme was strictly regulated, with minimal community participation, but no direct transfer of financial resources. Now, the government closely coordinates and monitors the scheme. Nonpoor, largely rural people are covered by the health card scheme. The poor, the elderly, children, and formal-sector workers are covered separately. Premiums and benefit packages are standardized. To facilitate portability of cardholders and risk sharing among provincial funds, risks are pooled at the central level, and 2.5 percent of total premiums goes to the central fund (started in 1995).

DEMOCRATIC REPUBLIC OF CONGO—BWAMANDA HOSPITAL INSURANCE SCHEME

Reference: Criel 1998.

Location: Northwest of the Democratic Republic of Congo.

Members: Roughly 60 percent of the population is covered. The target population is the 159,000 (1994) people living in the district.

Scheme description: The scheme was launched in 1986 by "district health authorities." Members pay a community-rated premium once a year. The household is the subscription unit. Risk coverage is limited to hospital care, with a 20 percent copayment rate.

Government mechanisms: *Minimal* (Criel 1998, p. 24). Under the Congolese decentralization policy, health districts were to be largely self-financed. The overall environment in which the initiative took place was characterized by the virtually total absence of the state, both in terms of resource allocation and in terms of planning, regulation, and control. This de facto vacuum left district teams with almost complete autonomy to manage (or not manage) the health systems for which they were responsible.

NOTES

1. Microinsurance is also referred to as *community-financed health insurance* and *mutual health insurance*. If a community-financing scheme includes prepayment, but no pooling, it is not an insurance scheme, but personal prepayment. For example, schemes that cover only preventive care (annual check-ups, prenatal visits) cannot be considered insurance and will not be discussed in this chapter.

2. Discussion in this paper will be limited to schemes that are community financed (via premiums collected from the beneficiaries) and which are owned and/or managed by an NGO or by a *governmental agency* at the district level or below. We have excluded schemes that are owned and/or managed by central or state governments (including some of the schemes reviewed by Bennett, Creese, and Monasch 1998).

3. We have not included efficiency and equity as goals in themselves; efficiency underlies the scheme's ability to maintain financial viability, and equity may be defined differently and given different importance from one microinsurer to another.

4. The parentheses within the quote are those of the original author.

5. Regulation is different insofar as it determines *how* an activity may be undertaken, but a private producer can react to regulation by choosing not to undertake the activity at all (Musgrove 1996, pp. 6–7).

6. See annex 11A for a description of evolving government mechanisms around the Thai Health Card scheme.

REFERENCES

Atim, C. 1999. "Social Movements and Health Insurers: A Critical Evaluation of Voluntary, Non-profit Insurance Schemes with Case Studies from Ghana and Cameroon." *Social Science and Medicine* 48(7):881–96.

Barr, N. 1998. *The Economics of the Welfare State.* Oxford: Oxford University Press.

Bennett, S., A. Creese, and R. Monasch. 1998. *Health Insurance Schemes for People Outside Formal Sector Employment.* Geneva: World Health Organization, Division of Analysis, Research and Assessment.

Chatterjee, M., and J. Vyas. 1997. *Organizing Insurance for Women Workers: The SEWA Experience.* Ahmedabad: Self-Employed Women's Association.

Criel, B. 1998. "District-Based Health Insurance in Sub-Saharan Africa: Part II, Case-Studies." *Studies in Health Services Organization and Policy* 10:1–91.

_____. 2000. "Local Health Insurance Systems in Developing Countries: A Policy Research Paper." Antwerp: Departement Volksgezondheid Instituut voor Tropische Geneeskunde. Commissioned by the Directorate-General International Cooperation, DGIC, Brussels.

Dave Sen, P. 1997. "Community Control of Health Financing in India: A Review of Local Experiences." Bethesda, Md.: Abt Associates Inc.

de Ferranti, D. 1986. "Paying for Health Care in Developing Countries." Washington, D.C.: World Bank.

Desmet, M., A.Q. Chowdhury, and K. Islam. 1999. "The Potential for Social Mobilisation in Bangladesh: The Organization and Functioning of Two Health Insurance Schemes." *Social Science and Medicine* 48(7):925–38.

Diop, F., A. Yazbeck, and R. Bitran. 1995. "The Impact of Alternative Cost Recovery Schemes on Access and Equity in Niger." *Health Policy and Planning* 10(3):223–40.

Eklund, P., and K. Stavem. 1995. "Community Health Insurance Through Prepayment Schemes in Guinea-Bissau." In P.R. Shaw and M. Ainsworth, eds., *Financing Health Services through User Fees and Insurance: Case Studies from Sub-Saharan Africa*. Washington, D.C.: World Bank.

Mills, A. 2000. "Reforming Health Sectors: Fashions, Passions and Common Sense." *Reforming Health Sectors*. London: M.A., Kegan Paul International.

Musau, S.N. 1999. "Community-Based Health Insurance: Experiences and Lessons Learned from East and Southern Africa." Bethesda, Md.: Abt Associates Inc.

Musgrove, P. 1996. *Public and Private Roles in Health: Theory and Financing Patterns*. Washington, D.C.: World Bank.

Pannarunothai, S., S. Srithamrongsawad, M. Kongpaen, and P. Thamwanna. 2000. "Financing Reform of the Thai Health Card Scheme." *Health Policy and Planning* 15(3):303–11.

Prasad, K.V.E. 1998. "Health Insurance for Tribals: ACCORD's Experience in Gudalur, Tamil Nadu." In W. van Ginneken, ed., *Social Security for All Indians*. Delhi: Oxford University Press.

Ranson, M.K., and K.R. John. 2001. "Quality of Hysterectomy Care in Rural Gujarat: The Role of Community-based Health Insurance" *Health Policy and Planning* 16(4):395–403.

Schneider, P., F. Diop, B. Sosthene. 2000. *Development and Implementation of Prepayment Schemes in Rwanda*. Bethesda, Md.: Abt Associates Inc.

Stinson, W. 1982. "Community Financing of Primary Health Care." *Primary Health Care Issues* 1(4):1–90.

van Ginneken, W., ed. 1997. "Social Security for the Informal Sector: Investigating the Feasibility of Pilot Projects in Benin, El Salvador, India and Tanzania." *Issues in Social Protection*. Geneva: International Labour Office.

World Bank. 1993. *World Development Report 1993: Investing in Health*. Washington, D.C.: World Bank.

_____. 2001. *World Development Report—2000/2001: Attacking Poverty*. Oxford: Oxford University Press.

WHO (World Health Organization). 2000. *The World Health Report 2000: Health Systems: Improving Performance*. Geneva.

CHAPTER 12

Regulatory Environment for Microinsurance and Reinsurance

Frank G. Feeley

The legal structure under which insurance and reinsurance schemes operate varies widely from country to country. Developed countries created insurance regulations as a form of consumer protection. The rules are designed to keep insurance companies solvent, to force them to perform on the insurance obligations they incur, and sometimes to provide partial protection to the insured if an insurer goes bankrupt. The rules are also intended to protect consumers from deceptive or discriminatory practices by insurers. These protections have been elaborated to a greater or lesser degree in different countries. The extent to which such regulations have been adopted in developing countries varies greatly with the colonial heritage, the level of private insurance activity in the economy, and the sophistication of the legal system.

The regulatory environment will be an important element in planning the reinsurance business. Regulations can determine the required amount of capital *(policyholder surplus),* influence corporate structure and management, and increase the cost of accounting and information systems. Such regulations may also govern the way in which reinsurers will interact with their clients, the microinsurance units that actually provide health coverage to enrolled individuals and families. Depending on the exact structure of the relationship with a microinsurer or community health plan, reinsurance might be classed as a primary insurer, rather than a reinsurer, thus bringing into play additional regulations. In certain circumstances, designating reinsurance as an insurer might reduce the burden of regulation on the individual microinsurers.

Understanding the applicable regulations is a key element in locating the first experiment with reinsurance. The regulatory regime may govern not only the

This chapter was prepared based upon the author's experience with health insurance and insurance regulation in the United States and other countries, including an outline prepared in 1995 of topics that might be regulated under voluntary health insurance legislation in the Russian Federation.

The author is indebted to discussions over the years on these matters with Professor Wendy K. Mariner, Boston University School of Public Health, and Nancy Turnbull, Harvard School of Public Health. The author is also grateful to Nicole Tapay, recently of the World Bank, now of the Organisation for Economic Co-operation and Development, for her comments on the draft.

site of the experiment but also the country where the reinsurer is incorporated. If successful, the reinsurer would want to expand and would have to consider the impact of regulation in each country before entering the new market. For this reason, we set out here a list of the regulatory issues that *may* be encountered. Not all issues will arise in each country.

In addition to looking at the regulations that may apply to reinsurance, we look briefly at the rules that may apply to the health plans reinsured by reinsurance and at the effect such rules might have on the relationship between reinsurance and the individual microinsurer. In the concluding section of the chapter, we look at the rules that apply to reinsurance in the Philippines, the current target for experimental operations. We have highlighted the salient points for the design of reinsurance and its operations.

BASIC REGULATIONS THAT MAY APPLY

In developing a strategy for regulatory compliance of reinsurance, first we have to understand the requirements an entity must meet simply because it is in the "business of insurance." These rules will determine corporate structure and capitalization. A reinsurer may choose, initially, to seek exemption from some or all of the rules applicable to ordinary insurance companies because of its extraordinary social purpose.

Licensing

In most industrial economies, the government must license a company before it can sell insurance products. The license is subject to periodic renewal and can be revoked for failure to meet certain financial and reporting standards. The license may be issued by an insurance commission or by a branch of the finance ministry. Such licenses are usually issued by the national government, but in the United States, state governments license insurance companies.

An insurance license may give a company the right to participate in the business of insurance generally, or it may be specific to certain products—for example, life insurance, casualty and accident insurance, or health insurance. Statutory definitions of the "business of insurance" differ, but generally state that *insurance* is any activity in which a company assumes risk by taking payments (premiums) from individuals or companies and contractually agreeing to pay a stipulated benefit or compensation if certain contingencies (death, accident, illness) occur during a defined period.

Ownership

The first question in applying for an insurance license is: What is the domicile of the applicant company? A series of questions follow:

- Can a company that is incorporated elsewhere obtain a license?

- If the insurance license is limited to domestic companies, can the local subsidiary of a foreign company obtain a license?

- If so, is there any ceiling on the percentage of the domestic company that can be owned by the foreign parent or foreign investors?

- Do the regulations prescribe how "ownership" or control is determined—by percentage of common stock or by some other means?

Some sophisticated jurisdictions have rules that apply to the parent or "holding" company to control transactions that might "milk" the locally licensed insurer or hide its true ownership.

Because of past insurance swindles, some jurisdictions have rules controlling who may become an officer or director of an insurance company. Individuals convicted of certain crimes, or involved in questionable insurance practices, can be barred from these positions. Under such laws, the applicant company must submit resumes of its candidate officers and directors, and often must supply affidavits concerning their prior conduct. The regulator may reject a candidate and force the applicant company to appoint another director or officer before approving a license.

In the case of a reinsurer, it is unlikely that directors or officers would not be found "fit" to run an insurance company. However, it is important to determine if all, or a certain percentage, of directors or officers must be citizens of the country granting the license. Such rules could limit the extent to which a reinsurer can operate in several national markets from a base in a single country, perhaps in Europe.

Solvency

Some of the most important rules—found in almost all regulatory systems—govern the solvency of the licensed insurance company. These rules will determine the amount of capital that must be raised to start the business. The rules may also determine the way in which capital is augmented as operations expand.

The first question is: What is the minimum capitalization required to obtain an insurance license? The statutory minimum may be far more than a single microinsurer can acquire. Although health insurance rules have recently been "reformed" in India, for example, they still require a minimum amount of capital that would preclude most microinsurers from obtaining a license.[1] In most markets, the minimum initial capitalization is unlikely to exceed the capacity of a reinsurer's investors and backers. However, aspects of the solvency rules could affect a reinsurer's start-up and growth.

Next, how is capital measured? The usual approach is to define and set minimum values for *policyholder surplus*, the amount by which net assets exceed liabilities. Such surplus can be invested by shareholders or accumulated from retained earnings. Depending on the rules, licensed companies may also include as surplus certain amounts that would normally be accounted for as debts or liabilities, as long as the lenders' interest is subordinated to the payment of obligations to policyholders.

Once past the initial hurdle of obtaining the requisite capitalization, a number of other rules may limit the operations of a licensed company:

- How must the capital grow as the company assumes additional liabilities? Must the company maintain a required ratio of surplus to liabilities or total assets? The reinsurer may need to negotiate contingent contributions of capital from its backers so that it can add capital as markets grow.

- Is the company required to discount its assets in any way? Called "risk-adjusted" or "risk-based" capital rules, these requirements force companies to discount the face value of certain assets to reflect risk or volatility. Equity shares or "junk bonds" are subject to a greater discount than bonds issued by highly rated governments and companies. Potential recoveries from reinsurance may be discounted to take account of the risk that a portion of the recoveries may be contested, or that the reinsurer may go bankrupt. Reinsurance receivables unpaid after a set period of time will usually be deemed uncollectible, and discounted 100 percent.

- Is the company required to post extra reserves for losses beyond those forecast by its actuaries? For example, regulators may adopt arbitrary ratios of reserves to collected premium when existing loss experience is limited.

To protect the solvency of licensed insurance companies, the regulator may limit the investments that can be used as company assets. A reinsurer is unlikely to select fly-by-night investments, but it might choose to place its assets in high-yielding, highly rated securities from another country. Such investments may not be on the list of investments permitted in a country where the reinsurer is licensed. The company's asset-management strategy must take such rules into account.

When underwriting results are poor—that is, the losses paid are greater than the amounts initially reserved—the policyholder surplus will be diminished. If surplus falls below the required level, the regulator will require the licensed company to obtain additional capital to comply with minimum surplus rules. If the company reports insufficient surplus at the time of a required financial statement, it may lose its license or be subject to a takeover by the insurance regulator. The reinsurer's arrangements with its investors must require infusions of additional capital quickly in such a situation to avoid intervention by the regulators.

Rate/Premium Setting

Some "tight" jurisdictions actually control the premiums an insurer can charge, reviewing the financial statements and rate calculations. The tightest jurisdictions may require prior approval by the regulatory agency before a company can change its rates (or sell a policy for the first time). In looser rate-regulation schemes, the insurer is required to publish its rates, including any range of discounts and surcharges that reflect variations in risk. The company may have to file these rates with the regulatory agency and give the regulator a chance to comment before the rates go into effect.

If coverage is characterized as reinsurance, not direct insurance, it is unlikely to be subject to rate review, even in jurisdictions that insist on prior approval of rates for direct insurers. Because a reinsurer's client is an insurance company, the client is assumed to be sophisticated and capable of protecting its own interests when purchasing reinsurance cover. In a tightly regulated jurisdiction, therefore, it would be important for a reinsurer to have its coverage classified as reinsurance—unless characterizing the coverage as direct insurance provides significant benefits to the microinsurers.

Jurisdictions that approve premium rates may have two (often conflicting) objectives:

- To protect the insurer's solvency and its ability to meet policyholder claims. In this case, the regulator wants to be sure that the premiums charged adequately cover the risk assumed. It may prohibit premiums viewed as too low. The regulator will favor higher rates within any band of uncertainty.

- To protect consumers (insureds) from price gouging and excessive rate fluctuations. If this is the objective, the regulator will try to force down rates. Since the reinsurer will not attempt to maximize returns to shareholders, it is unlikely to propose rates that would exceed reasonable levels in relation to the risk assumed. However, the jurisdiction may adopt arbitrary rules for rate determination such as maximum percentage increases in previous rates or unrealistic allowances for the cost of capital. Then reinsurance might encounter a problem, particularly if it initially sets rates too low and must revise them upward substantially once it has better actuarial data on the actual risk.

Sales

In many jurisdictions, licensed agents or brokers must sell insurance or reinsurance. If this rule applies, the reinsurer will have two choices:

- It can employ individuals holding the necessary licenses in the country where it operates. If the reinsurer planned to have an office and employees in the country, this would be only a minor inconvenience. But if the reinsurer hoped to serve the market from another jurisdiction, this requirement may add to operating costs.

- The reinsurer could sell coverage to microinsurers through agents or brokers who are already licensed and operating in the country. But it would then be expected to pay these brokers a commission, thus increasing its operating costs.

Required Reporting

Any country that licenses insurance companies will likely require them to file periodic financial reports. Timely reporting will be a major responsibility of company management and must be anticipated in designing the accounting and information systems of reinsurance. These designs, in turn, will determine a major portion of the operating costs. Questions reinsurers will want to answer are:

- How frequently must the reports be submitted—annually, semiannually, or quarterly?

- What kind of detail is required in the reports? Must the company show insured losses by line of business or location? This becomes an important issue for the reinsurer if it provides coverage to microinsurers in several countries.

- Must the reports show individual investment transactions or categorize investments in unusual ways?

- Are actuarial procedures prescribed for determining loss reserves, or does the company have discretion in selecting the most appropriate procedure?

- Must the required reports be prepared, or reviewed, by an independent auditor or actuary?

In countries that control licensed insurance companies tightly, or have had a recent insurance scandal, the regulatory agency may conduct periodic examinations of the financial reports, including reviews of accounting and loss records. The costs of such review are often imposed on the company in addition to any normal licensing fees. If the reinsurer is headquartered at some distance from the country where the licensed operation does business, the cost of such review could be substantial.

ADDITIONAL REGULATIONS THAT MAY APPLY

Besides the basic rules that apply generally to insurance and reinsurance companies, additional rules may apply to companies deemed to be writing health insurance. If reinsurance functions as a reinsurer, these rules would not be a problem in its own operations, but may affect its clients' operations. If reinsurance is characterized as a direct insurer of health plans that do not need their own insurance license, then reinsurers would be subject to these special rules.

Most of the regulations discussed below will develop only in countries with a history of private health insurance. The evils the regulations are designed to control may not seem as great when the health plans are organized at the community level and reinsured by a nonprofit or limited profit entity. However, if the regulatory scheme does not differentiate community health schemes and provide full or partial exemption from these rules, the cost of microinsurance—and reinsurance—is likely to increase.

Required Benefits

In more sophisticated jurisdictions, some advocacy groups force passage of laws that require health insurers to provide certain benefits. In the United States, for example, many states require insurers to cover treatment of alcoholism or to offer a certain minimum level of mental health services. Other laws may require the insurer to cover certain screening tests such as mammograms or Pap smears. Perhaps the rules require the insurer to offer important public health services—such as vaccinations and prenatal care—even if these services are already available from the limited government health services in a village. None of the countries likely to be targeted by reinsurance has the history of private health insurance seen in the United States. However, regulations should be quickly screened for any service mandates that would raise the cost of the benefit package.

One of the organizing principles of reinsurance is that local communities are in the best position to know what health benefits are needed, and thus a reinsurer should not be directive in designating the standard benefit package it will reinsure. If regulations do specify a minimum benefit package or mandate inclusion of certain benefits, the microinsurance plans may be forced to include services that potential consumers do not consider a priority. If that is the case, the plans will be more expensive than necessary and may not obtain a market share large enough to avoid adverse selection.

Limitations on Benefit Exclusions

Jurisdictions that have seen abuses by health insurers enact rules to prevent insurers from denying payment for a service on questionable grounds. For example, the rules may limit the insurer's ability to deny coverage on the basis of an insured's preexisting health condition. Most insurance regulators recognize that an insurer cannot pay the full costs of care if an insured can buy a policy at the last minute, knowing that major medical care is needed immediately. Thus, rules allow an insurer to deny coverage for preexisting medical conditions for some limited period (perhaps six months) after the policy is issued. Or, the rules require the insurer to cover the preexisting condition only if the insured has previous insurance coverage or is enrolled as a result of some event other than his illness—for example, taking a new job. Because it will likely be reinsuring the cost of major illness, the reinsurer has an interest in seeing that microinsurers avoid the adverse selection of individuals with immediate major medical needs. Very strict limits on benefit exclusions may raise the cost of premiums—and the reinsurance premiums that reinsurers must charge.

Regulations controlling benefit exclusions might also limit the ability of reinsurance and its community partners to design plans that exclude coverage of certain procedures or diseases. For example, a community plan might decide that the costs of HIV/AIDS treatment are so high as to make a plan covering HIV/AIDS unmarketable. If a jurisdiction has rules that prevent an insurer from denying coverage for antiretroviral treatment, the community plan might become unworkable. Similarly, rules that focus on plans offered to the upper middle class might forbid exclusion of cancer treatment and other major diseases requiring tertiary care. Plans in poor communities, on the other hand, might want to exclude such conditions to keep coverage for accidents and infectious disease more affordable.

In setting its reinsurance premiums and advising participating microinsurers, reinsurers will need to know if applicable regulations prohibit the exclusion of benefits the microinsurers did not plan to cover.

Restrictions on Underwriting and Risk Selection

Underwriting is the process by which an insurer decides if it will take a risk. In health insurance, this means the insurer decides that the potential insured does not present a high risk of incurring large medical bills. In addition to barring coverage for preexisting conditions, insurers may completely deny coverage to certain classes of individuals they think are high risk.

Policymakers are understandably anxious to provide fair access to health insurance and to limit insurers' underwriting practices. Microinsurers will have a similar desire to provide community members with equitable access to policies. But national rules intended to provide fair access may create problems for microinsurers.

For example, many small community insurance plans are based on ethnic, religious, or affinity groups. If these groups bar membership to those outside the group, could they be accused of discriminating in the provision of insurance? If so, reinsurance and the schemes it reinsures may have to use a broader definition of "community" in developing the microinsurance plan. Similarly, many plans may be intended to cover children and working parents of reproductive age. Does the jurisdiction have age discrimination laws that would limit the microinsurer's ability to exclude older individuals with high-cost chronic diseases? Such regulations might be avoided by charging an age-related premium, but the actuarial information on which to base such premium differentials is likely to be limited.

Countries can pass rules limiting an insurer's ability to deny coverage if the medical history of the insured indicates conditions such as positive HIV status, prior treatment for mental illness, or recent history of cardiac disease. To keep premiums affordable, community plans may want to exclude certain individuals who have medical histories that suggest a high probability of future expensive medical treatment. If the decisions are not arbitrary, such discrimination may be a reasonable way to offer a plan that meets the most pressing community needs at an affordable cost. However, reinsurance and its clients must be sure that the underwriting rules applied do not violate these restrictions.

Countries with substantial experience with private health insurers may limit undesirable underwriting practice by requiring insurers to accept all applicants who apply on an annual open enrollment date and by insisting that premiums be based on a community rating system. The idea of annual open enrollment should not create great problems for established health insurance programs. However, during start-up, the microinsurer will want to enroll new plan members over an extended period of time but may exclude individuals whose medical histories suggest high medical expenses in the very near future. Requiring a plan to wait for the next annual enrollment period to add members will slow its growth, but requiring it to take everyone, whenever they apply, could destroy the plan through adverse selection.

Community rating is an appealing concept in practice. If required, it could create problems for reinsurance, particularly if the reinsurer is deemed to be a direct insurer. The reinsurance concept assumes that different communities will want different benefit packages and may have different medical costs, depending on the providers available, the insureds' disease profile, and the desired benefit package. If required to charge a standard community rate across all these plans, reinsurance would run the risk of losing money in higher cost locations. If reinsurers were allowed to argue that each plan is entitled to a different community rate, it could stay within the regulations, but could incur major accounting and legal costs in justifying the rate differences.

Restrictions on Provider Selection

When insurers and health professionals clash over the selection of providers to participate in a particular insurance plan, provider groups pressure the regulators to limit the insurer's ability to choose providers. In the United States, disputes over the narrowing of managed care networks led to the introduction of *any willing provider* laws. These laws specify that an insurer must extend provider status to any provider in a certain category if the provider meets minimum quality standards and agrees to accept the rates and conditions of payment offered by the insurer.

If such a regulation is introduced in a jurisdiction where reinsurance works, it could limit the use of plan structures that may be highly desirable. For example, community health plans may be formed around a single provider (as has happened with some hospitals in Africa). The provider itself may even sponsor the plan. If the plan otherwise meets the local community's needs, it would be unfortunate if rules require the plan to extend provider status (and payments) to a hospital that is accessible to only a few insureds. In addition, community health plans may want to select providers competitively, contracting only with providers that deliver good service at the lowest prices. The health plan's bargaining power is reduced if it is forced to make payments to other similarly qualified providers.

Just as microinsurers will want to choose a benefit package that best meets perceived local needs, they may want to limit the types of providers with which they contract. Although unlikely to be a problem in most rural areas, any rule requiring an insurer to include certain types of providers in a plan might conflict with the general principle of community determination. For example, in a moderately developed country, a plan might include limited mental health services but refuse provider status to individuals not qualified as medical doctors. In some U.S. states, psychologists and social workers obtained legislation entitling them to provider status under state-licensed insurance plans. Such a rule is not likely to affect reinsurance clients in remote communities and underserved populations. But if a company reinsures plans for the informal sector in large urban areas with a developing cadre of mental health professionals, such rules might drive up the cost of benefits.

Restrictions on Marketing

As discussed above, insurance regulations may require that licensed brokers or agents, who usually take a commission, sell policies. Community plans targeted by reinsurers will not want to restrict community sales in this way or incur these expenses. In addition, reinsurers would like to avoid—where possible—payment of an agent's or broker's markup on its reinsurance premium.

More sophisticated jurisdictions may have other rules that control marketing of the primary health insurance policy. Where private health insurance is still limited, such rules may not yet have developed. However, reinsurers should review the regulatory regime to make sure that marketing practices are not controlled by rules such as those that:

- Specify policy language or the clarity with which insurance policies are written. Traditionally, insurance policies have been written with opaque language that well-educated citizens find difficult to comprehend. If too many people find that the policy denies benefits they thought were covered, the regulators may adopt language giving standard benefit definitions or specifying the format for a "consumer-friendly" policy.

- Control the advertising claims that can be made about a policy. Adopted to prevent an unscrupulous insurer from misleading the customer, such rules are unlikely to be problematic for community health insurers if they sell by word-of-mouth instead of through print and electronic media ads.

- Mandate audits of sales activities. If the regulator is sufficiently skeptical of an insurer's marketing practices, it might enact regulations subjecting the insurer to an audit of its market conduct. In addition to reviewing policy language and advertising, the auditors might also review the way the insurer determines premium rates or makes underwriting and benefit decisions.

None of the above regulations would be a reason for a reinsurer to stay out of a market. However, if such regulations are in force, they may raise the operating costs of whoever assumes the responsibilities of a primary insurer, be it the microinsurers or the reinsurer.

Some specific comments on the regulatory environment in which the pilot of the reinsurance of microinsurance units might be conducted in the Philippines are offered in chapter 22 of this volume, which provides a comprehensive assessment of the planned pilot.

NOTE

1.   Conclusion based on inquiries of the Economic Section, Embassy of India, Washington, D.C., in the fall of 2000.

CHAPTER 13

Role of Subsidies in Microinsurance: Closing the "Recovery Gap"

Reinhard Busse

N o matter how well reinsurance mechanisms deal with insolvency risks associated with randomly fluctuating expenditure, microinsurance units may encounter a *recovery gap,* a systematic excess of expenditure on benefits over income (Preker, Langenbrunner, and Jakab, chapter 1, this volume). Because the recovery gap is not random, reinsurance cannot solve it. Solutions for this financial problem should therefore be sought outside the context of risk management—through subsidies.

This chapter draws heavily on Western Europe's experience with social health insurance.[1] It describes reasons for the recovery gap, including uninsurable health expenses, and offers a model for analyzing the role of subsidies financed from taxation, foreign donors, or other sources in filling the gap.[2] It examines the role and extent of tax subsidies in West European countries, addressing such questions as whether tax subsidies increase systemic equity and whether they are only a short-term measure or are needed permanently. Two reasons argue for drawing on the West European experience, even though we are discussing seemingly different circumstances of microinsurers in low- and middle-income countries:

- Most health insurance funds started out as a kind of microinsurance.

- Long-term dependence on tax subsidies can best be estimated by studying well-developed systems in countries with a long history of social health insurance.

From this experience come some lessons for low- and middle-income countries embarking on the insurance route.

WHENCE THE RECOVERY GAP?

Where does a recovery gap come from? Both theory and history hold some answers.

In projecting an insurance scheme's income, five main factors come into play: the contribution rate or per capita premium, the contribution base, the

The author acknowledges, with thanks, the helpful comments on a draft of this chapter from Joe Kutzin, World Health Organization Senior Resident Advisor, MANAS Health Policy Analysis Project, Bishkek, Kyrgyz Republic; and from Michael Cichon, Chief, Financial, Actuarial and Statistical Branch, Social Protection Sector, International Labour Office.

declaration rate, the collection rate, and the expenditure. Errors in estimating any of these can result in a deficit.

Microinsurers have two options for calculating an income that meets their needs, either as a per capita premium or, more commonly, as a percentage of the contribution base, the *contribution rate*. The contribution base is usually work-related income but may also include other income (for example, from investments) or assets.

Box 13.1 presents some simple formulas for calculating the necessary per capita premium and contribution rate. The formulas take into account factors such as the beneficiaries' honesty in declaring their income *(the declaration rate)* as well as the microinsurer's ability to fully collect the premiums or contributions *(the collection*

BOX 13.1   CALCULATING A MICROINSURER 'S PREMIUM OR CONTRIBUTION RATE

The basic formula for calculating the *premium* is:

(1a) Necessary per capita premium = total expenditure – copayments – other income/
number of beneficiaries.

Using an easy example of 1,000 currency units (CU) expenditure, CU100 in copayments (assuming no other income), and 100 beneficiaries, this would result in a premium of CU9.

The formula for calculating the *contribution rate,* given by Cichon and others (1999) is:

(2a) Necessary contribution rate = total expenditure – copayments – other income/
contribution base.

Assuming the same expenditure, copayments, and number of beneficiaries, and a contribution base of CU10,000 (an average of CU100 per person), this would result in a contribution rate of 9 percent.

Taking both the declaration rate and the collection rate into account, the formulas are as follows:

(1b) Necessary per capita premium = total expenditure – copayments – other income/
number of beneficiaries x collection rate.

Retaining the values of (1a), a collection rate of 90 percent would increase the necessary premium to CU10; one of 80 percent, to CU11.25. (Note: As the premium is independent of the beneficiaries' income, the declaration rate does not enter the formula.)

(2b) Necessary contribution rate = total expenditure – copayments – other income/
contribution base x declaration rate x collection rate.

Retaining the values of (2a), a declaration and collection rate of 90 percent each would increase the necessary contribution rate to 11.1 percent; rates of 80 percent, to around 14.1 percent (that is, by more than half).

(Box continues on the following page.)

BOX 13.1 (continued)

Adjusting for Income Deficits

If the necessary premium/contribution rate is below these levels (that is, if the actual premium/contribution rate is lower than necessary), a new variable—a deficit—has to be introduced in the formulas:

(1c) Actual per capita premium = total expenditure – copayments – other income – deficit/number of beneficiaries x collection rate.

Building on (1b) but assuming an actual per capita premium of only CU9, the deficit would reach CU100 under the 90 percent collection rate and CU212.50 under the 80 percent rate.

(2c) Actual contribution rate = total expenditure – copayments – other income – deficit/contribution base x declaration rate x collection rate.

Building on (2b) but assuming an actual contribution rate of only 9 percent, the deficit would reach CU211.11 under the 90 percent and CU500.63 under the 80 percent assumption for declaration and collection rate.

Adjusting to Cover Indigents

The effects of including indigents can be demonstrated by the calculations for the per capita premium (1a) and the contribution rate (2a). Let us assume that, in both cases, the number of beneficiaries is increased by 20 indigents whose health needs are comparable to those of the other 100 members. The result is stable per capita expenditure.

As the 20 new members can pay neither a premium nor copayments, total expenditure would increase to CU1100 from CU900. Adding the 20 indigents would *either* result in an increase in each of the original beneficiaries' premiums to CU11 (and the necessary contribution rate to 11 percent) *or* cause a deficit of CU200 (potentially adding to the deficit resulting from imperfect declaration and collection rates). Subsidies can solve this kind of recovery gap, which is caused by adding health coverage for indigents.

---

rate). The two rates will fluctuate between a maximum of 100 percent (meaning that all income is declared or collected) and a theoretical 0 percent. As can be seen from the formulas in the box, if these factors do not reach 100 percent, premiums or contributions will have to increase—or a deficit will result.

Thus, misjudging the declaration and the collection rate can easily lead to a deficit—if the actual rates are less than 100 percent. Although such deficits constitute a certain type of "recovery gap," they do not qualify for subsidies to cover them. They should be addressed by tackling the reasons for the shortfalls.

As candidates for generating a real recovery gap, the expenditure and the contribution base deserve close attention.

On the expenditure side, Dror has pointed to several problems (chapter 5, this volume). A recovery gap could reflect:

- Demand-side expectations of increased benefits without any corresponding increase in the premium on the income side

- Supply-induced moral hazard and monopolistic pricing if competition between suppliers is weak or nonexistent

- Pressures from inflation or from a pandemic (for example, HIV-AIDS).

If expenditure is not driven by providers' unrealistically high income expectations, a recovery gap resulting from the other reasons given should be considered a candidate for subsidies. (A liberal attitude may be justified when assessing whether income expectations are "unrealistic." After all, highly trained professionals are expected to work in low-income rural areas where the income differential between them and the insured population may, of necessity, be high.) The expenditure side, not further explored here, is a topic all by itself (Dror, chapter 5, this volume).

Regarding the contribution base, a distinction has to be made between a recovery gap that relates to the whole insured population and a gap that is concentrated in certain segments of the insured population. In the first instance, the economic base is too weak in comparison to expenditure (see box 13.1).

The second case, concentration in certain population segments, was not originally a problem in Western Europe because social health insurance was work related. All participants were employed, even though their incomes, number of dependents, and health status might have been different.

Gradually, coverage was expanded to nonworking population segments throughout Western Europe, achieving population-wide coverage only in Switzerland (1996), Belgium (1998), and France (2000). Since 1968, introduced under the Exceptional Medical Expenses Act, the Netherlands' universal Algemene Wet Bijzondere Ziekenkosten (Exceptional Medical Expenses) has covered long-term care and populationwide prevention programs, mainly "uninsurable" services.

The creation of social health insurance schemes covering most or all of the population put pressure on planners to find ways of including everyone without creating a recovery gap. Contributing members were not always willing to see their contributions used to cover noncontributing members' health costs.[3] A deficit resulting from adding insurance coverage for indigents is a prime candidate for subsidies. Subsidies can avoid overburdening the contributing population (leading to decreasing acceptability of the whole scheme) and the exclusion of individuals who cannot (fully) contribute to financing.

The four factors addressed so far—declaration rate, collection rate, expenditure, and contribution base—all relate to the inability to raise contributions for various reasons. Another reason for a gap between health insurance fund income and expenditure is an "unwillingness" to set a high enough contribution rate to cover spending. Who among the decisionmakers is unwilling? Although health insurance funds in most West European social health insurance countries are "self-governing," the government or legislature exerts the decisive influence in setting contributions. In France, by law, contribution rates are negotiated between the government and representatives of employees, employers, and the social security organizations, but the government makes the final decision. In the Netherlands, the Board for Health Care Insurance (College voor zorgverzekeringen, CvZ) runs the central funds required under AWBZ and the Sickness Funds Act (ZFW) and recommends the next year's contribution rates to the Ministry of Health. The Ministry of Health then sets the rates.

Only Germany and Luxembourg have delegated power to decide upon contribution rates to self-governing bodies—Luxembourg, to the Union of Sickness Funds, and Germany, to the individual funds. However, their decisions are subject to governmental approval. For regionally operated funds in Germany, "the government" is the statutory health insurance unit within the Länder ministry responsible for health. An independent agency, the Federal Insurance Office, is charged with the supervision of countrywide health insurance funds. The health insurance funds are legally obliged to calculate a contribution rate that is neither too high nor too low to cover all expenditure and to keep reserves at the required level (Social Code Book V, Article 220). The government may refuse approval if the rate does not meet this requirement, but it can also act if a health insurance fund does not suggest a rate change when it should. Similarly, under supervision of the Federal Office for Social Insurance, Swiss insurers are allowed to set their own community-based premiums.

Needless to say, neither the unwillingness to set an appropriate contribution rate nor regulations preventing microinsurers from doing so—although leading to a recovery gap—justify subsidies. The deficit should be addressed instead by changing the regulatory framework or the supervision of the fund's decisions.

CLOSING THE RECOVERY GAP: A MODEL

At first glance, closing the recovery gap through tax subsidies is a straightforward affair. But a closer look reveals many possibilities, each with a different rationale and potentially different implications (figure 13.1).

Subsidies can be paid into the system in three ways: to individuals (Si in figure 13.1), to the social or community-financed microinsurance unit (Sf), or to providers (Sp).

Paying Subsidies to Individuals

The first option is paying subsidies directly to the needy, usually defined in terms of low income but sometimes including individuals in poor health (Si). The subsidy, in extreme cases amounting to the entire contribution, enables individuals to acquire health insurance coverage they could not otherwise afford.

FIGURE 13.1   Role of Taxes and Tax-Financed Subsidies in Financial Flows under Social Health Insurance or in Community-Financed Microinsurance Units

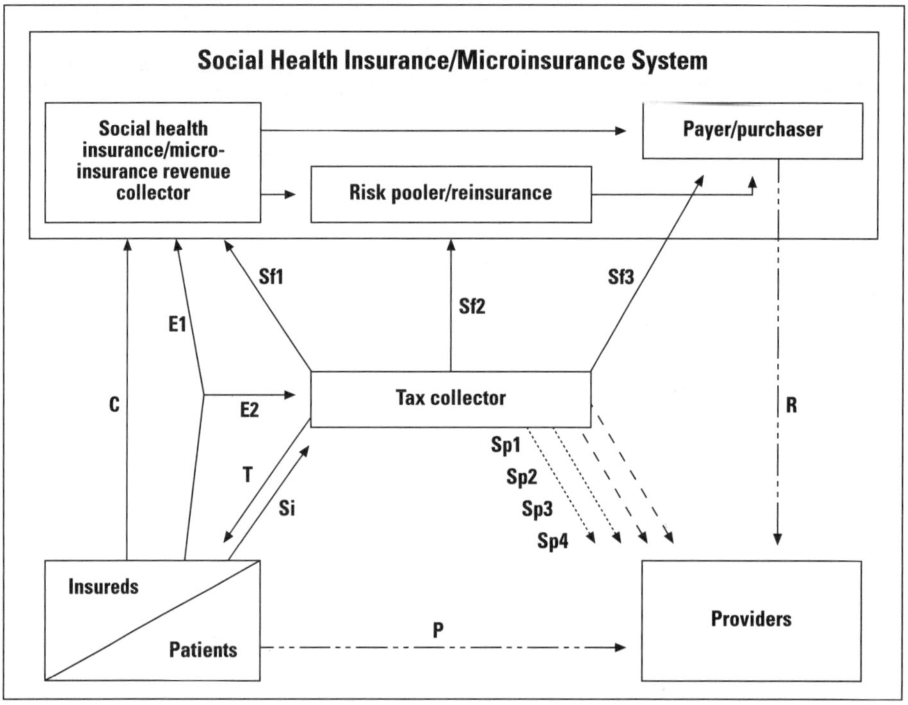

C   Contributions (both income and nonincome related).
E   Earmarked/hypothecated health taxes.
P   Private expenditure (cost sharing for social health insurance/microinsurance services; voluntary health insurance; and out-of-pocket for nonsocial health insurance/microinsurance services).
R   Provider payment/reimbursement (directly under contract model or indirectly under patient reimbursement model).
Sf1   Tax-financed contributions, for example, for nonsalaried persons.
Sf2   General subsidies for pooled social health insurance/microinsurance finances/reinsurance.
Sf3   Subsidies for individual funds/community schemes.
Si   Subsidies to individuals to purchase insurance.
Sp1   General, unspecified subsidies to providers.
Sp2   Nonservice payments (for example, for investments).
Sp3   Reimbursement for nonsocial health insurance/microinsurance services (for example, public health).
Sp4   Reimbursement of services for nonsocial health insurance/microinsurance-covered persons.
T   Taxes used for health care (general).

This kind of subsidy can be targeted directly to needy individuals. However, direct subsidies also have disadvantages: having to define limits for entitlement, verify that applicants fulfill these limits, and ascertain that recipients of a subsidy use it for the intended purpose—here, to buy health insurance. Thus, a fairly extensive monitoring mechanism is needed—which may be available in Switzerland but not in every country introducing health insurance.

FIGURE 13.2   Tax Subsidies in Dutch Social Health Insurance, 1980–2000
(percent of total income)

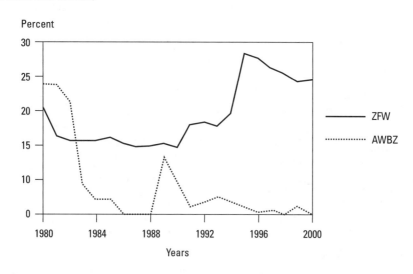

Note: These are payments into the pooled fund, Sf2 in figure 13.1.
Source: F. Bertens, personal communication, January 26, 2001.

Paying Subsidies into Funds or Microinsurance Units

Paying contributions for the needy directly into the social health insurance fund or microinsurance units (Sf1) may therefore be more appropriate. Many Central and East European countries have chosen this option. In this case, the subsidies must cover 100 percent of the contributions for the needy or the same problems arise as with subsidies to individuals.

This option, too, has disadvantages. People who do not have to contribute might feel less ownership in the insurance fund. People outside the subsidized group might feel unfairly treated if their incomes are only slightly higher. A second set of concerns is related to the ability (and willingness) of the subsidy payer (whether finance ministry or outside donor) to pay the amount needed as long as it is needed.

Many of these disadvantages are circumvented if the subsidies are paid into the pooled financial resources of the social health insurance or microinsurer (Sf2) instead of to individuals. Every individual must join the scheme if such a subsidy is to close the recovery gap for the entire covered population (and not just forestall contribution increases for people who can afford insurance). This means that the contribution amount should not be set so high as to prevent the poor from joining, as could happen under a per capita premium (instead of an income-dependent contribution). If the contribution is income differentiated, paying a subsidy into the financial pool—or to reinsurance—is a flexible possibility for closing the recovery gap.

Sometimes a subsidy payment to the purchasing fund (Sf3) is appropriate, for example, if income and risk differences between funds or microinsurers are insufficiently offset through the pooling mechanism. Examples include funds/microinsurance for only the self-employed when most other insured individuals split the contribution with a third party (usually their employer). Without a subsidy, the self-employed would have to pay much more than wage earners. Sf3 may also be relevant in case of large regional differences in per capita income that are not mediated via the pooling mechanism (for example, to maintain compliance with the system in high-income areas). Sf3 would then subsidize regionally organized purchasers located in low-income areas. Again, the choice is between subsidizing service provision or purchase. In either case, geographic targeting may be easier for most countries than targeting based on individual income or risk profiles.

Paying Subsidies to Providers

Providers are the third group of subsidy recipients. These subsidies can serve many purposes:

1. General, unspecified uses, including debt coverage (Sp1)

2. Specific, but not service-related, uses, often for investments (Sp2)

3. Reimbursement for services outside the benefit package such as public health measures (Sp3)

4. Reimbursement for services provided to uninsured persons such as the needy (Sp4)

Options 1 and 4 point toward deficits in the system while 2 and 3 can be effectively integrated into the overall financing. Sp1 subsidies decrease the chances of bringing providers into a system where they agree with the funds on volume and reimbursement levels that do not endanger systemic sustainability. Sp4 subsidies sound an alarm that other subsidies in the system are not targeted in a way that ensures the poor the same entitlements as everybody else. They will be better served by Si- or Sf1-type subsidies. Sp4 might also cost the subsidy payer more than would the other types because no insurance contributions are paid for those individuals, and the full reimbursement cost falls on the subsidy payer (with the possible exception of out-of-pocket user fees).

Sp2 subsidies enable providers to offer facilities in remote areas, where microinsurers are often based. Without subsidies, the investment costs might prove too high for a prospective investor to locate in areas lacking the "guaranteed" purchasing power promised by wealthier urban areas. Additionally, Sp2 subsidies help hold down reimbursements, thereby alleviating one potential source of a recovery gap. Sp3 subsidies provide an option for restricting the social health insurance/microinsurance benefit package to insurable services, that is, excluding the uninsurable services that should be promoted as a matter of public health (for example, immunizations).

CLOSING THE RECOVERY GAP: EUROPE'S EXPERIENCE

West European countries have taken different approaches to dealing with recovery gaps.

The Netherlands

As the first universal social health insurance scheme, the Dutch AWBZ is a good place to start. Before AWBZ, much of the care it now covers was funded from general revenue. The new insurance scheme saved the government a good deal of money, and part of those savings was recycled into the AWBZ Fund as a structural subsidy. Over the years, this government subsidy has changed many times, as benefits have been added or removed from the ambit of the Act. The AWBZ Fund therefore consists of both contributions (C) and government subsidy (Sf2) in figure 13.1.

At first, the health insurance scheme for the elderly and the voluntary health insurance scheme were partially funded by the government. On April 1, 1986, both funds were taken over by the General Fund for the sickness fund scheme. When the Medical Insurance (Access) Act and the Act governing the Joint Funding of Elderly Sickness Fund Patients went into force on the above date, the ZFW was amended to the effect that the government would pay an annual grant into the pooled fund (Sf2) toward the cost of financing sickness funds scheme for all. The grant amount, determined annually, has fluctuated widely as benefits and population groups have been included or excluded from the two schemes (figure 13.2).

France

France, with its state-fixed social insurance contributions, provides an example of a different type of recovery gap. The social security system ran a deficit throughout the 1990s, and health care was the main source. Political unwillingness to adjust the contribution rate to need was based on the notion that social contributions were increasing labor costs, thereby dampening employment. In an effort to address these structural problems leading to financial difficulties, Prime Minister Alain Juppé, in December 1995, presented a plan to reform social security financing.

Widening the contribution of the General Social Levy Tax was a main proposal. This tax, levied on all types of income (savings, subsidies, pensions, stocks), was set at 1.1 percent in 1991. Initially allocated to the family allowances branch, revenue generated by this tax was earmarked for health in 1996. Additionally, employee payroll contributions for health were largely replaced by an increase in the earmarked health tax, starting in 1998. The payroll contribution rate decreased from 5.5 percent to 0.75 percent, and the earmarked health tax increased from 3.4 percent to 7.5 percent—thereby reducing the overall contribution/tax rate from 8.9 percent to 8.25 percent but widening the contribution/tax base. The employer contribution was maintained.

A social debt-reducing fund (Caisse d'Amortissement de la dette sociale) was also created. It manages a new income tax, the Social Debt Tax (Remboursement de la dette sociale), to pay off the social security system's deficit (Lancry and Sandier 1999, pp. 443–70). Since 1996, this new 13-year tax, set at 0.5 percent of total income, has been levied on everyone but recipients of government social assistance and disability pensions.

Now France has three different sources of social security financing: social contributions (C), the earmarked health tax (E1), and the social debt-payment tax (E2) in figure 13.1. E2 is a mechanism through which social health insurance financing (originally contribution based) has been made partly tax based. Future debate will revolve around the collective choice between proportional taxes, notably the earmarked health tax, and progressive taxes such as the income tax (Bouget 1998).

Switzerland

While the Netherlands fills the financial risk pool with tax money and France has shifted a good part of its financing from contributions to earmarked taxes, Switzerland takes yet another approach. Instead of paying subsidies into the social health insurance system, Switzerland gives them directly to individuals, on a means-tested basis, to enable them to purchase health insurance (Si in figure 13.1). Before the introduction of the current system of compulsory insurance in 1996, health insurance funds received subsidies amounting to about 30 percent of their expenditure (Sf3). Premiums for persons in poor health nonetheless became so costly that such people could no longer acquire any health insurance, especially in high-expenditure cantons. The new act made health insurance compulsory, introduced community rating by canton, and cut off direct subsidies to the health insurance funds. Subsidies to individuals are calculated in different ways from canton to canton but can include a full premium subsidy, depending on the insurance policy chosen (Minder, Schoenholzer, and Amiet 2000).

How Much Subsidization from Taxes?

In all these experiences, some degree of tax subsidization is present, but just how much is hard to tell. International statistics are often fuzzy on sources of health care funding, for example, whether expenditure through taxation includes tax-financed payments to social health insurance (Sf in figure 13.1) or whether these are included as social health insurance expenditures.

Austria and Switzerland, for example, finance a large part of hospital care directly through taxation—and have therefore relatively low figures for the social health insurance expenditure share. In the Netherlands and other countries, hospital care is financed exclusively by the health insurance funds, which receive substantial subsidies from general taxation. Tax subsidies paid into the joint health insurance funds' pool (Sf2) are also substantial in Belgium and Luxembourg. In Belgium, about 60 percent of all subsidies are paid into the social health insurance scheme's pooled finances (Sf2), and the rest goes directly to providers, mainly to cover investments (Sp2). In Austria and Germany, the social health insurance schemes receive no tax subsidies—with the small but noteworthy exception of the farmers' funds in both countries (Sf3). Besides the special taxes mentioned earlier, France also uses direct tax subsidies to funds with low-income/high-need members, such as the farmers' fund.

To estimate the degree to which countries rely on wage-based social health insurance contributions, two factors have to be combined: the percentage of social health insurance income from contributions (C/C + E1 + Sf) (figure 13.1; data for Western Europe, table 13.1) and the percentage of overall health expenditure covered through social health insurance (C + E1 + Sf/C + E + P + T).

Based on that calculation, Germany and the Netherlands are the only countries in Western Europe that cover more than 60 percent of all health care expenditure from wage-related contributions. Until 1997, France was the country that relied most heavily on wage-related contributions but, since its shift to a wider contribution base, that share has dropped below 60 percent. Austria and Luxembourg finance a little less than 50 percent, and Belgium less than 40 percent, of total health care expenditure from wage-related contributions. In some respects, Belgium is closer to a "mixed" system of funding, as taxes accounted for 38 percent and social security contributions for 36 percent in 1994 (Crainich and Closon 1999, pp. 219–66).

TABLE 13.1   Tax Financing in West European Social Health Insurance Systems, 1999–2000

	Austria	Belgium	France	Germany	Luxembourg	Netherlands	Switzerland
Extent of taxes for social health insurance financing (if available: percent of fund income)	Generally no (except 23% for farmers fund, that is, 0.5% of total)	Yes, 35–40%	Yes (up to 8%); plus special taxes (up to 34%)[a]	Generally no (except 52% for farmers' funds, that is, < 1% of total)	Yes, max. 40[a]	Yes, AWBZ < 1%, ZFW 25%	Only indirect subsidies (that is, to insureds, not to funds)

a. Supplement of 250 percent on pensioners' contributions, 10 percent on other contributions.
b. On car insurance, alcoholic drinks, and pharmaceutical marketing.
Source: Author's calculations, based on various sources.

Central and Eastern Europe

To include Central and East European countries in the comparison, both direct, wage-related contributions and the overall social health insurance contributions to total health expenditure have to be considered. For example, in both the Czech Republic and Slovak Republic, the state pays contributions for all nonwage earners (Sf1 in figure 13.1). This group encompasses more than 50 percent of the population, including not only pensioners and the unemployed but also nonwage-earning spouses and children, persons covered as dependents in Western Europe (Busse 2000; Hlavacka and Skackova 2000). Wage-related contributions cover around 65 percent of total health care expenditure—as much as or slightly more than in Germany or the Netherlands and more than one-and-a-half times as much as in Belgium. This apparent contradiction results from the state's low contributions, a major source of those countries' financial difficulties.

DO MORE SUBSIDIES MEAN MORE EQUITY?

When evaluating equity in health care financing, an analogy can be made to taxation systems. In a *progressive* tax system, the proportion of income paid in taxes rises as income rises. In *a regressive* system, the proportion falls as income rises. And so it is with health care—the proportion of income paid for health care rises as income rises in progressive funding and falls in a regressive system.

In Western Europe, social health insurance is slightly less progressive than general taxation, but much more progressive than private financing arrangements (Wagstaff and others 1999; van Doorslaer, Wagstaff, and Rutten 1993). In poorer countries, with very different taxation systems and revenue-collection performance, these findings may not be applicable. In either setting, however, private out-of-pocket spending is the most regressive form of health care financing.

Differences in tax loads within tax-financed systems depend on the mix between (progressive) income taxes and (regressive) indirect taxes as well as their completeness of collection. Equity differences among social health insurance countries depend on the extent of the tax-financing component and its progressivity, the proportion of private direct payments, and differences in social insurance contributions. In West European social health insurance countries, there is no direct correlation between the extent of tax subsidies and "financing fairness," as measured in the *World Health Report 2000* (WHO 2000). Belgium and Luxembourg, with high subsidies, rank almost equal with Austria and Germany. This finding suggests that it is not the extent of tax subsidies that makes health care financing more or less equitable but the exact design and mix within different categories of funding.

Equity differences in social insurance contributions depend on the extent to which contributions are income-based (instead of per capita premiums); the relative tax burdens of rich and poor (through income ceilings or no-claim bonuses); the extent of contribution pooling and adjustment for differing risks;

and the extent to which benefits are fully covered or require cost sharing (Normand and Busse 2002). When considering these points, special attention has to be given to the inclusion or exclusion of dependents—equity decreases if per capita premiums are charged for dependents as well as members (as in the Netherlands). Conversely, the inclusion of dependents might increase inequity if there is a ceiling on contributory income—a "millionaire" with a nonworking spouse pays only once, while a middle-class, double-income couple pays twice.

CONCLUSIONS

The European experience suggests several important lessons for countries embarking on the insurance route. First, no matter how skillfully the social health insurance or community-financed health system is designed, no matter how long it has been in operation, and no matter how rich the country is, some sort of subsidization will always be needed to complement the main system of finance. Subsidies are the only way of ensuring adequate population coverage, stimulating delivery in otherwise underserved areas, or encouraging the delivery of certain, often public health–related, services. In Europe, the extent of subsidization varies from modest amounts to 50 percent of total finance.

Second, there is no single, perfect way to put subsidies into the health finance system. Based on a country's needs, administrative capacity, banking system, and political priorities, subsidies can be given directly to individuals to acquire health insurance, paid into a financial pool (through mechanisms including reinsurance), or given to providers to cover investments or uninsurable services. In reality, a balanced mixture between these options has to be found, and adjustments may be necessary if the desired propoor effect is not achieved (as in Switzerland).

Third, subsidies do not guarantee social fairness or improved access for the poor. How the money for subsidies is raised and how it is spent are both important. Depending on the means used, fund raising or spending can worsen the situation of the poor if the subsidy system is not carefully designed.

NOTES

1. Using the social health insurance definition in the System of National Accounts, microinsurance also falls into this category if "the programme is operated on behalf of a group and restricted to group members" (SNA 1993, annex IV, para. 4.111). As long as they are not "imposed and controlled by government units" (SNA 1993, annex IV, para. 4.130) as in Western Europe, they would, however, be classified as "private social insurance."

2. The model incorporates elements from other health financing frameworks (OECD 1992; Kutzin 2001).

3. For the largest group of indigents, the pensioners, contributions vary from country to country in Western Europe, both in the amounts paid and in the agency responsible for paying them. In most cases, pensioners pay the same rate on their pension

as employees pay on their income (or, in Switzerland, the same per capita premium). This amount may be split between the pensioner and the statutory pension fund (substituting for the employer, as in Germany and Luxembourg) or it may be placed entirely on the pensioner (as in the Netherlands). The contribution rate may, however, also be lower or higher. In Belgium, pensioners pay only the employee's part of 3.55 percent. In Austria, pensioners pay more, with a contribution rate of more than 11 percent. Because pensioners themselves pay only as much as working members on average (3.75 percent), two-thirds of the contribution falls on the pension funds (European Commission 1999). These arrangements are feasible only if a fund has enough nonpensioner members to cover additional expenditures. A fund with only pensioners—or a microinsurer with only indigent members—would not be viable.

REFERENCES

Bouget, D. 1998. "The Juppé Plan and the Future of the French Social Welfare System." *Journal of European Social Policy* 8(2):155–72.

Busse, R. 2000. *Health Care Systems in Transition—Czech Republic*. Copenhagen: European Observatory on Health Care Systems. Also available at www.observatory.dk.

Cichon, M., W. Newbrander, H. Yamabana, A. Weber, C. Normand, D. Dror, and A. Preker. 1999. *Modelling in Health Care Finance: A Compendium of Quantitative Techniques for Health Care Financing*. Geneva: International Labour Office.

Crainich, D., and M-C. Closon. 1999. "Cost Containment and Health Care Reform in Belgium." Chapter 4 in E. Mossialos and J. Le Grand, eds., *Health Care and Cost Containment in the European Union*. Aldershot: Ashgate.

European Commission, Directorate General for Employment and Social Affairs. 1999. *MISSOC [Mutual Information System on Social Protection in the European Union]—Comparative Tables*. Available at http://europa.eu.int/comm/employment_social/soc-prot/missoc99/english/f_tab.htm. Last accessed on July 19, 2001.

Hlavacka, S., and D. Skackova. 2000. *Health Care Systems in Transition—Slovakia*. Copenhagen: European Observatory on Health Care Systems. Also available at www.observatory.dk.

Kutzin, J. 2001. "A Descriptive Framework for Country-Level Analysis of Health Care Financing Arrangements." *Health Policy* 56(3):171–204.

Lancry, P.J., and S. Sandier. 1999. "Twenty Years of Cures for the French Health Care System." Chapter 9 in E. Mossialos and J. Le Grand, eds., *Health Care and Cost Containment in the European Union*. Aldershot: Ashgate.

Minder, A., H. Schoenholzer, and M. Amiet. 2000. *Health Care Systems in Transition—Switzerland*. Copenhagen: European Observatory on Health Care Systems. Also available at www.observatory.dk.

Normand, C., and R. Busse. 2002. "Social Health Insurance Financing." Chapter 3 in E. Mossialos, A. Dixon, J. Figueras, and J. Kutzin, eds., *Funding Health Care—Options for Europe*. Buckingham: Open University Press.

OECD (Organisation for Economic Co-operation and Development). 1992. *The Reform of Health Care: A Comparative Analysis of Seven OECD Countries*. Health Policy Studies No. 2. Paris: OECD.

SNA (System of National Accounts). 1993. *System of National Accounts 1993*. Brussels/Luxembourg, New York, Paris, Washington: Commission of the European Communities, International Monetary Fund, OECD, United Nations, World Bank.

van Doorslaer, E., A. Wagstaff, and F. Rutten. 1993. *Equity in the Finance and Delivery of Health Care: An International Perspective*. Oxford: Oxford University Press.

Wagstaff, A., E. van Doorslaer, H. van der Burg, S. Calonge, T. Christansen, G. Citoni, U.-G. Gerdtham, M. Gerfin, L. Gross, U. Häkinnen, P. Johnson, J. John, J. Klavus, C. Lachaud, J. Lauritsen, R. Leu, B. Nolan, E. Perán, J. Pereira, C. Propper, F. Puffer, L. Rochaix, M. Rodrígeuz, M. Schellhorn, G. Sundberg, and O. Winkelhake. 1999. "Equity in the Finance of Health Care: Some Further International Comparisons." *Journal of Health Economics* 18:263–90.

WHO (World Health Organization). 2000. *The World Health Report 2000—Health Systems: Improving Performance*. Geneva: WHO.

CHAPTER 14

Linking Ability and Willingness to Contribute to Microinsurance

Logan Brenzel and William Newbrander

As more and more health systems require direct financial contributions from households, an important policy question arises: How should health services be priced? Studies of willingness to pay can help answer this question.[1]

Willingness to pay can be assessed either by evaluating past health care utilization and expenditure information or by using a contingent valuation methodology. In the latter approach, people are asked about the maximum amount they would be willing to pay under a variety of hypothetical scenarios that reflect current market conditions (Olsen and Smith 2001). A substantial literature reviews the reliability of responses and possible biases that arise with the contingent valuation approach (Wouters, Adeyi, and Morrow 1993; Russell, Fox-Rushby, and Arhin 1995). However, contingent valuation is currently the most widely accepted approach for ascertaining willingness to pay for services in the health sector.

Contingent valuation studies have been conducted in industrial countries to evaluate individuals' willingness to pay for improvements in health status (Whittington and others 1990; Johannessen, Jonsson, and Borquist 1991, 1993; Neumann and Johannessen 1994). In developing countries, this tool has been used to evaluate willingness to pay for improvements in health services, including quality upgrades (Donaldson 1990; Weaver and others 1996; Mills and others 1994; Arhin 1995; ESHE 2000). Willingness-to-pay responses in these cases are usually linked to the types and quality of services, the health facility providing services, geographical area, and household income.

This chapter explores the utility of employing willingness-to-pay methodologies for determining contribution rates (premiums and copayments) for community-based health insurance schemes, called microinsurance units. The chapter also addresses the relationship between willingness to pay and the affordability of contributions to microinsurance. Issues such as implications for enrollment, on-time payment, and seasonality are discussed. The chapter closes with a discussion of microinsurers' willingness and ability to pay for reinsurance.

For reviewing the draft of this chapter, the authors thank Guy Carrin, Health Economist, World Health Organization, Geneva, and Dr. Benito Reverente, Chief of Party, Management Sciences for Health, the Philippines. We also acknowledge, with thanks, contributions from Jean-François Outreville of the United Nations Office at Geneva.

THE APPLICATION OF WILLINGNESS TO PAY TO MICROINSURANCE UNITS

Microinsurers' Rate-Setting Experience

Figure 14.1 illustrates factors important for determining microinsurance premium and copayment rates. Copayments are often included in the design of microinsurance as a strategy for managing risk and reducing the effects of moral hazard. They also add to the resource base of the insurance fund. Contribution levels are related to the cost of the benefit package(s), administrative costs, cost-recovery targets, expected utilization, other market prices, and affordability to consumers. Contributions will influence utilization rates through the price elasticity of demand. Utilization will affect estimates of administrative costs and the unit cost of benefit packages. The interactive nature of these factors makes pricing very important in designing health insurance schemes.

Empirical evidence shows that contribution rates have been set for microinsurance on the basis of the cost of benefit packages, utilization rates, household size, affordability, and other market prices, particularly user fees (Musau 1999; Atim 1999; Schneider, Diop, and Bucayana 2000). Most schemes arrived at contribution rates by making assumptions about the utilization of outpatient services and hospitalization rates. Few schemes had cost data available for benefit packages and services, so these figures had to be estimated as well. Affordability

FIGURE 14.1   Factors Affecting Contributions to Microinsurance Units

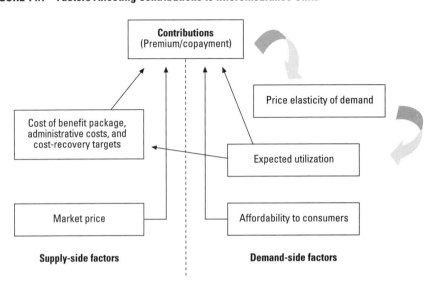

was usually measured either in comparison to daily wages or estimates of household income. None of the schemes evaluated had access to actuarial information or more comprehensive database information on patients.

Willingness to Pay and Contribution Levels

The contingent valuation (willingness-to-pay) methodology rarely has been used to determine actual contribution rates for microinsurance. Instead, other approaches such as focus groups or household surveys have been used to ascertain population interest in community-based health insurance as well as how much individuals could foresee paying for health insurance (Hailemariam and Brenzel 1998; Musau 1999; Atim 1999).

There are several reasons to expect that individuals would be willing to pay for health insurance, particularly if membership in an insurance scheme guarantees the enrollee access to quality care. First, there is significant evidence that individuals and households are willing to pay for quality improvements associated with health care (Wouters, Adeyi, and Morrow 1993; Arhin 1995; Weaver and others 1996). If microinsurers' benefit packages ensure that beneficiaries receive access to high-quality health care services in cases where these services were previously unavailable because of financial barriers, it seems clear that individuals would be willing to pay for health insurance at the community level. The popularity of community insurance schemes also suggests willingness to pay.

Second, because of their proximity to the community, it is thought that the design of microinsurance and user-fee systems will be responsive to the preferences, needs, and demands of the local population (Carrin, de Graeve, and Deville 1999). Involvement of the population in the organization and financing of microinsurance links the health insurance schemes to consumer preferences. The principle is that the community sees advantages in voluntary prepayment for services as a mechanism for ensuring stable financing and improved provision of services. In other words, individuals may be willing to pay for insurance designed with community needs in mind.

Third, many community-based schemes are founded on existing social solidarity mechanisms, such as the *eder* (burial) societies in Ethiopia (Hailemariam and Brenzel 1998) and the *engozi* (health transport) societies in Uganda (Musau 1999; Walford and others 2000). Therefore, community-based health insurance offers another way of pooling resources for the benefit of the larger group. Experience with social risk-sharing strategies may increase the population's willingness to pay for health insurance.

However, even if communities are prepared to be involved in managing a community scheme, they may have very limited understanding of insurance or prepayment mechanisms (Ron 1999) or have different concepts of risk and risk management than the designers of these schemes. Education of the population on the concept of insurance and risk management is imperative to improve the quality of responses relating to willingness to pay for insurance as well as to engender realistic expectations about microinsurance. The potential cultural and social barriers to insurance will need to be overcome (chapter 19, this volume). If the willingness-to-pay methodology is used to determine contribution rates, one must be careful to specify clearly a feasible and acceptable benefit package, or series of packages, so that the results of the willingness-to-pay survey will make sense in a particular context (Carrin, De Graeve, and Deville 1999).

Willingness to Pay and Pooling Issues

One of the most difficult obstacles for any health insurance scheme is adverse selection. Adverse selection occurs when more sick than healthy individuals enroll in a health insurance plan, affecting the fund's financial viability. This problem arises because of asymmetry of information about a member's health status. Adverse selection can be significantly reduced if enrollment is mandatory instead of voluntary (so that healthy individuals cannot opt out of the scheme). To reduce this problem, enrollment can also be based on affinity groups such as community groups, employment groups, or social groups. In addition, enrollment can be based on families within certain groups.

However, solidarity is not always present in groups, which may lead to nonpooling of resources, depending on how the health insurance fund is managed. For instance, in China, some members of the group were systematically excluded from health insurance schemes, which contributed to adverse selection (Bloom and Shenglan 1999). The choice of groups to insure, and whether they represent homogeneous or heterogeneous risks, is particularly important (Mintz 1999).

Most willingness-to-pay studies show a positive relationship between income and willingness to pay for high-quality health care services. While microinsurance may be offered at the community level, the actual enrollment of members may be skewed toward certain subgroups within the larger population, and these subgroups may not be identical in terms of risk for high-cost health events. Therefore, microinsurers will have to take household income into account by including some sort of sliding scale for poorer families. However, microinsurers run into the same problems that routine health services have in classifying patients as poor or nonpoor.

For instance, the Gomoshasthaya Kendra (GK) scheme in Bangladesh established fee structures according to household ability to pay. Premiums were based on socioeconomic status, with symbolic payments made by the poorest income group (Desmet, Chowdhury, and Islam 1999). After 15 years of operation, this health insurance scheme still has not reached its main target group (poor households), despite the sliding scale for contributions. In surveys, the contribution levels were most frequently cited as the reason for nonsubscription (Desmet, Chowdhury, and Islam 1999). Similarly, in the Democratic Republic of Congo, a study showed that the very low-income group (<US$20/month) and the very high-income group (>US$200/month) were overrepresented in the nonsubscriber group for the Bwamanda hospital insurance scheme compared with other income classes (Criel, van der Stuyft, and van Lerberghe 1999).

Willingness-to-pay studies can provide insight into the community's heterogeneity vis-à-vis socioeconomic status, use of facilities, willingness to participate in a health insurance pool, and willingness to pay certain premiums for a range of benefit packages. This information is useful in determining whether pooling should be at the level of the community or among a group of communities.

THE AFFORDABILITY OF MICROINSURANCE UNITS

In health care, affordability is a relative term that refers to the ability of individuals and households to finance health care within their means. Health expenditures are considered unaffordable when people are deterred from using services for financial reasons or when people spend so much on health care that they lack the resources to pay for other essential commodities or services (Russell 1996).

Research and policy discussion have tended to assume that willingness to pay is similar to ability to pay (Russell 1996). However, the affordability of health care is a critical issue, particularly when consumers are expected to finance a range of essential services, including health, education, and water, out of pocket.[2] Although individuals may be willing to pay for health services, this does not imply that they can afford user charges, premiums, and copayments.

> [F]amilies do, on occasion, encounter great difficulties in paying for health services. They persist in using services because they do not see that they have any choice if they are to save their relatives. The money used to pay for health care may otherwise have been used for food, agricultural development or education. Payment for health services is thus made at considerable social cost to the family and can scarcely be said to represent a "willingness" to pay in the normal sense of the word (Waddington and Enimayew 1989).

Consumers may delay seeking care, choose cheaper health care alternatives, reallocate resources away from other goods and services, or borrow to finance the care they need. The more serious the illness, the more likely are households to incur debt or forgo essential services to finance care (Russell 1996; Desmet, Chowdhury, and Islam 1999; Ron 1999). In China, people have to choose between borrowing to pay for health care or going without. Illness has become a major cause of impoverishment, as health care costs have risen faster than disposable income (Bloom and Shenglan 1999).

In addition to contributions for services, households also pay for transport and other costs such as food for the patient and accommodations for caretakers in the event of hospitalization. The loss of income resulting from illness can also be devastating to a household. Defaulting on loans in Bangladesh is thought to relate more to lost income from illness than to health care costs (Desmet, Chowdhury, and Islam 1999).

The affordability of premiums and copayments is related to the total amount of the expected payment, frequency of payment, and timing of the payment cycle. Affordability is also related to the social acceptance of prepayment, concepts of risk, and cultural beliefs about risk aversion (chapter 19, this volume). Microinsurers usually rely on monthly contributions or annual contributions made at the time of the year when cash availability is high. A one-time annual payment reduces microinsurers' administrative costs and managerial requirements but may limit wider participation across income groups if cash availability is low. Frequent payments might be more affordable, but they raise administrative requirements and costs.

Affordability may be relative to the way resource-allocation decisions are made in households. If women earn a large share of household income but do not have control over the way this income is spent, a health service may not be affordable in this context. Studies conducted in many cultures demonstrate that income control by women results in different patterns of household resource allocation than income control by men (Brenzel 1996).

Finally, prepayment through microinsurance spreads payment over a year so that financial barriers are reduced or removed. In the Kisiizi Hospital Scheme, it was found that many patients no longer borrowed to pay for health care, and fewer patients were in debt because of illness (Musau 1999; Walford and others 2000).

To extend access to services to the widest population and to remove financial barriers to health care, microinsurers may need to be partially subsidized to cover contributions from the poorest households (Busse, chapter 13, this volume). Subsidies can come from donor organizations, nongovernmental organizations, and missions that also provide technical assistance in fund management and operation, or from ministries of health that are concerned about guaranteeing access to care and about accountability of funds to consumers who prepay into them.

WILLINGNESS TO PAY AND REINSURANCE

Little empirical work has been done on willingness to pay for reinsurance of microinsurers. In rare cases, funds have established some type of contingency or reserve fund in case of shortfalls. Microinsurers' lack of reserves seems to indicate that the costs of providing coverage far exceed income from premiums and copayments; premiums cannot be raised because of affordability issues; current management of insurance funds, including risk-management strategies, precludes setting aside reserves or contingencies—or some combination of the above.

According to Atim (1999), reserves should represent between three and six months' expenditures to provide reasonable coverage for unexpectedly high expenses associated with increased hospitalization during an epidemic. He found a ratio of net reserves to monthly expenditure of 1.46 for the scheme in Ghana (Nkoranza), and a ratio of 5.46 for the scheme in Cameroon (Mutuelle Famille Babouantou de Yaoundé). Nkoranza was deemed not to be in a good financial position.

In Uganda, there is interest in setting aside contingency funds or reserves, or even in purchasing reinsurance, but microinsurers are precluded from doing so because malaria epidemics have depleted their fund balances. In addition, most funds' low cost-recovery rates deter private reinsurance companies. The government recently abolished user fees and is increasing district and health subdistrict budgets to make up for the difference in income. The availability of extra Ministry of Health resources to fund or cofinance reserve funds for microinsurers is probably limited at best.[3]

Individual consumers are probably not aware of the need for reinsurance as part of their contributions to a health insurance fund. However, some patients have prepaid for services that are not available when they need them because of financial shortfalls in insurance funds. In these environments, consumers might be willing to pay a small fee to insure against this type of occurrence. In willingness-to-pay surveys, this notion could be built into the contingent valuation technique by asking individuals if they would be willing to pay for guaranteed access to a high-quality package of health care services.

Fund managers and community-management committees are the real consumers of reinsurance. Their incentives to purchase reinsurance depend on the consequences of financial failure. If the ministry of health or donor agencies agree to finance deficits, microinsurers have little incentive to procure reinsurance. If, however, the fund managers are obligated by law to provide services to members regardless of the microinsurer's financial position, they would either have to procure reinsurance or set aside a reserve fund to cover financial shortfalls.

We explored the additional cost requirement for reinsurance (as a part of premiums) for a typical African microinsurer.[4] From facility statistics, each member is assumed to make one outpatient visit per year at a cost of US$1.79 per visit, and have a 6 percent hospitalization rate at a cost of US$18.71 per hospitalization. The health insurance scheme's administrative costs are about US$2.31 per family of six, resulting in a total cost of US$22.81 to the fund to provide care to a family of six. The premium paid for a family of six per year is US$24.23, resulting in a 6 percent margin between fund revenues and expenses. If health care costs for all families in the scheme were 5 percent higher than expected, the fund would run a deficit of approximately US$5 per family per year. A reinsurance rate of 25 percent of the premium would be required to cover this deficit. However, the new premium would rise to approximately US$31 per year per family, and this figure seems high relative to household income, particularly in rural areas. This example highlights both the financial vulnerability of microinsurers and their need for some form of protection, either through reserve funds or reinsurance, as well as the potential financial burden of reinsurance for rural families.

The issue of affordability to households of increased premiums to cover the cost of a reserve fund or reinsurance is a vexing one and must be considered when final premium rates are set. However, there may be limits on solidarity within communities to pool funds, and arguments about affordability may hide this fact.

CONCLUSIONS

This chapter highlights the role that willingness-to-pay studies can play in determining contribution levels for microinsurance and identifies their possible application in addressing pooling and enrollment issues. Responses to willingness-to-pay surveys are generally related to the quality of health services and choice of health care providers. These factors are inextricably linked to the design and development of benefit packages that form the basis of contingent valuation surveys. These factors also play a role in determining contribution rates.

Willingness-to-pay responses are positively related to household income. If the contingent valuation methodology is used to determine contribution rates for microinsurance, survey responses must come from a cross-section of the population within a community to capture variation in amounts individuals are willing to pay. This information may be used to develop a range of benefit packages, from a basic minimum package affordable to the poorest households, to a more comprehensive package that wealthier households could afford. Ability to pay may be a better predictor than willingness to pay of probability of enrollment, as well as continuity and sustainability of prepayment.

This chapter also highlights the narrow margin that exists between revenues and expenditures for some microinsurers and the vulnerability of these funds to external shocks such as epidemics. Reinsurance, while protecting schemes against catastrophe loss, may render premiums unaffordable to families. Instead of passing on the full cost of reinsurance to members through increased premiums, schemes need to consider other mechanisms for financing reinsurance, either through a sliding scale or subsidy from government or donors.

One crucial issue is whether replication of community-based schemes should be encouraged. Many such schemes may be successful, but the possibilities for pooling resources and spreading risks are limited. So, too, are the administrative capacities to launch, manage, and maintain funds.

NOTES

1. In theoretical terms, the area under the demand curve represents how much a consumer would be willing to pay for a service, while holding the level of satisfaction constant.

2. Even if people are willing to pay for microinsurance, this does not necessarily guarantee that they will commit funds or be able to afford prepayment over the long term. Lack of empirical evidence curtails further exploration of this relationship.

3. Personal communication, Uganda Community-Based Health Financing Association.

4. This example is based on financial figures for the Kisiizi Hospital Health Scheme in Uganda for 1999, as reported in Musau (1999). The average outpatient cost per visit was estimated to be Ush 2,100 (US$1.79) using reported exchange rates. The scheme assumes an average of one outpatient visit per member per year. The average inpatient cost for the scheme was estimated to be Ush 22,000 (US$18.71). Administrative costs for the scheme are approximately Ush 3 million, and there are 6,600 members, resulting in Ush 455 per member or Ush 5,523 (US$2.31) per family. The total annual cost of providing care to a family of six under the scheme (US$22.81) represents the sum of outpatient costs (US$1.79), hospitalization (US$18.71), and administrative costs (US$2.31).

REFERENCES

The word *processed* describes informally reproduced works that may not be commonly available through libraries.

Arhin, D. 1995. "Health Insurance in Rural Africa." *The Lancet* 345:44–45.

Atim, C. 1999. "Social Movements and Health Insurance: A Critical Evaluation of Voluntary, Non-profit Insurance Schemes with Case Studies from Ghana and Cameroon." *Social Science and Medicine* 48:881–96.

Bloom, G., and Shenglan, T. 1999. "Health Prepayment Schemes in China: Towards a More Active Role for Government." *Social Science and Medicine* 48:951–60.

Brenzel, L. 1996. "Female Decision-Making Power and the Intrahousehold Allocation of Food and Medical Care Resources in Ghana." Paper prepared for the Annual Meeting of the Population Association of America. New Orleans, La.

_____. 1999. *Results of Health Care Financing Studies in Ethiopia*. Arlington, Va.: BASICS Project.

Carrin, G., D. de Graeve, and L. Deville. 1999. "Editorial: Introduction to Special Issue on the Economics of Heath Insurance in Low and Middle Income Countries." *Social Science and Medicine* 48:859–64.

Criel, B., P. van der Stuyft, and W. van Lerberghe. 1999. "The Bwamanda Hospital Insurance Scheme: Effective for Whom? A Study of Its Impact on Hospital Utilization Patterns." *Social Science and Medicine* 48:897–911.

Desmet, M., A.Q. Chowdhury, and K. Islam. 1999. "The Potential for Social Mobilization in Bangladesh: The Organization and Functioning of Two Health Insurance Schemes." *Social Science and Medicine* 48:925–38.

Donaldson, C. 1990. "Willingness to Pay for Publicly-Provided Goods: A Possible Measure of Benefit?" *Journal of Health Economics* 9:103–18.

ESHE (Essential Services for Health in Ethiopia). 2000. *Estimating the Willingness and Ability to Pay for Health Services in Ethiopia*. Draft. Addis Ababa: ESHE Project and the Health Care Financing Secretariat, Ministry of Health, Federal Democratic Republic of Ethiopia.

Hailemariam, D., and L. Brenzel. 1998. *Feasibility of Community-Based Health Insurance in Ethiopia*. Arlington, Va.: BASICS Project.

Johannessen, M., B. Jonsson, and L. Borquist. 1991. "Willingness to Pay for Antihypertensive Therapy: Results of a Swedish Pilot Study." *Journal of Health Economics* 10:461–74.

_____. 1993. "Willingness to Pay for Antihypertensive Therapy: Further Results." *Journal of Health Economics* 12:95–108.

Mills, A., J. Fox-Rushby, M. Aikins, U. D'Alessandro, K. Cham, and B. Greenwood. 1994. "Financing Mechanisms for Village Activities in The Gambia and Their Implications for Financing Insecticide for Bednet Impregnation." *Journal of Tropical Medicine and Hygiene* 97:325–32.

Mintz, P. 1999. "Managing Acute, Chronic, and Catastrophic Health Care Costs: Experience and Policy Issues in the U.S. Context of Managed Care and Comparative Analysis of the Chilean Regulatory Framework." World Bank, Washington, D.C. Processed.

Musau, S.N. 1999. *Community-Based Health Insurance: Experiences and Lessons Learned from East and Southern Africa*. Technical Report No. 34. Bethesda, Md.: Abt Associates, Inc., Partnerships for Health Reform Project.

Neumann, P.J., and M. Johannessen. 1994. "The Willingness to Pay for in Vitro Fertilization: A Pilot Study Using Contingent Valuation." *Medical Care* 32:686–99.

Olsen, J.A., and R.D. Smith. 2001. "Theory versus Practice: A Review of 'Willingness-to-Pay' in Health and Health Care." *Health Economics* 10:39–52.

Ron, A. 1999. "NGOs in Community Health Insurance Schemes: Examples from Guatemala and the Philippines." *Social Science and Medicine* 48:939–50.

Russell, S. 1996. "Ability to Pay for Health Care: Concepts and Evidence." *Health Policy and Planning* 11(3):219–37.

Russell, S., Fox-Rushby, J., and Arhin, D. 1995. "Willingness and Ability to Pay for Health Care: A Selection of Methods and Issues." *Health Policy and Planning* 10(1):94–101.

Schneider, P., F.P. Diop, and S. Bucayana. 2000. *Development and Implementation of Prepayment Schemes in Rwanda*. Technical Report No. 45. Bethesda, Md.: Abt Associates, Inc., Partnerships for Health Reform Project.

Waddington, C.J., and K.A. Enimayew. 1989. "A Price to Pay: The Impact of User Charges in the Ashanti-Akim District, Ghana." *International Journal of Health Planning and Management* 4:14–47.

Walford, V., and others. 2000. "Uganda Community Health Financing Project: Output to Purpose Review." Report to Department for International Development (DfID), Institute for Health Sector Development, London, U.K.

Weaver, M., R. Ndamobissi, R. Kornfield, C. Blewane, A. Sathe, M. Chapko, N Bendje, E. Nguembi, and J. Senwara-Defiobona. 1996. "Willingness to Pay for Child Survival: Results of a National Survey in the Central African Republic." *Social Science and Medicine* 43(6):985–98.

Whittington, D., J. Briscoe, X. Mu, and W. Barron. 1990. "Estimating the Willingness to Pay for Water Services in Developing Countries: A Case Study of the Use of Contingent Valuation Surveys in Southern Haiti." *Economic Development and Cultural Change* 37:293–311.

Wouters, A., O. Adeyi, and R. Morrow. 1993. *Quality of Health Care and Its Role in Cost Recovery with a Focus on Empirical Findings about Willingness to Pay for Quality Improvements, Phase 1: Review of Concepts and Literature and Preliminary Field Work Design*. Bethesda, Md.: Abt Associates, Inc., Health Financing and Sustainability Project.

CHAPTER 15

Creating a Favorable Market Environment for Microinsurance at the Community Level

William Newbrander and Logan Brenzel

Microinsurance units provide an opportunity to extend access to health services by spreading costs and risks over a wide group within a community. Because there is an implicit allocation of resources from healthy to sick individuals and from wealthier to poorer households, community-based health insurance can contribute to equity in health care financing. Microinsurers also provide an opportunity to increase appropriate use of cost-effective health services by covering basic promotive and preventive care while facilitating access to necessary curative services (McPake, Hanson, and Mills 1993).

This chapter identifies some of the market forces affecting development of microinsurers, discusses ways of creating a more favorable environment for them, and examines the potential market for reinsurance among microinsurers, highlighting factors enabling or hindering growth of reinsurance. Alternative formats for reinsurance for microinsurers are also proposed.

LINK BETWEEN MARKET FACTORS AND DEVELOPMENT OF MICROINSURANCE UNITS

The number of microinsurers in developing countries has grown tremendously in recent years, as has interest in microinsurance. This growth is partly a response to fiscal situations in most public health systems that preclude universal coverage of the population. Another part can be attributed to the increasing involvement of grass-roots movements in health care delivery. There is little direct empirical evidence, however, about the factors impelling growth in the number of schemes or about the proportion of population covered by any particular scheme. Nor is it known whether these factors overlap or are entirely distinct. Nevertheless, factors that may be leading to growth should be identified.

First, the extent to which microinsurance development and demand for community-based insurance schemes have traditionally responded to market

The authors acknowledge, with thanks, contributions from Jean-François Outreville of the United Nations Office, Geneva. For reviewing a draft of this chapter, the authors thank Guy Carrin, Health Economist, World Health Organization, Geneva, and Dr. Benito Reverente, Chief of Party, Management Sciences for Health, the Philippines.

forces is unclear. This is particularly true in the early stages of microinsurance development, which often arises because governments or donors want to launch a pilot experiment to resolve a financing or access issue. Governments have promoted microinsurance as either a solution to lack of financing or a way to extend access to the rural population. Donors have promoted microinsurance as part of an agenda to increase community participation in health services financing and management so as to alleviate some of the pernicious problems associated with inadequate access and low-quality services. Mission facilities and nongovernmental organizations (NGOs) have promoted microinsurance as a way of sustaining their health facilities despite reduced financial support from abroad.

On the supply side, three other factors may affect the proliferation of microinsurers: the willingness of providers and facilities to participate in schemes; the willingness of community management committees to support the development and implementation of schemes; and the financial and general management capacity available in a locality. Often, providers are reluctant to be involved in setting up schemes, since they change the way in which services are financed and may pose financial hardships for patients. For instance, an insurance feasibility study in Ethiopia showed that hospital physicians were not entirely in favor of introducing health insurance, and this group posed a potential obstacle to the implementation of the scheme (Hailemariam and Brenzel 1998).

Operating a successful microinsurance unit requires sophisticated management skills at both the facility and community levels, skills that are often in short supply in developing countries, especially in the health sector. Managing schemes is often more complex than managing a hospital. The fund manager or the management committee play a critical role in ensuring the scheme's financial sustainability. A project supporting insurance schemes in Uganda has recognized the difficulties of attracting and retaining management staff and is thinking of designing robust management systems that can operate with limited management capacity (Walford and others 2000). Community participation and scheme management are also necessary to create community ownership of the scheme and commitment to its success.

On the demand side, several factors relate to the creation of schemes. First, factors affecting households' disposable income (macroeconomic policies, crop failures, or agricultural policies) are linked to willingness to pay for health insurance (ESHE 2000). Some schemes have come into existence or perished as a result of economic and political factors (Creese and Bennett 1997). Clearly, the external environment influences demand for schemes as well as scheme design. However, the health sector has limited leverage to manipulate external social and economic factors.

Significant work has been done to evaluate whether demand exists for community-based health insurance (Creese and Bennett 1997; Brenzel and Newbrander, chapter 14 in this volume). In addition, the rising price of health care, either as a result of user fees or an increasing private sector role in service delivery, may make prepayment schemes attractive to households. Health insurance is more likely to be accepted in an environment where patients are familiar with user fees and accustomed to paying for health care. However, an environment where user fees are lower than expected premiums provides little incentive for people to join schemes. In that case, the user fee system should be modified before community-based insurance is introduced.

The perceived quality of health services offered through microinsurance is a key factor in the demand for services and, by extension, the demand for microinsurers. Household characteristics, including income, education, gender of the household head, and number of dependents, influence a household's demand for alternative financing through prepayment schemes. Finally, design features such as size of the premium, frequency of payment, coverage of household members, and choice of provider influence interest in schemes. Rural risk sharing appears to be targeted more toward the rural middle classes than the rural poor (Creese and Bennett 1997).

CREATING A FAVORABLE ENVIRONMENT FOR GROWTH IN MICROINSURANCE

Uncontrolled proliferation of poorly designed microinsurance, particularly with respect to risk-management strategies, increases the likelihood that they will fail and that people will become skeptical about using them. Governments cannot abdicate their responsibility for ensuring access to high-quality health services for the population by delegating the financing of services to the schemes themselves. Instead, governments must continue to oversee the design and implementation of schemes, and ensure their financial viability, as part of a holistic health-financing strategy.

The most critical factor for enabling proper growth in the number of micro-inisurers is the regulatory environment. Currently, many microinsurers skirt the regulations and requirements of national insurance industries because they classify themselves as schemes, funds, or programs. As a result, they are not required to meet the standards set by national insurance commissions, established generally to oversee casualty, auto, and life insurance. In classifying themselves as schemes, they are not required to charge higher premiums to cover the additional costs associated with reinsurance and guaranteed payment of claims. This strategy leaves scheme members without legal recourse if a fund becomes insolvent. The fund, therefore, is not legally accountable to its members. However, if the fund is managed by a community committee, fund members may be able to influence its operations through peer pressure or other means.

This situation allows ministries of health to become proactive in setting policies and establishing procedures to ensure the schemes' financial viability. This oversight can give people confidence that their resources will not be squandered and that services will be available when needed. Ministries of health need to explore building linkages between microinsurers and national insurance regulations.

Another factor that will enable the growth of microinsurance is building the capacity to design and manage schemes. Governments and donors need to provide training in fund management, computer database management, and financial and administrative control. A recent evaluation of schemes in Uganda, supported by the United Kingdom's Department for International Development (DfID), attributed the schemes' success in part to the efforts of the central team to improve management capacity and systems (Walford and others 2000).

From a consumer's perspective, health insurance is complicated, requiring several layers of understanding and decisionmaking. The marketing function of health insurance schemes is often overlooked, although it can play a tremendous role in increasing the coverage of schemes and people's interest in them (Hailemariam and Brenzel 1998). The successful operation of microinsurers and attenuation of moral hazard are dependent on consumer education about the purpose of the scheme; the prices (premiums and copayments); schedule and place of payment; the package of services covered and excluded and the rationale for this distinction; coverage or noncoverage of household members; and procedures for obtaining health services and reimbursement.

Finally, improving existing schemes' financial viability may enable proliferation of other schemes. Improved viability can come about through better risk management, increased coverage, and government subsidies. Although difficult to design and implement, strategies for curbing adverse selection, moral hazard, cost escalation, and cheating on membership will improve financial viability. These strategies include requiring mandatory enrollment of groups; creating a gatekeeper function; instituting copayments and a waiting period before entitlement to benefits; issuing identification cards; tracking benefits and treatment costs and introducing cost-containment measures; controlling the use of technology and treatment practices; and limiting the services covered.

Expanding membership not only enlarges the risk pool, thereby reducing the probability of adverse selection, but also brings in additional revenues. The risk of financial insolvency generally decreases with the number of enrollees representative of a cross-section of the population as a whole. Sufficient scale allows the scheme to keep the cost of insurance *(load)* low relative to payouts to make the premiums affordable (Bovbjerg 1999). However, some schemes are limited by the size of the population that can be covered as a result of geographical constraints or competition for the same pool of members. For instance, in the Philippines, the small population limits risk pooling and cross-subsidization among income groups (Ron 1999). Hence, microinsurers in poor, rural areas are viable but on a limited scale and primarily among mission and NGO facilities that are well established in these areas.

Subsidies may become a more important feature of microinsurance in the future as a means of offsetting some membership costs for households and enrolling members who would otherwise be excluded because of inability to pay or preexisting conditions. The best subsidy program would target specific population groups in specific schemes such as the poorest households or those affected by HIV/AIDS. To implement this type of program, criteria should be developed for the types of services to be covered, target populations, and efficiency standards (Walford and others 2000). In Rwanda, donor organizations and NGOs are beginning to finance poor households' premiums, and they are considering doing the same for people affected by HIV/AIDS.

PROTECTION AGAINST FINANCIAL INSOLVENCY

In the life cycle of microinsurers, the first few years are usually characterized by large claims and limited revenues until utilization patterns even out and enrollment reaches a critical threshold. As a result, many schemes have been subsidized through the initial phases to cover expected deficits or unanticipated losses from high-cost, low-probability events. Subsidies to the fund, from ministries of health or donors, have traditionally been used to protect insurance schemes against financial insolvency. In Uganda, DfID provided grants as a stop-gap measure to keep the schemes going, particularly in the initial period. However, this type of stop-gap financing by donors or governments creates disincentives for the health facility or third party to control utilization and costs if they can expect all losses to be covered. For this reason, few schemes have developed reserve or contingency funds to cover unexpected losses.

THE NEED FOR REINSURANCE FOR MICROINSURERS

Reinsurance is one approach for coping with financial risks, since it spreads risk among a group of insurers. Insurers seek to reinsure for two primary reasons: to protect their financial assets from unforeseen losses from high-cost cases and to underwrite more risks than they could by relying on their own surplus.

Insurers face financial risk even after pooling individual risk because rare high-cost events could still bankrupt a scheme. In the United States in 1987, 1 percent of the population accounted for 30 percent of total health expenditure, while 50 percent of the population spent only 3 percent of total health expenditure. Risk can be mitigated by enrolling a large enough population so that, in the aggregate, the magnitude of these expenditures can be anticipated (Bovbjerg 1999). In small schemes, however, the ability to predict financial losses is limited.

For community-based schemes, the most common sources of unpredictable financial risk are epidemics and disease outbreaks that result in much higher than predicted utilization of health services. For instance, malaria epidemics in Uganda around the Kisiizi, Ishaka, Bushenyi, and Nyakibale Hospital Schemes have had a big financial impact. An evaluation of these schemes recommends some form of reinsurance to cope with these losses (Walford and others 2000). The treatment and care of HIV/AIDS patients is another high-cost and somewhat unpredictable need. The growing prevalence of HIV/AIDS in rural areas, particularly in Sub-Saharan Africa, represents a high-risk scenario for health insurance schemes, unless a mechanism such as direct subsidies or reinsurance is established to handle treatment costs.

REINSURANCE OPTIONS FOR MICROINSURANCE UNITS

Reinsurance is provided through one of the following mechanisms. First, some companies focus exclusively on reinsurance, operating outside the organization seeking to transfer risk. Second, a primary insurer may have reinsurance branches or departments, as do large insurers with multiple products. Finally, associations or cooperatives may provide reinsurance.

Usually, the establishment of a national reinsurance company in a developing country is associated with a system of compulsory cessions from the *primary* (direct) companies operating in the market. The *quota-share* system (redistribution of proportional business) is the most suitable in these countries, at least during initial market development.

National reinsurance institutions have the following advantages (UNCTAD 1973):

- Reinsurance institutions are generally created to expand the market's retention capacity.

- The overall risk-bearing capacity is enhanced and surpluses, up to a ceiling, are redistributed among the national ceding companies.

- A national reinsurance institution can effectively promote sound market development because it has a broad knowledge of market conditions, which the direct companies, operating on their own, cannot acquire.

Regional or Subregional Cooperation

Insurance companies in a region or subregion are said to have formed a *regional insurance* pool when they decide to cooperate by setting up an administrative framework or scheme by which they systematically cede or retrocede a portion of their business for distribution among the participating companies in accordance with an agreed system.

Regional pools, formed purely as reinsurance pools, are different from national insurance pools in several ways. Although many regional pools benefit from some sort of governmental support, most companies decide voluntarily to participate. The decision depends largely on the company's confidence in the pool's other members and management.

One of the most difficult problems in operating a regional pool arises from its member companies' use of a variety of currencies. Currency fluctuations can complicate balance settlement among the pool's participants.

The arguments in favor of the formation of a reinsurance institution at the national level also apply at a regional or subregional level. Regional reinsurance organizations such as the Asian Reinsurance Corporation and the Africa Reinsurance Corporation have played an important but limited role in the development of local insurance markets in their area of expertise.

The International Reinsurance Market

In the middle of the nineteenth century, the first specialized reinsurance company was created, in Germany. Subsequently, other specialized reinsurers were established in Europe and North America. The emergence of specialized institutions signaled the internationalization of this type of activity.

Traditionally, few major markets could offer reinsurance facilities on an international scale. Today, reinsurers from fewer than 10 countries still dominate the international reinsurance scene. However, increased demand for reinsurance all over the world has spurred a tremendous expansion in the number of reinsurers (chapter 3, box 3.1, this volume).

New markets have sprung up, particularly in free zones and in countries that offer offshore facilities. Captive insurance companies, created to cover their principals' risks, enlarged the scope of their activity to encompass reinsurance of open market business. A number of reinsurance companies were also established in developing countries nationally or regionally. Large primary insurers have further enlarged this market.

Today, the volume of international reinsurance is quite large, although its exact magnitude is unknown. According to Standard & Poor's, the first 125 reinsurers wrote reinsurance policies with premiums of US$72 million in 1999. As mentioned by Outreville (chapter 3, this volume), this market is in the hands of a few companies. The top 30 companies wrote nearly 75 percent of all net premiums in 1999. The largest 15 companies are based in only four countries (box 3.1).

POSSIBLE FORMATS FOR REINSURANCE FOR MICROINSURANCE UNITS

Microinsurance units can reinsure by pooling reinsurance, by accepting reciprocal arrangements, by obtaining subsidies, or by joining a regional or international insurance pool.

Pooled Reinsurance

In insurance, pooling is a means of gathering individual member companies' risks and redistributing them on a broader plane, thus leveling liabilities and premiums. Pools can apply to both direct insurance and reinsurance. Each company's share is determined by criteria specified in the pool agreement, which takes into account each member's risk-retention capacities.

Provided that the pools are adequately organized and properly managed, they can be an excellent means of serving the interests of both the country and the participating insurance companies. All the members' retention capacities are better utilized, and terms, conditions, and rates tend to be coordinated.

The proper functioning of any pool requires that no individual member company try to use the pool for its own profit to the detriment of the other members. A pool therefore imposes discipline on the local market. Among other prerequisites, pooled business must show some uniformity, and members should follow the same ethical and business principles. For this reason, such pools are almost always national or subregional, confined to a limited area with similar market conditions.

For developing countries, contributions into a reinsurance pool, independently managed by an umbrella organization for a group of microinsurers, might be an effective mechanism where there are many small community or NGO-based funds, as in Uganda or the Philippines.

Reciprocity

Reciprocity between one company and another will stabilize the portfolio results provided that a prudent policy is followed in accepting reciprocal arrangements. The probability is small that adverse results in a company's own net business will coincide with an overall adverse result from the reciprocal exchanges accepted from the various territories.

Proportional reinsurance treaties, in particular quota-share arrangements, are generally the most suitable for attracting reciprocity, especially when the arrangement is reasonably balanced between the two companies. However, many companies that accept reciprocity from other companies cannot thoroughly investigate the business offered.

Subsidies from Government or Donors

As another possible strategy, microinsurers that cannot afford reinsurance might be able to arrange for financial cover from either the government or donor organizations in the event of a deficit or unanticipated financial loss. However, this approach is not sustainable, may give negative performance and risk-management incentives, and may perpetuate poor microinsurance designs. Instead of using scarce public resources or donor funding to cover deficits, these resources can be better spent on developing management capacity and management systems and on improving scheme design to reduce financial risk.

Cross-National Reinsurance

Because one country may have too few microinsurers to support reinsurance at the national level, cross-border or regional reinsurance pools for microinsurers might be considered. This might make sense for countries with small populations and few microinsurers.

FACTORS FACILITATING REINSURANCE FOR MICROINSURERS

Scale, financial viability, and government regulation all influence the environment in which reinsuring microinsurers will or will not attract prospective reinsurers.

Reinsurers will be interested in reinsuring microinsurers only if enough of them have large enough enrollments. Without sufficient scale, reinsurers will have difficulties predicting financial losses, setting accurate reinsurance rates, and determining whether to extend proportional or quota-share contracts.

Government and donor support is essential both in promoting the need for reinsurance and in supporting the smaller insurance efforts of communities and NGOs. The government has an interest in ensuring that microinsurers do not threaten access to health services because of unanticipated financial losses. If a microinsurer fails, the government and public health system will have to provide the needed services. Thus, the public sector has a compelling interest in the success and viability of microinsurance, to which reinsurance contributes. Donors can help by providing technical assistance for establishing reinsurance pools to strengthen microinsurers' operations.

Government regulation should be developed to ensure that microinsurers and insurers have sufficient funds and reserves to pay claims and cover any unexpected loss. Regulations can also give legal status to microinsurers and reinsurance funds or companies.

Donors and the government can assist by ensuring sound financial management of microinsurers and routine monitoring of utilization and the cost of services. Payments to providers should be monitored to reduce the risks of uncontrolled cost escalation. The insurer needs to know that prices are reasonable and customary. The price of obtaining reinsurance must be affordable and must not threaten the schemes' financial viability. Finally, schemes that find reinsurance difficult to afford should consider setting up reserve and risk funds before participating in reinsurance.

Reinsurance, though unquestionably required for large insurers, poses other challenges for microinsurers. One challenge is to ascertain the necessity and viability of market creation for reinsuring microinsurers within or across countries. Fraud must also be thwarted. For instance, in South Africa a number of private medical aid schemes have used reinsurance to remove significant reserves from insurance companies for transfer to parent companies and shareholders (van den Heever 2001). Hence, decisionmakers must be cautious in ascertaining the need for and designing reinsurance mechanisms.

REFERENCES

Bovbjerg, R. 1999. *Covering Catastrophic Health Care and Containing Costs: Preliminary Lessons for Policy from the U.S. Experience*. Washington, D.C.: Urban Institute.

Creese, A., and S. Bennett. 1997. "Rural Risk-Sharing Strategies." In G. Schieber and A. Maeda, eds., *Innovations in Health Care Financing: Proceedings of a World Bank Conference, March 10–11, 1997*. World Bank Discussion Paper No. 365. Washington, D.C.: World Bank.

ESHE (Essential Services for Health in Ethiopia). 2000. *Estimating the Willingness and Ability to Pay for Health Services in Ethiopia*. Addis Ababa: Essential Services for Health in Ethiopia Project and the Health Care Financing Secretariat, Ministry of Health.

Hailemariam, D., and L. Brenzel. 1998. *Feasibility of Community-Based Health Insurance in Ethiopia*. Arlington, Va.: BASICS Project.

McPake, B., K. Hanson, and A. Mills. 1993. "Community Financing of Health Care in Africa: An Evaluation of the Bamako Initiative." *Social Science and Medicine* 36:1383–96.

Ron, A. 1999. "NGOs in Community Health Insurance Schemes: Examples from Guatemala and the Philippines." *Social Science and Medicine* 48:939–50.

UNCTAD (United Nations Conference on Trade and Development). 1973. *Reinsurance Problems in Developing Countries*. New York: United Nations.

van den Heever, A. 2001. Personal communication with member of the Republic of South Africa Council for Medical Schemes.

Walford, V., R. Basaza, A. Magezi, A. Masiko, G. Noble, F. Somerwell, J. Thornberry, and R. Yates. 2000. "Uganda Community Health Financing Project: Output to Purpose Review." Report to Department for International Development (DfID), Institute for Health Sector Development, London.

CHAPTER 16

Minimum Accounting and Statistical Framework

David M. Dror

Microinsurers exercise several roles, all of them requiring data.[1] The focus here is on the data necessary in the relationship between reinsurer and microinsurer. In this context, the main purpose of a statistical and accounting framework is to provide the data required to operate the reinsurance model. This chapter defines this cluster of data. The framework also provides microinsurers with the information they need to fulfill their other roles.

DATA NEEDS

What data are needed and what for? A short recapitulation of the reinsurance model may help answer this question. As described in chapter 7 of this book, the model allows microinsurers to cede to a reinsurer those risks exceeding a predefined reinsurance threshold, provided that the risks are "insurable."[2] This transaction requires that both the microinsurer and the reinsurer know what benefits the microinsurer covers, which of them are considered insurable, what the average cost of each benefit is (and of the package as a whole), which distribution laws best describe the cost-generating events, and who is entitled to benefits. On the income side, both parties need to know the microinsurer's income and the expected balance between income and expenditure for each accounting period. The complexities of each data element are discussed in the following sections.

IDENTIFICATION OF THE BENEFIT PACKAGE AND ITS COST

In the basic contract between an affiliated microinsurer and the reinsurer, the microinsurer is responsible for all expenditure on uninsurable benefits and on insurable benefits up to a specified reinsurance threshold, responsibility that cannot be cancelled unilaterally during the life of the contract (Dror 2000). To

The author acknowledges with thanks the useful comments offered by Robert Fonteneau, Senior Specialist, Caisse Nationale d'Assurance Maladie, Paris, detailed to the Social Protection Sector, International Labour Office, Geneva, and Professor Ruth Koren, Medical School, Tel Aviv University.

implement this model, both microinsurer and reinsurer must have access to credible data identifying the amounts for which each party will be responsible. These include, first of all, data for calculating the average cost of the package (assumed to be the reinsurance threshold in chapter 7). The total cost of benefits for the accounting period must also be known.

How can the average cost be determined? First, the benefit package has to be defined, and records kept on its cost. Benefits are, as a rule, identified both by the service provided and by the diagnosis. The definition of the benefit package could theoretically rely on a list of service types (for example, consultations, diagnostic services, imaging, medicines, hospitalization, and surgical procedures). Excluded services could also be specified. Some rationing rules may impose limitations not in terms of service type but in terms of diagnosis. In that case, those exclusions also have to be specified (for example, restorative plastic surgery may be covered but not aesthetic plastic surgery; or, some schemes in Africa exclude HIV/AIDS-related treatment).

Defining a benefit package by service type or by diagnosis does not, in and of itself, provide information on the cost of that package. Obtaining cost data is not a straightforward exercise for several reasons. For one, individual microinsurers' accounting records are often partial and may vary from one provider to another depending on the information that the service provider delivers with the bill. Second, each microinsurer's caseload may be too small in the short term to provide a reliable estimate of average cost. Therefore, estimates of the average have to be obtained through alternative methods such as aggregating the caseloads of several small microinsurers that are similar in terms of their geographic location, sociodemographic profile, or economic situation.

Aggregated data can be useful for estimating purposes, as seen in an example from Uganda. Data collected from Kisiizi Mission Hospital covered utilization and cost information for 30 small microinsurers (each with 15 to 57 households with an average of five persons per household) for a period of three trimesters in 1999. The provider's records included identification of each patient's microinsurer. The available records, although far from complete, included a sufficiently large caseload to obtain a reliable estimate of both the incidence and cost of the benefits. Although the individual microinsurers were unable to identify exactly what their benefit package included, the ex post composition of their average package is described in figure 16.1.

Analysis of these data also reveals large gaps in risk profiles between the individual microinsurers in the pool of 30 microinsurers for which an average was calculated (figure 16.1). This figure depicts observed incidence, which is directly related to cost. As can be seen, because any one of the three microinsurers' incidence can vary by more than 50 percent from the average, a reliable average is preferable to data from a single microinsurer.

Another way of estimating the average cost is by observing one microinsurer over a longer period of time. Such estimates have been done in the Philippines, where the ORT Health Plus Scheme has kept data for a larger population (more

FIGURE 16.1   Average and Specific Risk Profiles

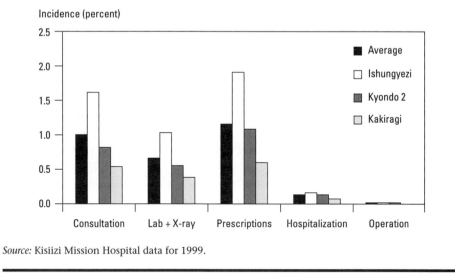

Source: Kisiizi Mission Hospital data for 1999.

than 2,500 insureds) over a longer period (more than five years). This observation method is not entirely error-free, however, given changing individual and provider utilization patterns (and thus expenditure patterns) over time. Inpatient admissions in ORT illustrate this point (figure 16.2). As can be seen, despite the

FIGURE 16.2   Inpatient Admission, 1997–2000

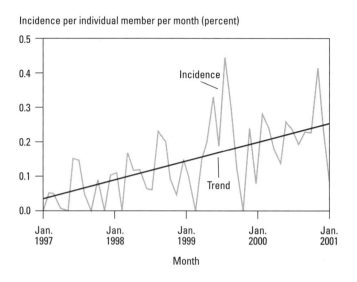

Source: ORT Health Plus Scheme (La Union, Philippines) data.

expected random fluctuations in the incidence, there is an evident and significant upward trend in utilization ($r = 0.6$, $p = 6.5$ x 10^{-6}) from about 0.03 percent to 0.25 percent (incidence per member per month) for the period from January 1997 to January 2001. This example justifies the admonition that historical data must be viewed with caution and cannot be taken as the sole source for a reliable estimate of average cost.

A third method of approximating average cost is extrapolation based on national utilization and epidemiological data. Any extrapolation from national data depends on the ability to arrange local information in terms of the parameters known to influence the burden of disease such as age and gender, distribution, income, geographical locations, and lifestyles. Obtaining these data at the level of the microinsurance unit requires an elaborate information system, which is normally nonexistent at the community level.

When extrapolation from epidemiological data is used, the outcome is incidence data. These data can be converted to cost estimates when two more pieces of information are available: unit costs and the intensity of health care, both of which need to be cross-checked with local providers (see also Haggerty and Reid, chapter 18, this volume).

In conclusion, reinsurance contracts require reliable estimates of the average cost of the benefit package, which are hard to obtain at the level of a single microinsurer. Three approaches have been described for estimating the average, each with its shortcomings. In view of the difficulties described, the initial estimates of average costs might be inaccurate and will have to be adjusted through analysis of data over longer periods of time. In the short term, however, this risk of error must be recognized when calculating the premium.

ESTABLISHING THE INCOME SIDE

The income side has to cover the average cost of benefits plus administrative costs plus the reinsurance premium (if reinsured). For most microinsurers, contributions from members are the largest and most stable source of income. Payment of contributions is one of the two fundamental components defining the relationship between microinsurers and their members (the other is the benefit package). For the individual, paying a contribution differs fundamentally from paying for services in that payment falls due before anyone knows whether the events covered will occur. This prepayment is a standard rule in insurance. Implicit in prepayment is the understanding that the contribution amount, based on averages and set up front, is independent of future consumption by any specific individual. The contribution must be paid even if an individual stays healthy and needs no care during the accounting period. For this reason, the periodicity of contribution payment is disconnected from the time and place of direct service delivery.

Although the system is called "prepayment," it seems fair to say that the term really means an individual's obligation to pay contributions for the entire period, instead of actually paying in advance. Since most people cannot pay the full contribution for the entire period up front, most insurers agree to shorter-than-annual periodicity of payments (monthly, quarterly). The down side of this system is that, although the obligation to pay the premium is absolute, compliance may drop over time if members think their chance of getting benefits drops. Microinsurers operating under voluntary affiliation and with membership composed of low- and irregular-income earners may have to exercise flexibility in scheduling payments. Flexible periodicity is not a problem as long as the compliance rate is kept at acceptable levels. For instance, ORT (the Philippines) allows members to be in arrears for up to three months but still maintains a high compliance rate of about 85 percent (Yamabana, chapter 21, this volume).

Accounting for members' contributions requires that the microinsurer know at all times the number of active members and the demographic composition of the membership. Estimating the number of members into the future would require adjustments to reflect two distinct influences: an upward or downward trend and fluctuations around that trend, which can be quite pronounced when the claim load is low (Dror 2001). Also, a significant change in the number of dependents (who do not pay contributions), or in the composition according to age and gender, may have major implications for income. These changes are illustrated in figure 16.3, based on ORT membership data for the period from January 1995 to May 2001. A clear upward trend in membership (both as individuals and in terms of families) can be seen, with significant fluctuations and short time spans when membership declined. This pattern suggests a high turnover of membership, estimated

FIGURE 16.3   ORT Membership Information

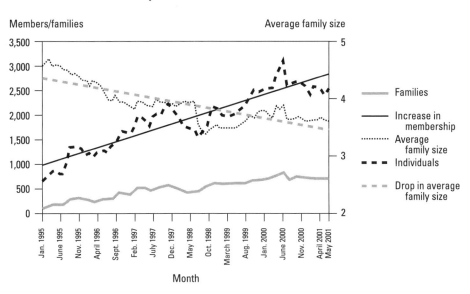

Source: ORT Health Plus data.

in the actuarial review to be on the order of 35 percent a year (Yamabana, chapter 21, this volume). These fluctuations in membership weaken the microinsurer's ability to reliably project its future income. Another interesting feature emerging from the same data is the demographic change in membership, with a drop in the average size of families (from a high of 4.71 to a low of 3.39 persons per family). Without data on age and gender of all members, it would be difficult to understand the full impact of this change, even though it is bound to influence the microinsurer's income as well as the balance between income and expenditure.

Based on impressions from the field, it appears that many microinsurers do not keep information on age and gender for all members. This problem seems to be linked to the fact that the basic subscription unit is the household or the family rather than the individual (the norm in national health systems in industrial countries). The microinsurer's rationale for minimal record-keeping may be a short-term gain in administration, but it is a long-term loss of essential information for proper scheme management.

These problems are all the more relevant when considering that fluctuations in membership and in premium payments are not normally reinsured. Hence, the fluctuations pose a financial risk for the microinsurer, one that can hardly be reduced without analysis of reliable records.

The subscription unit defines the contribution rate payable by each individual as a paying member or as a dependent (for whom partial or no payment may apply). As the applicable contribution rate may differ for members of one and the same subscription unit, the microinsurer must figure out the contribution rate that applies to each individual, a task that can become elaborate. This method requires that microinsurers publish a schedule of contribution rates and qualifying conditions. This is rarely done, with two consequences. First, members in a similar situation may pay different rates. Second, microinsurers may not know how much each member should pay.

BALANCE BETWEEN INCOME AND EXPENDITURE

The next issue is how high contributions should be. Most industrial countries distribute the cost of benefits over the entire covered population, in a manner known as *income rating*, whereby the same contribution rate applies to all insured. This way, each person pays the same percentage of his or her income. Because microinsurers do not normally have information on their members' income, they would be unable to apply income rating. Alternatively, if income has to be high enough to cover expenditures, total contribution revenues should equal expenditures not covered by other income (provided that the amount of "other income" is known). As reinsurance can deal with above-mean expenditures, the calculation should be based on the expected mean costs of the benefit package, not on actual costs in any single period. It has been shown why it is difficult to calculate the mean, and in reality microinsurers rarely do it.

As microinsurers often do not have good knowledge of the expenditure side or the overall amount of other income or even the exact number of members, they have difficulty determining income on the basis of expenditure. Instead, it is not rare to see contributions set arbitrarily or by reference to a comparator. A comparator could be, for example, the cost of one consultation in a government service, other microinsurers' premiums, a study or a survey of costs, or a vote by the microinsurer's general assembly. Whatever system is used to set contributions, information on the way contributions were set is rare, and a validation at the end of the accounting period of the assumptions that led to setting the contribution rates is even more rare.

An example, again from Kisiizi, Uganda, illustrates the possible effect of setting contribution levels without taking account of the expenditure level. The ratio between income and expenditure is shown in figure 16.4. Two levels are shown: income relative to actual expenditure of the specific microinsurer and income relative to the estimated average cost, over the entire period for which data were available. Income varies between 30 percent and 200 percent of actual cost. When calculated in relation to the average, however, the resemblance between the microinsurers is high, ranging from 44 percent to 62 percent of average cost. Seeing that the microinsurers' income is within a similar range of average cost suggests that the huge difference between the microinsurers relative to actual costs is due to accidental clustering of cost-generating events.

In this example, the contributions are clearly too low to cover the cost of the benefit package offered, which means that all 30 microinsurers are bound to

FIGURE 16.4   Contributions and Expenditure

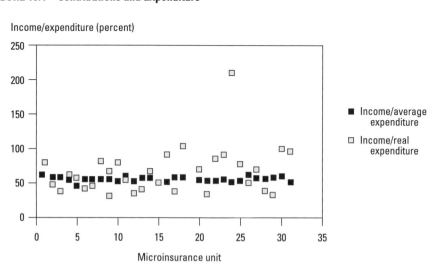

Source: Based on Kisiizi Mission Hospital data for 1999.

become insolvent as soon as the provider ceases to subsidize the cost of care. This situation would force the membership to agree to pay more, reduce the package, or consider other alternatives.

The microinsurer need not know, and indeed often does not know, whether the contribution level accurately reflects members' willingness and ability to pay.[3] In the Kisiizi example (box 16.1), one way of proceeding would be to explore alternative packages that can be maintained with existing contribution levels (figure 16.5).

Some microinsurers accept payments in kind. For instance, Peso-for-Health (the Philippines) allows members who cannot pay premiums in cash to provide work or goods worth the same amount as the contribution due. This ad hoc

---

BOX 16.1   FINDING THE MOST SUITABLE COMPOSITION FOR THE BENEFIT PACKAGE

In discussions, members and leaders of the microinsurance units in Uganda expressed a strong preference for including hospitalization and surgery in the package. They maintained that these events were totally beyond the reach of individual households (even though they could not provide cost details). The composition of the Kisiizi package was established ex post, based on hospital data as shown in the figure.

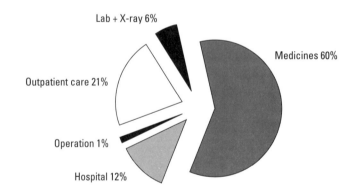

Source: Kisiizi Mission Hospital 1999.

The most striking feature is the large share of medicines in the total cost (60 percent of the total, compared with about 20 percent in industrial countries). Members did not seem to know first that unit cost for prescriptions varied enormously (from Ush 150 to 20,000), putting the expensive prescriptions at a cost level comparable to surgery; and second, that the probability of having to pay for medicines was much higher than the risk of incurring inpatient care costs.

The gap in people's perception about affordability of inpatient care and medicines is striking. It seems to tally with the relatively high unit cost of hospitalization and surgery but to overlook the unusually low prevalence of surgery.

(Box continues on the following page.)

BOX 16.1 (continued)

Further analysis of the Ugandan data reveals that, with the same resources, if the microinsurers in Kisiizi had to survive without a hospital subsidy, they could have responded to members' insistence on including inpatient care in the benefit package by introducing some rationing. The analysis of three comparable options for package composition with rationing is presented in figure 16.5: excluding inpatient care (status quo); paying only 50 percent for medicines[4]; or excluding medicines altogether. Needless to say, other rationing options can be explored.

Bearing in mind that contributions covered only about 50 percent of the cost, the three alternative options were considered from the point of view of closing the recovery gap. The last solution seemed to close this gap the most, but it shifts the most expensive share of the package to the members. This is undesirable, as the microinsurers would lose their attraction for members. Similarly, excluding inpatient care (the first option on the graph) is also undesirable, because the inpatient benefit represents a low-probability, low-elasticity event that can be insured and reinsured, but also because no single household (and probably no single microinsurer) can afford to self-insure this risk. The most balanced rationing option seems to be the second option, covering medicines at 50 percent and retaining coverage of surgery and hospitalization.

FIGURE 16.5   Alternative Composition of Benefit Package

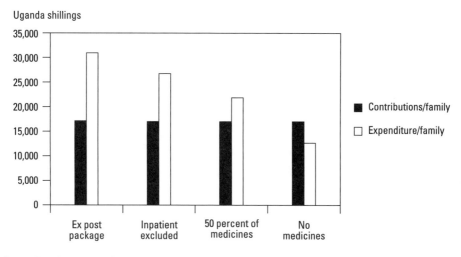

Uganda shillings

■ Contributions/family
□ Expenditure/family

Source: Based on Kisiizi data.

arrangement does not change the need to register the cash value of these pay-ments to guarantee members the same entitlements for their in-kind payment.

Whatever system is used to determine premiums, total income is made up of all sources.[5] When total income is recorded, it can then be compared with the expenditure side to determine the microinsurer's business results.

OTHER INFORMATION NEEDED TO CALCULATE VARIANCE

The reinsurance model proposes that the calculation of the premium (chapter 7, annex 7B, of this volume) is proportional to the standard deviation of each microinsurer's expected cost of benefits (for insurable items only). This standard deviation can be calculated provided that cost-generating events are indepen-dent (or alternatively, a quantitative estimate of their correlation is available), their probability is known, and the distribution of unit costs is also available.

The complexities of obtaining these data are similar to those described earlier for calculating average cost. Utilization data, if available, are unreliable for small caseloads, and historical data may mask time trends. Often records are so scant, particularly for low-frequency events, that it is difficult to estimate their probability and hence the standard deviation. In the absence of solid data, other methods have to be used, notably those described by Auray and Fonteneau in chapter 8 of this book.

The laws that best describe the distribution of unit cost and probability have not yet been validated. They will have to be proven by experience, especially when the lowest possible reinsurance premium is set and when the reinsurer's own business results are highly sensitive to errors in estimating variance.

GENERAL MANAGEMENT INFORMATION

In addition to accounting information, microinsurers need general information on providers, staff, and members.

Provider-Linked Information

When microinsurers reinsure, they become more viable not only for their mem-bers but also for providers, who have a self-explanatory interest in working with solvent clients.

At the same time, microinsurers often function in a scarce-supply environ-ment. As they move toward financial stability and as they attract more members, they would become larger purchasers of services. Besides size, microinsurers' bar-gaining power also depends on knowing from whom they can buy services, what services providers can offer, and at what cost. The reinsurer also has an interest in solid information on providers because of the importance of holding down costs.

Last, insofar as microinsurers can negotiate better rates for the entire group than any single member can do for him- or herself, microinsurers can improve members' welfare by negotiating with providers. For this purpose, microinsurers need to keep a database identifying the providers in their catchment area and their service capacity.

Staff, Management, and General Information

Microinsurers need to estimate their expected business results. For this purpose, besides tracking contributions and other income, they have to track and report benefit costs and other expenditures.[6]

Their relationship with a reinsurer may force microinsurers to shift their subscription unit from family to individual to overcome two main problems. First, family subscription cannot provide accurate demographic, morbidity, and utilization information. Second, there is a high risk of free riding of unaffiliated family members.

Just as microinsurers need to be able to identify their members, so too the reinsurer must be able to identify each microinsurer. The microinsurer identifier would have to be recognized as part of each individual's unique identification to allow studies of regional phenomena.

Other general information may include details on its ownership, management, and accreditation.

DATA TEMPLATE

The data needs described in this chapter require expertise usually unavailable to single microinsurers. Also, some of the more complex data elements are analytical and serve the reinsurer's needs more directly than those of the microinsurer or its members. Therefore, it seems fair that the reinsurance facility should provide an integrated framework for recording and analyzing the data needed. This database can also generate standard reports for various purposes.

A survey of published material aiming to serve microinsurers (Atim 2000; Cripps and others 2000; ILO-STEP 2000; GTZ and others 2001) and validation with several microinsurers in the field has led to the conclusion that such a framework is at present unavailable. The existing sources do not address the data needs of reinsurance operations. It has therefore been necessary to develop such a framework. The framework, in the form of a user-friendly computer application called the *Social Re Data Template,* is described in appendix A of this volume.

For microinsurers, this data template can release operators from doubts associated with implementing an information system. At the same time, the framework leaves sufficient flexibility to allow each microinsurer to define its contractual relationships with members around a clear list of benefits due and contributions payable. The template provides internal automatic validations, audit trails, and checks to endow the system with data consistency, integrity, and security that cannot be achieved in manual bookkeeping. Furthermore, since the ultimate purpose is to pool the resources and manage the risks of many microinsurers through reinsurance, aggregating similar risks can be simplified by standardized data structure.

The data template feeds data into a computational tool, called the *Social Re Toolkit*, with which the reinsurance premium can be calculated (appendix B, this volume).

CONCLUSIONS

The reinsurer needs some information to operate the reinsurance model presented in Bonnevay and others, chapter 7, this volume. With the information most microinsurers can currently provide, the reinsurer has to content itself with less than full information. This means that two basic parameters of the reinsurance contract, the reinsurance threshold (based on the mean expenditure) and the premium (based on the variance), will have to be determined initially through approximations rather than from verified data.

This situation requires remedial action from the very start. On the one hand, the reinsurer must keep higher reserves to cover errors in the approximations; on the other, the microinsurers must agree to implement a system to collect data that will provide all the information necessary to improve the original estimates as fast as possible.

The data requirements must include all the elements of information to enable calculation of the benefit costs and verification of their average and standard deviation. Such requests include data on both expenditure and income.

On the *expenditure side,* detailed utilization information would be broken down into records of:

- *Incidence of* cost-generating *events* in terms of identifying the individual, gender, and age. Such a data frame will provide not only accurate and updated estimates but will also allow extrapolation of incidence resulting from changes in the size and characteristics of the insured population.

- *Cost associated with each event* both in terms of the unit cost and in terms of the total number of units served, plus an indication of the diagnosis. This will allow improvements in the estimate of the unit cost distribution function, helping identify cost indicators by diagnosis, which can enable more accurate extrapolations from national and regional data. Last, these data are necessary for rate negotiations between the microinsurers and health care providers.

On the *income side,* the data must provide an accurate record of the contributions paid by each member so that both recovery and compliance rates can be assessed accurately.

NOTES

1. They manage health plans, purchase services from providers on behalf of their members, manage assets, and sometimes also operate for-profit business enterprises (for example, a local pharmacy).

2. For a distinction between insurable and uninsurable events, please see Vaté and Dror, chapter 6, this volume.

3. Willingness to pay is probably linked to the level of confidence in the microinsurer's ability to meet its obligation in the future, and the relevance of its benefits in the eyes of the catchment population. Ability to pay is quite complicated to measure, but if potential members consider the premium too high, fewer of them will subscribe, and the microinsurer might be more exposed to the negative effects of small group size, to a high turnover of members, or both.

4. Payment of 50 percent for medicines does not necessarily mean 50 percent of each prescription. It may mean varying levels of payment, for example, covering more than 50 percent for expensive medicines and nothing for the cheapest prescriptions. This may be more realistic in the real-life scenario in which some medicines cost as much as surgery.

5. Microinsurers' income may come from many sources besides premiums: matching contributions (in industrial countries, frequently the employer pays a matching contribution); subsidies from a government unit; external budgetary support (either to meet general operating costs or for a specific kind of activity, for example, vaccinations); grants from NGOs; income from user fees; revenues from sales of goods and services or from civic activities (for example, lotteries and games of chance); interest income; and the like.

6. Including salary costs of their staff. A survey of the staff employed by microinsurers in the Philippines shows more than 30 different professional categories (for example, doctor, nurse, pharmacist, clerical staff, health worker, bookkeeper, cashier, driver, education coordinator, promoter, computer operator, and medical secretary).

REFERENCES

Atim, C. 2000. *Training of Trainers Manual for Mutual Health Organization in Ghana*. Bethesda, MD: Abt Associates, Inc., Partnerships for Health Reform/USAID and DANIDA Health Sector Support Office.

Cripps, G., J. Edmonds, R. Killian, S. Musau, P. Satow, and M. Sock. 2000. *Guide to Designing Community Health Financing Schemes in East and Southern Africa*. Bethesda, MD: Abt Associates Inc., Partnership for Health Reforms, and USAID Regional Economic Development Services Office in East and Southern Africa (REDSO/ESA).

Dror, D.M. 2000: "Reforming Health Insurance: A Question of Principles? *International Social Security Review* 53(2):75–99.

_____. 2001. "Reinsurance of Health Insurance for the Informal Sector." *Bulletin of the World Health Organization* 79(7):672–78.

GTZ (German Technical Corporation) and others. 2001. *Infosure*. 1st Ed. Wiesbaden: Universum Verlagsanstalt.

ILO-STEP (International Labour Organisation/Strategies and Tools against Social Exclusion and Poverty). 2000: *Mutuelles de santé en Afrique: Characteristiques et en place: Manuel de Formation*. Geneva: ILO/STEP.

PART 4

Toward a Reinsurance Pilot in the Philippines

CHAPTER 17

Social Health Insurance in the Philippines: A Review of the Context

Jonathan Flavier, M.D., Elmer S. Soriano, M.D., and Anne Nicolay

The Philippines is the second largest archipelago in the world (after Indonesia) with more than 7,000 islands. Its population, about 75 million people (1999 projection from the 68.6 million of the 1995 census), grows at an average annual rate of 2.3 percent (1990–95) (PSY 1999, p. 1-4, table 1.1, and p. 1-10, table 1.2). In 1998, the per-capita gross domestic product (GDP) was PHP 35,486 (box 17.1).

The net growth rate was 1.5 percent during the decade from 1989 until 1998 (PSY 1999, pp. 3-12–3-13, table 3.5). The 1999 human development index (HDI)[1] of the Philippines, with a value of 0.749, lies in the middle-income group (rank 70 out of 162, Norway rank 1: 0.939, world average 0.684) (UNDP 1999). Despite the prevalence of poverty, the literacy rate is high for a developing country, with 95 percent of the adult population functionally literate in 1997 (World Bank 2000).

Governed by the president, the Philippines is a democratic and republican country, divided into 16 administrative regions, administered by regional directors. The 16 regions are further subdivided to create the local government units (LGUs), consisting of 78 provinces (headed by governors), 1,524 municipalities (headed by mayors), and 41,940 barangays (headed by village chairpersons). Each region, province, city, and municipality is given a class rating ranging from one to six, based on the average annual income of the area over the previous three years, the population, and the land area.

The 1997 Asian economic crisis may have had a lesser impact on the Philippine economy than on some neighboring countries. Nevertheless, there were tangible negative effects. Unemployment increased from 7.9 percent in 1997 to 9.6 percent in 1998 (PSY 1999, p. 11-4, table 11.1), and the economy has been struggling with the effects of inflation (5.9 percent in 1997, 9.7 percent in 1998, and 11.5 percent in 1999) (PSY 1999, p. 2-28, table 2.11). Foreign investment has decreased, and there has been a net outflow of capital.

The authors acknowledge, with thanks, the useful comments on an earlier draft by Dr. Madeleine R. Valera, Director III, Quality Assurance Research and Policy Development Department, Philippine Health Insurance Corporation, Manila, and by Marilyn E. Lorenzo, Director, Institute of Health Policy and Development Studies, National Institutes of Health, University of the Philippines, Manila.

BOX 17.1   THE VALUE OF THE PHILIPPINE PESO

The value of the Philippine peso has fluctuated widely over the past decade. These tables are included to help readers gauge relative values cited in the text.

Exchange Rate: Philippine Peso/U.S. Dollar

PHP/US$1.00	1990	1991	1992	1993	1994	1995	1996	1997	1998	1999	2000[a]
Average	24.31	27.48	25.51	27.12	26.42	25.71	26.22	29.47	40.89	39.09	44.19

a. The exchange rate on December 31, 2000, was PHP 49.9980, reflecting the worsening of the political situation, before the resignation of President J. Estrada in January 2001.
Note: Averages are based on reference rates from December 13, 1984, to December 3, 1992. Values for 1992 are weighted average rates under the Philippine Dealing System, starting August 4, 1992.
Source: Bankers' Association of the Philippines.

Purchasing Power Parity (PPP)

1990–98	PPP$ used for health expenditure per capita:	PPP$/$ = 3.875
1998	PPP$ used for GNP per capita:	PPP$/$ = 3.548

Note: The PPP is a value that weighs a currency to account for different economic settings of different countries. It gives comparable values to countries having a different economic reality.
Source: World Bank, Web site statistics (per country).

Overall, the health status of the Philippine population has improved over the past 50 years but slowed down during the 1980s. Recent estimates suggest that in 1990–95, the infant and under-five years mortality rates[2] (IMR and U5MR, respectively) declined from 57 to 49, and 80 to 67 deaths per 1,000 live births, respectively (PSY 1999, pp. 9-16–9-17, tables 9.8 and 9.10). During the same period, the maternal mortality rate (MMR) decreased from 209 to 180 per 100,000. Despite all the progress in infectious disease control, pneumonia, tuberculosis, and diarrhea remain major causes of morbidity in all age groups, accounting for 39 percent of total deaths in 1995 (PSY 1999, p. 9-23, table 9.16). With increasing life expectancy, chronic diseases are growing in importance. Heart and vascular diseases and malignant tumors are leading causes of death, accounting for 47 percent of all reported deaths in 1995 (PSY 1999, p. 9-23, table 9.16) (tables 18.3 and 18.4, this volume).

HEALTH CARE DELIVERY

Public hospitals, 36 percent of all hospitals in 1998, provide slightly more than half of all beds in the country's 1,713 hospitals (PSY 1999, p. 9-24, table 9-17). In 1997, at the primary and municipal levels, 2,405 rural health units each served about 30,000 people; the 13,096 barangay health stations had catchment populations of around 5,300 each (PSY 1999, p. 9-29, tables 9.23 and 9.24). Many of the facilities are in poor physical condition and lack essential equipment. The distribution of the hospital system is tilted in favor of urban areas (GTZ 2000).

Decentralization of health care delivery to LGUs, based on the Local Government Code of 1991, fragmented the original national health care system, partly because the new structure does not include the old "district," which was the operational level of the previous health system. The devolution also affected the continuity of technical guidance[3] from the Department of Health (DOH) to the different levels of LGUs.

Because the structure of public health delivery is organizationally complex, it is difficult to operate. The DOH still funds tertiary hospitals at national and regional levels, while 72 provincial governments fund and manage the provincial and district hospitals. More than 1,600 municipalities and cities independently manage and finance their respective rural health units and barangay health stations. The DOH regional and provincial offices provide the LGUs with technical assistance and guidance in the implementation of national policies and delivery of efficient and effective medical services. The DOH must license all health care facilities, and the Philippines Health Insurance Corporation (PHIC) reimburses only claims made by accredited providers.

Private hospitals, also concentrated in cities, are subject to the same licensing and accreditation rules as public hospitals. They must set aside at least 10 percent of bed capacity for charity patients and are forbidden to refuse service to patients who cannot put up monetary deposits. Nonetheless, these facilities are not subsidized by the government and are taxed exactly like private corporate institutions, even though they pursue a social mission and follow directives given by the DOH. To overcome this tax disadvantage, private hospitals have nursing/teaching schools attached, which allow for some tax relief. Both the establishment and operation of private hospitals are closely regulated. On the other hand, the establishment of private outpatient facilities, which offer consultations, diagnostics, surgery, and laboratory services, is not subject to any regulatory framework; all they need is a business license issued by an LGU. Some information is available on some private clinics (139), ambulatory surgical clinics (8), and dialysis centers (18) accredited by the DOH, but no comprehensive information is available on the number of private facilities or where they operate.

According to data on utilization of health services, first-referral hospitals are underutilized while secondary and tertiary hospitals are swamped (box 17.2).[4] Utilization of primary health care services is reported only by public facilities. Lack of health facilities and professionals in rural and remote areas limits their residents' access to health care. The poor also have limited financial access to secondary and tertiary health care.

In 1997, 2,582 doctors, 1,370 dentists, 4,096 nurses, and 13,275 midwives were practicing in the public sector (PSY 1999, p. 9-28, table 9.22). However, up to 10 percent of the doctors, dentists, and pharmacists, 20 percent of the nurses and medical technicians, and 35 percent of the midwives practice in rural areas—

BOX 17.2   NEED VERSUS DEMAND FOR HOSPITALS

According to the utilization data, demand is lower than supply for first-referral hospitals but higher than supply for secondary and tertiary hospitals. This situation illustrates the analysis presented in chapter 2 (this volume) that a gap between needs, demand, and supply explains, in part, exclusion from health care (figure 2.1, three-circle diagram). Another, more complex, issue entails establishing the meaning of this ex-post account: Are secondary and tertiary hospitals swamped because primary hospitals cannot deliver good medical care (that is, a gap between needs and supply)? Or does differential pricing create a disincentive to use primary facilities (that is, a gap between needs and demand)? Or maybe people simply harbor (unjustified) distrust toward primary facilities?

Increasing the overlap between needs, demand, and supply—without subsidizing only supply or only demand—could increase overall access to care (chapter 2, this volume). An effective corrective intervention to increase overlap would require answers to these questions.

---

where more than half of the population resides (box 17.3). The national capital region alone accounts for about 43 percent of all—private and public—doctors (Development Academy of the Philippines 1994b). This uneven distribution of medical personnel results in inequity.

BOX 17.3   DOCTORS PER CAPITA—INCOME RELATED?

Two factors influence access to health care in the Philippines: income and distance from facilities (and from urban centers, where most facilities are located). Do the data reflect these two factors? Assuming that the number of physicians per capita (PPC) provides a quantitative indicator for access to health care, what can be said about relative access in different provinces? This was explored by compiling data from PSY 1999. Figure 17.1A shows a weak and insignificant correlation between average income and PPC in 12 rural regions.

At incomes between PHP 75,000 and PHP 100,000 (the most prevalent range in the rural Philippines), comparing the number of PPC in two regions with the same average income shows a twofold difference. These facts show that income is not the only, and probably not the main, factor opening access to health care in rural regions. In fact, this finding suggests that in some places, better utilization of available economic resources can increase access to health care.

Figure 17.1B compares Manila with rural regions. The trend line here is the same as the one in figure 17.1A, extrapolated to the average income level in Manila. There are almost twice as many PPC in the capital as could be expected from the extrapolation. The difference between the capital and rural regions clearly reflects much more than the (big) difference in household resources, which confirms Manila residents' advantage in this regard, resulting from policy choices.

FIGURE 17.1A   Correlating Physicians and Income (without CAR and NCR)

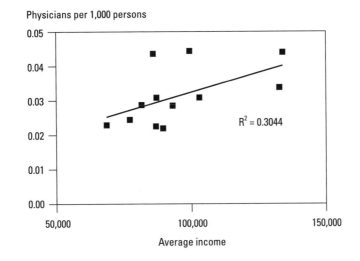

NCR National Capital Region.
CAR Cordillera Administrative Region.
Source: Development Academy of the Philippines 1994.

FIGURE 17.1B   Correlating Physicians and Income (Provinces and Manila)

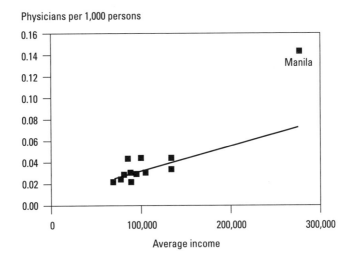

Sources: Development Academy of the Philippines 1994; PSY 1999.

HEALTH SERVICES FINANCING AND SPENDING

The share of gross national product (GNP) devoted to health care expenditures rose from 2.86 to 3.43 percent from 1991 to 1999. This percentage increase is significant, but the absolute amount of spending is still below the minimum target of 5 percent of GNP set by the World Health Organization. Compared with the 2.3 percent average annual population growth rate, the 14.8 percent rise in health spending (6.4 percent in real terms—1985 prices) allowed an increase in current per-capita health expenditures from PHP 575 in 1991 to PHP 1,449 in 1999. In real terms, per-capita expenditures increased from PHP 334 in 1991 to PHP 459 in 1999, an average annual growth rate of 4 percent. Total health expenditure in 1999 amounted to PHP 108.3 billion (NSCB 2001).

During the same period, the proportion of total expenditure devoted to curative care decreased slightly, while the share of expenditure on public health increased. Nevertheless, curative care still absorbs the major part of health expenditure—76 percent against 12 percent spent on public health. Other expenses (including general administration and operating costs, as well as research and training) remained fairly constant at about 11 percent of total health care spending (figure 17.2).

In 1999, the government, social health insurance institutions, and private sources shared the burden of total health expenditure, with respective contributions of 37.9 percent, 4.6 percent (and trending down), and 57 percent, respectively (figure 17.3 and box 17.4). Contributions from voluntary health insurance schemes, other funds, and direct foreign grants to health care delivery are not accounted for.

The share of all *government* levels (national and local) in overall health financing remained fairly constant from 1991 to 1999. Reflecting decentralization, however, the national share declined from 34.7 to 20 percent while the local government's share rose from 3.9 percent to 17.9 percent during this period. Transferred facilities receive less money from the LGUs than they did from the DOH, and the reduced allocations do not cover their operating costs.

FIGURE 17.2   Health Expenditure, by Use of Funds, 1999

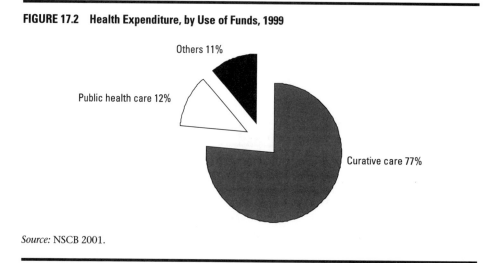

Source: NSCB 2001.

FIGURE 17.3   Health Expenditure, by Source of Funding, 1999

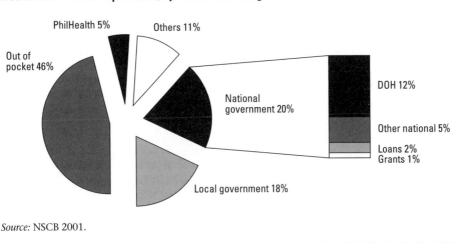

Source: NSCB 2001.

BOX 17.4   INSURING PREVALENT RISKS

Figure 17.2 shows that 77 percent of health expenditure is devoted to curative care; most of the care is for contagious conditions (chapter 18, this volume, table 18.3). This leads to the conclusion that when the probability and distribution pattern are known, these events can be insured because they are, broadly speaking, "insurable" events (chapter 6, this volume). At the same time, infectious diseases can provoke large variations (for example, because of an epidemic), and their large share in overall health expenditure suggests they may be prevalent. Therefore, reinsurance can provide a mechanism to flatten cost fluctuations and homogenize this type of risk.

Private sources of funding also remained constant at a hefty 57 percent of all funding. Out-of-pocket expenditure is a substantial 46 percent (NSCB 2001). Private health insurance, health maintenance organizations, and employer-based plans covering mid- to high-income populations represent 10 percent of all health expenditures. They offer comprehensive benefit packages, and premiums are risk-related. Local health care financing schemes are not accounted for.

HEALTH INSURANCE

The National Health Insurance Program (NHIP), implemented by PhilHealth, aims for universal coverage by 2010 but in 2001 covered only 43 percent of the population (PHIC 2001).[5] Coverage of the formal sector seems fairly extensive, but coverage of indigents and workers in the informal sector is still very limited. For-mal sector premiums, 2.5 percent of salaries between PHP 3,000 and PHP 7,500, are divided equally between employer and employees. Indigents' premiums, PHP 1,188 a year, are copaid by the LGU where they reside and the national govern-ment, according to sliding contributions. Over a maximum of five years, the LGU and the national government will split the costs (50–50). At the end of 2000, 347,000 indigents were enrolled in the PhilHealth program, about triple the num-ber at the end of 1999 (PHIC 2001).

Self-employed individuals (including those in the informal sector) pay a yearly premium of PHP 1,200 (the equivalent of a premium based on a PHP 48,000 yearly income). This program, launched in October 1999, enrolled almost a half-million members in its first year. At this initial stage, most current enrollees are probably self-employed, with incomes above the poverty line, and not members of the informal sector per se. These members were simply transferred from the former Social Security System to the new PhilHealth program. Getting the un-salaried poor members of the informal sector into social health insurance cover-age remains a challenge.

The PhilHealth benefit package concentrates on hospitalization and hospital-dispensed outpatient care but provides some outpatient benefits for indigents treated at public rural health units. In 2000, PhilHealth spent 79 percent of its collected contributions on claims reimbursement (fund utilization). Over the same year, the overall program utilization rate[6] was 3.6 percent: 5.6 percent for public servants, 0.6 percent for indigents, and 3.2 percent for the privately employed (including people paying as individuals, not as employees). To increase its mem-bership base, PhilHealth is developing additional benefits, mostly for outpatient care, and is studying possibilities for interfacing with local community schemes as a sustainable outreach strategy.

HOUSEHOLD INCOME, ABILITY TO PAY, AND HEALTH EXPENDITURES

The national average household income of PHP 123,168 a year varies from a low of PHP 67,772 in a predominantly rural region to a high of PHP 270,993 in the national capital area (table 17.1).[7] Nationally, almost half the income earners are on wages and salaries. The capacity to pay also varies widely among regions and between urban and rural areas—an average rural family earns only 41 percent of an urban family's income (table 17.1). An average annual income of about PHP 73,000 leaves rural families with monthly incomes of just greater than PHP 6,000, about PHP 1,200 per capita.

A typical household devotes 2 percent of its income to health care expendi-tures—about the same amount it spends on alcohol and tobacco (PSY 1999, p. 2-23, table 2.8). Of these family health expenditures, 46 percent goes for hospital services, 26 percent for services to nonhospital facilities such as freestanding clinics,

TABLE 17.1   Household Income, 1998

Location	Average annual income (in PHPs)
Philippines	123,168
Standard deviation (σ)	48,577
Urban	178,121
Rural	73,319

Source: National Statistics Office, 1997, in PSY 1999.

and 28 percent for drugs and other medical products as part of self-care (table 17.2). Assuming that the 2 percent share of income reflects the household's ability and willingness to pay for health services, the PhilHealth program addressed to the informal sector targets people who earn PHP 60,000 a year or more.

The prohibitive share of family expenditures spent on drugs reflects the oligopolistic structure in drug importing and retailing, where a single provider dominates each market (Zuellig for importing and Mercury for retailing). Local production also offers high-cost drugs, because of supposedly high costs of marketing and raw materials. Generic drugs' market share is low. The NHIP's benefit package for hospitalization puts a ceiling on drug prices. The local schemes that offer such a package also severely limit the drug benefit. Although the DOH and the LGUs provide public health care services with some drugs for chronic and acute diseases, drug purchases hit hard on household budgets.

TABLE 17.2   Family Out-of-Pocket Health Expenditures, 1994

Type of care	Amount (billion PHPs)	Percent share
Total hospital services	11.9	46
Government hospital	9.0	35
Private hospital	2.9	11
Total nonhospital services	1,506.0	26
Nonhospital MD facilities	5.3	20
Other professional facilities	381.0	1
Dental facilities	648.0	3
Traditional health care	471.7	2
Total drugs and self-care	7.3	28
Drugs and other nondurable purchases (self-care)	7.1	27
Vision aides and other medical durables (self-care)	0.2	1
Total curative care	25.9	100

Source: Development Academy of the Philippines 1994a.

THE COMMUNITY-BASED HEALTH CARE ORGANIZATION MARKET

The delivery and financing of government health services are far from reaching the entire population. Geographical and financial access to health services remains an issue for about half the population. To make up for low geographical or financial access, alternative ways of providing and financing health care services have emerged from the Philippines' traditional self-help schemes. These funds target people with earnings above the poverty line but below PHP 60,000.[8] This population segment, an estimated 19 million individuals (by deduction) comprising roughly 25 percent of the Philippine population, is the potential market for community-based or decentralized health care organizations (CBHCOs). So far, the national programs have not succeeded in finding ways of locating and motivating the informal sector or people with low incomes but above the poverty line and willing to pay. Likewise, determining the exact size of the informal sector and its capacity to contribute to national health insurance is problematic for the state. PhilHealth's indigent program strains the LGU budgets that share the subsidies with the national government.

In view of market imperfections, the weakness of national health service delivery and financing, and the strength of the private sector, individuals play a large role in their health care. Their financial participation in health care expenditure is high (46 percent of the total) and, through some civil society organizations, they try to make up for unavailability or inaccessibility of government services. Although the private sector has a role to play, government still has an obligation to fulfill its responsibilities for providing basic health services for the very poor and the underserved.

In financing services, organizations such as CBHCOs and their external supporters are noteworthy stakeholders who can help lighten the burden of administrative costs and logistical difficulties in providing people with basic services. Their potential contribution is not limited to paying fees but could extend to participation in decisionmaking and setting health program priorities. There are several examples of successful government–market–civil society cooperative efforts. One of them is the Partnership for Community Health and Development, implemented by the DOH with support from the World Bank (Flavier 1998). Judging by the more than 500,000 health volunteers thought to be working in the Philippines, civil society is emerging as a major player in the health system. Community-based organizations may be the vehicle by which PhilHealth, the DOH, and international development partners can facilitate the expansion of access to health care and encourage communities to participate in health program management.

CBHCOs: WHAT TYPE OF PARTNERSHIP IN HEALTH CARE FINANCING AND DELIVERY?

One strategy toward universal coverage (prescribed in Philippine RA7875 NHIP) is to have community groups play a predominant role in providing health insurance coverage for the informal sector. For the past five years, the DOH and the PHIC have been pursuing this idea, with the support of GTZ through the Social Health Insurance Networking and Empowerment (SHINE) project. One activity has been to establish and to update a census of community and local groups involved in health care provision or financing, to collect and analyze information, and to work closely with them. Despite their name, community-based health care organizations encompass schemes of various origins. Some are initiated and managed by health care providers, LGUs, communities, nongovernmental organizations, or people's organizations (POs). Some deal with health care provision or health care financing, and seldom deal with health insurance or a prepayment system.

Thirty-eight of the 66 community-based health care schemes in the SHINE database were selected, using a five-point purposive sampling criteria that mostly ensured differentiation and sampling balance among selected schemes.[9] The survey instrument was based on a WHO format and reworked with representatives from local health insurance schemes, SHINE-GTZ technical assistance, and some PhilHealth and DOH participants to make it more responsive to and useful for Filipino realities. The questionnaire included queries related to the socioeconomic environment and the nature and scope of scheme activities. The survey consisted of reviews of records and interviews of scheme managers, health and local authorities, and members, when possible. The survey task force consisted of 20 persons from PhilHealth, 6 from the DOH, and 4 from the SHINE project. The task force was divided into groups of one to three persons who gathered data at the study site for two to three days. Data sets from 35 CBHCO schemes were accepted, organized, and analyzed. Because consistency of the data collected was sometimes questionable (data could vary from one source to another), the survey analyst made some judgments and interpretations that are reflected in the information generated.

Of the 35 CBHCO schemes analyzed, 55 percent were in rural areas, 11 percent in urban areas, and 34 percent in mixed settings. The 35 schemes were classified into three general primary roles and any combination of the three, according to the selection criteria. Only schemes scoring above a threshold number of points were classified into the different roles. Schemes that scored lower, indicating a weaker component, were disqualified. The sample was too small for statistical generalizations.

The different roles are: health care services providers (three schemes); administrative intermediaries with strong information, education, and communication activities (five); and health care financing schemes (four). Mixed roles are distributed as follows: health care providers–administrative intermediaries schemes (four); health care providers–financing schemes (two); health care financing schemes–administrative intermediaries schemes (nine); schemes involved in all three (four); and unclassified (four). Hence, 19 schemes (54 percent of the sample) have a health care financing component in their activities. Various CBHCO roles seem responsive to local realities, as more CBHCOs functioning as health service providers are found in areas where health services from government or the private sector are scarcer. More CBHCOs providing health financing mechanisms and health care benefits are found in areas with lesser resources to pay for health care services, and with prior experience in risk pooling and risk sharing.

SELECTED SURVEY RESULTS

We review here selected aspects of the CBHCOs: benefit packages, income (contributions and other), membership, and management. The aim is to extract the basic information most needed for reinsurance. All issues related to health care quality, provider accreditation, pricing services, and the like are equally important, but we do not address them here, partly to allow concentration on some basic financial information but also because most schemes have not reached a level of systemic sophistication that would give them much to share on these topics. In some cases, analysis covers both the whole sample (35 schemes) and the subsample, including schemes with a major health care financing component (19 schemes).

Benefit Packages

The benefit packages offered by local schemes are usually more sensitive to their members' needs, and package changes are not uncommon (box 17.5). Of the 23 respondents (65 percent), 15 schemes reported that the benefit packages were derived from members' needs; 18 (78 percent) reported changes in their benefit package, indicating responsiveness to members' needs. Twenty-eight percent of the respondents changed their packages at their members' request or for increased coverage (39 percent). In practice, however, it is difficult to assess how closely the packages correspond to local realities because the questionnaire addressed only general aspects of the benefits, not the details. The benefit package can include coverage for outpatient and inpatient treatment (both including drugs) and/or diagnostics.

Twenty-five schemes reported offering their members some health care services; some schemes provide the services for free. Eighty percent of those 25

BOX 17.5   GROUP SIZE AFFECTS BENEFIT PACKAGE

Membership of 1,000 members or less was reported by 57 percent of the microinsurance units. Small microinsurers are particularly prone to insolvency because of larger expected statistical fluctuations in the number of claims (chapter 5, this volume). The exposure of small groups to statistical fluctuations is aggravated in the case of benefits that are low frequency and expensive, particularly when unit cost is highly variable (table 17.3 and box 17.4). A typical example of a high-cost, low-frequency benefit is surgery: 11 schemes (even those with smallest membership) opted to include it in their package. (The available data do not indicate whether any of the small schemes ran into insolvency resulting from outlier hospitalization or surgery costs). This choice may reflect the need to resort to high-cost care rather than to preventive care, which attracts lower resources (only 11 percent, compared with 77 percent for curative care; see figure 17.2). It may also reflect a benefit package designed to respond to community perceived priorities, rather than to community willingness to pay.

schemes provide outpatient care packages, 68 percent inpatient care packages, and 56 percent diagnostics. A closer look at benefits showed that 24 percent of the schemes (6) offer a comprehensive outpatient care package, 32 percent (8) a comprehensive inpatient care package, and 56 percent (14) a diagnosis and laboratory package. On partial packages, 56 percent (14 schemes) offer a partial outpatient care package and 36 percent (9) a partial inpatient care package. Only 8 percent (two schemes) offer a comprehensive package of outpatient and inpatient care as well as diagnostics.

Only 19 schemes have a health care financing component in their activities. The information these schemes provided on their benefit package is gathered in table 17.3. Standardizing information on benefits is difficult because they work differently from one scheme to another and can take different forms (for example, discounts, cash benefits, health care cost reimbursements). The packages presented cover a year. The numbers in table 17.3 are raw, as they do not take into account

TABLE 17.3   Benefit Packages

| | Benefits (in PHPs) | | | | | | Scheme beneficiaries | |
Service	Minimum	Maximum	Average	Median	Std. dev. (σ)	Number of respondents[a]	Member only	Member and dependents
Primary health care	—	—	—	—	—	1	1	3
Drugs, outpatient	1,500	1,500	1,500	1,500	0	2	1	4
Consultation, outpatient	50	1,350	700	700	919	2	2	5
Drugs, inpatient	300	12,510	3,748	1,250	4,882	6	1	7
Surgery	1,000	30,000	15,473	15,445	14,591	4	2	3
Room and board	55	1,350	525	400	504	5	1	2
Professional fees	900	21,240	7,830	1,350	11,616	3	1	4
Rehabilitation	—	—	—	—	—	0	—	1
Diagnostics and laboratory	130	11,535	3,893	1,953	5,301	4	—	4
Other services								
Hospitalization (mostly cash benefits)	300	70,000	11,589	4,000	22,209	9	1	3
Dental	—	500	500	—	—	1	—	1

— Not indicated.

a. The number of respondents is constrained by the completeness of the answer (some schemes did not make a complete answer; and as the benefits are not always predefined, some schemes could not answer this question).

Note: The data above show huge differences between the minimum and maximum unit cost of some benefits: 24-fold for professional fees, 30-fold for surgery, 40-fold for inpatient drugs, and 90-fold for diagnostic services. This variability, especially of expensive benefits, adds variance to the expected expenditure. The consequence of increased variance is a decrease in the value of the *security coefficient*, resulting in decreased cost-effectiveness of the insurance transaction (chapter 16, this volume). Therefore, benefits that are both variable and expensive would be the first candidates for reinsurance.

Source: SHINE-GTZ 2001.

the various rules on waiting periods and ceilings. Some numbers suggest actual expenditure in place of a predefined package. Most of the time, benefits go to members as well as their dependents (but the response rate to this question is low).

Waiting periods between enrollment and eligibility for benefits are common; only 11 percent of respondents reported no waiting period. For the others, waiting periods' median values grow higher with health care costs: 7 days for outpatient services, 11 days for maternity care, 15 days for inpatient care, 37.5 days for surgery, and (surprisingly) 90 days for medicines (drugs). The average values are one month for outpatient care, three months for maternity care, two months for inpatient care, four months for surgery, and 2.5 months for medicines (drugs).

Of the 21 respondents, most schemes (38 percent) pay providers directly, similar to service insurance provision. Others (33 percent) pay providers directly or reimburse members (often this dual system reflects flexibility for emergencies). Only 9.5 percent of the schemes reimburse the patient as with indemnity insurance, and 14 percent have alternative benefits such as loans or cash benefits.[10]

Two CBHCOs indicate extreme hospitalization benefits between about PHP 3,000 and PHP 75,000, while PhilHealth can go up to PHP 150,000. With the study limitations in determining support value, the "health care financing" subsample has a ratio of 78 percent.[11] Compared with the more than PHP 5,000 average value per claim of PhilHealth, the CBHCOs have an average value per claim three times lower, PHP 1,671.

Income

Contributions. Across the whole sample, the average annual income, as reported by the municipal planning and development offices, is PHP 49,000, 28 percent lower than the minimum per-capita income reported in national statistics and 18 percent lower than the income necessary to pay for PhilHealth membership (PHP 60,000), given the reported household expenditure on health (2 percent). Most contributions are made in monetary terms (67 percent of the respondents), but 6 respondents (22 percent) said they could accept payments in kind. The CBHCO contribution amounts to 0.7 percent of average household income, markedly lower than the 2 percent average Philippine household expenditure on health. The highest share reported is around 3 percent.

For 24 respondents (69 percent of the sample), the yearly contribution ranges between PHP 6 and PHP 1,980, with a PHP 350 average and a PHP 109 median value; 16 schemes (67 percent of the respondents) reported a contribution lower than PHP 196, and 20 (83 percent of the respondents) indicated a yearly contribution lower than PHP 501. Most contributions are flat fees (47.2 percent). Only 14 percent of the schemes apply income-related fees; mixed and other types of fees complete the sample. Culturally, assistance to neighbors and solidarity in times of need is frequent (68 percent of the respondents), but prepayment or preparation for future needs is not. Exemptions are few, mainly for scheme employees and indigents (8 percent of the schemes) and for the elderly (3 percent).

Premiums are paid by different sources. Individual members are the main payers (63 percent), followed by government (17 percent), the organization itself (10 percent), and donors (10 percent).

Findings of this survey suggest that NGOs, cooperatives, and POs can absorb a transaction load of collecting from members that government agencies cannot. Private schemes (NGOs, POs, cooperatives) collect more frequently than smaller schemes. Premiums are collected any time from weekly to yearly. CBHCOs (NGOs and cooperatives) collect monthly, and POs as frequently as weekly. Perhaps some functional synergies in CBHCOs allow them to maintain cost-efficiency despite their higher transaction volume. Overall, monthly and yearly collections are the preferred collection frequencies (44 percent and 42 percent, respectively) and on regular collection schedules (more than half of the cases). Members pay their premiums or contributions directly to the CBHCO (52.6 percent) or through community-based collectors (57.9 percent). In the other cases, the premiums are collected by CBHCO staff (26.3 percent), through salary or dividend deductions (15.8 percent), and through the local government offices (10.5 percent). Compliance data are not available.

User fees, subsidies, other income resources. The data on total scheme revenues and expenses are indicative, not exact. Of the 13 respondents, overall revenue per capita for the most recent year (1999 or 2000) ranges from PHP 1 to PHP 959, with a median of PHP 194. Average revenue per capita amounts to PHP 284 (with a standard deviation of PHP 338). Revenues include contributions, subsidies, and other income. Overall, revenues from contributions amount to 37 percent, subsidies 61 percent, and other income 2 percent. However, once the largest subsidized scheme is excluded from the sample, the subsidy share falls to 4 percent, while the contribution and the other revenue shares increase to 88 percent and 7 percent.[12] Financial assistance is not reported as regular income, and other types of subsidy exist. Of the 19 respondents, 11 schemes (58 percent) indicated that they had financial assistance from foreign donors, 4 (21 percent) reported financial assistance from technical clubs and others, and 3 (16 percent) reported assistance from NGOs and other private sector sources. Schemes classified as focusing on administrative tasks (such as community development, training and organization, networking and advocacy, health awareness and education, or other development objectives) rely more heavily on external funding than do those involved more specifically in health financing, as it seems that their own funds are insufficient.

Social capital generation is high among CBHCOs, as indicated by the fact that 85 percent of CBHCO workers are reported as volunteers (chapter 19, this volume). Only 170 staff members are salaried, compared with 1,004 community health workers and volunteers. Some remuneration is foreseen, however, for some types of work such as collecting contributions. In any case, the voluntary human resource contribution allows these schemes to stretch their limited funds.

As for copayments, 67 percent of the schemes had none; 22 percent had arrangements with PhilHealth; and 22 percent had arrangements supplemented by schools or businesses. The response rate to this question was low (26 percent).

Membership

Overall, membership varies greatly according to amount and type of premium and benefits. Where the premium is higher and the benefit package wider, the schemes attract low- to upper-middle-income groups, and the benefits offered complement those offered by the national health insurance scheme. Lower premiums enhance access by lower-income groups. Forty-four percent of the overall survey membership belongs to the formal sector, and 52 percent to the informal sector, but these figures should be read with caution, as some are drawn from approximate statistics.

Twenty-one respondents reported a total of 100,000 beneficiaries, but one scheme alone (LGU-led) reported 62,000 beneficiaries. Reporting schemes serve between 37 and 62,000 beneficiaries, with a median of 800 beneficiaries. Forty-three percent of the schemes have fewer than 500 members; 57 percent, fewer than 1,000 beneficiaries; and 76 percent, fewer than 2,100 beneficiaries. The average CBHCO serves more than 4,000 beneficiaries; excluding the biggest LGU scheme lowers the average to fewer than 2,000 beneficiaries.

Data on dropout rates and population coverage are too unreliable for publication. A third of the 29 respondents said they kept membership rosters so that providers and the scheme administrators could identify their members. Another third said they use identification cards. Four (14 percent) schemes said they used both a membership roster and an identification card. Only five use scheme passbooks, supplemented, in two cases, by an additional means of identification.

The data show that CBHCOs provide health services and health financing services either to people who cannot afford the PHIC premium of PHP 1,200 (33 percent of the schemes) or to the formal sector as a complement to PhilHealth subscription (44 percent of the schemes). The average contribution is PHP 350. In most cases, membership is voluntary (96 percent of the respondents). Family and individual memberships predominate. The few group memberships (from villages, companies, or other organizations) are exceptional in the sample. Membership is paid per individual in 56 percent of the schemes or per family in 39 percent.

Factors sustaining membership are hard to derive. Major contributing factors reported were: "satisfaction with benefits" (56 percent of the schemes); "solidarity with community/organization" (25 percent); and "positive, courteous, and competent attitude from the health care providers" (17 percent). Members drop out for several reasons: most commonly, a "tight financial situation" or a "transfer out of the area," far ahead of "nonuse of benefits," or "nonpayment of loans."

Management

CBHCOs have been operating for an average of 11 years, excluding the average 2.2-year start-up phase. Of the 17 respondents, members own the funds in 58 percent of the cases. In two cases, local government or fund directors hold minority shares.

Nonfinancial resources. Salaried staff members and volunteers usually work together (75 percent of the schemes reported some of each). The ratio of volunteers to salaried employees is 6 to 1, which emphasizes the large human subsidy transferred to most schemes. Volunteer staffing is not listed as a financial asset. Sometimes public servants or persons regularly employed outside the scheme run operations.

The fund manager's education varies from one CBHCO to another (but is based on a very low response rate). In 40 percent of the schemes reporting, the manager had attended NGO seminars and courses, 20 percent had a college degree, 20 percent had an elementary school degree, and 20 percent had no education degree.

A third of the respondents indicated that the provider-scheme initiators often invested in equipment and supplies—land and other real estate or, in fewer cases, building space and the space within buildings. These contributions are not quantified.

Financial resources. With regard to financial management, schemes were reported to have competent fund managers and administrators as well as efficient collecting agents (and, through their direct contact with people in the community, even recruiters for PhilHealth). Administration absorbs 20 percent or more of total expenditures in 6 CBHCOs (out of the 14 respondents), and hidden costs often crop up (43 percent of the respondents have no administrative expenditure). Thirty-six percent of them have reserve funds (minimum of PHP 16,500, maximum of PHP 900,000, median of PHP 121,631, and standard deviation of PHP 366,102). Of the 19 schemes, only 37 percent rely on government to provide audit functions. The rest are overseen by their boards, managers, or their own staff.

No LGU-owned funds showed commingling of funds. This indicates the use of financial control systems typical of government agencies, more stringent than the systems used by some cooperatives, NGOs, and POs that did report commingling of funds. All in all, only 16 schemes (out of 33 respondents) reported using the funds only to finance health care. Based on 18 respondents, the average value of the funds is PHP 1.9 million. Seventy-five percent of all funds are kept in banks (54 percent in savings accounts, 13 percent in current accounts, and 8 percent as time deposits).

Management systems. Of the 21 respondents, 14 schemes (67 percent) said they have a personnel system; 14 schemes, an accounting system; and 15 schemes (71 percent), a management system for membership, contribution collections, and claim processing (see box 17.6 for a discussion of gaps in information). Twelve schemes had all three systems. However, the sophistication of these systems is not clear, for example, whether they are computerized or manual and what data level they can process. Asked whether the membership records are computerized, only 3 of 7 respondents said yes, and only 14 of 29 respondents had a membership roster. Because each scheme has its own way of reporting, generalizations for this review are impossible without a case-by-case study.

BOX 17.6   INFORMATION: (ALMOST) AS IMPORTANT AS MONEY

Financial performance monitoring information is inadequate or lacking at the level of single microinsurance units. For instance, many microinsurers cannot identify each beneficiary. Each microinsurer also needs epidemiological risk profiling of its beneficiaries, which requires estimates of disease prevalence by age and gender (chapter 18, this volume). Without such information, it is impossible to assess the cost of benefits, provide sufficient funding, or prioritize risks. Nor can risks be insured or reinsured unless the microinsurer can provide reliable information (chapter 6 and 16, this volume). Appendix A (Data Template) provides a user-friendly framework to help microinsurers gather needed information.

RISKS AND OPPORTUNITIES

Risks and opportunities have been evaluated based on the survey and the prospect of social reinsurance and interface with PhilHealth. While the discussion is based on the survey results, other important factors must be considered, such as the independent nature of the local schemes and the political factors that may frustrate attempts to provide these schemes with standardized tools and umbrella protection through, for example, social reinsurance. All of these should be rationalized under an umbrella to achieve a common purpose such as social reinsurance. Success will hinge on offering the right incentives, preserving the schemes' autonomy, and allowing them a voice in management through representation in mid- and top-level organizations. Putting all the necessary conditions in place will take time. Also the role of and interaction with the PHIC need to be determined; PhilHealth's role could be joint for social reinsurance and interfacing with the microinsurers (for example, financial and statistical reporting).

Main Financial Problems and Potential Solutions for Local Schemes

CBHCO beneficiaries pay an average of 29 percent of PhilHealth's annual premiums, according to the survey. A premium midway between PhilHealth's and the lower CBHCO charges might be feasible.

Excluding the most heavily subsidized scheme from the sample, most of the other CBHCOs' revenues come from member contributions. If the membership base were solid, member contributions might be a sustainable revenue source, but the base is not solid; it is very unstable. Revenues are also too low to cover catastrophic or simultaneous claims and could cover maximum hospitalization benefits for only 1 percent of the beneficiaries. Social reinsurance may be called for in this situation. Since only five of the CBHCOs with financing roles reported that they set aside reserve funds, other possible sources of payments for reinsurance may have to be identified, for example, administrative and operations funds or even premium increases, which might, however, cost them members.

For so many small initiatives, premium collection and administrative costs have become a financial burden. The nature and content of CBHCO health financing and services (outpatient and medications) expose them to higher risk of moral hazard. Because of the nature of the package, abuse is easier and more difficult to control than fewer and less frequent hospital benefits. Additionally, a drug package could threaten financial viability—if drugs are provided as a true benefit package—because of their high cost. CBHCO participation in the collection effort, their closeness to the community, and their pool of community-based workers might be mitigating factors to hold down administrative and monitoring costs.

Intrinsic Capacity to Pool with Other Schemes

Many CBHCO schemes are stand-alone initiatives, said to be resistant to (unrelated) superseding bodies. Others belong to networks with common statistical and financial reporting forms. During workshops in 2001, four CBHCO representatives said they would like to link up with each other in cooperative arrangements. Dealing with individual schemes would not be impossible, but the formation of federations or second-tier associations of CBHCOs would lighten the administrative load. The Organization for Educational Resources and Training/ORT Health Plus Scheme (ORT/OHPS) scheme in La Union, Peso-for-Health in Negros Oriental, and Botika Binhi in Quezon City and Caloocan are examples of the way cooperative arrangements can be built up from the community level.

There are also some national federations such as the network of midwife-managed reproductive health clinics initiated by the JSI Research and Training Institute. Over the past decade, NGOs have worked with the JSI Research and Training Institute to develop and organize clinics owned and managed by midwives. Already, 240 community-based Well-Family Midwife Clinics are operating around the country (JSI 2000). Their standardized reporting and uniform franchise format made it easy for PhilHealth to tap into this network in 2001 to begin to expand services with a low-risk maternity care package. Recognizing the unmet health financing needs of coop members, the National Confederation of Cooperatives (NATCCO), a network of more than 1,000 cooperatives covering 1.5 million individuals, has embarked on a three-year program to promote this coop-based social health insurance through its network. Standardized training modules, software, and information-management systems are being developed for social health insurance. Risk sharing among cooperatives within NATCCO has been implemented through regional liquidity and loan insurance funds. Considering the financial stability and managerial sophistication of many network coops, NATCCO has the potential to become a major partner of PHIC in serving the informal sector.

The DOH is in the process of aggressively organizing interlocal health zones, district health systems made up of several LGUs, into a sustainable local health system to ensure that devolution of health services works. The CBHCOs can fit into this system by linking up with the LGUs and local PhilHealth offices to increase synergy. Several provinces have already been modeling such systems.

CONCLUSIONS

The current Philippine health care system is characterized by an inadequate health care provider network, particularly in the remote areas and island communities, and by inadequate health care financing. The national health insurance scheme was set up in 1995, but the country has many poor people who cannot pay the premiums set by PhilHealth and who, culturally, are averse to prepayment schemes. PhilHealth's benefit package and premiums are suitable for people who have access to health care providers and can pay the premium for a basic package. Hence, with current arrangements and the single-insurer model, universal coverage cannot be attained, and the strategic policy priority is not financially viable.

Attempts are now being made to shift from a monolithic to a composite system—which recognizes the contribution and role of various stakeholders in achieving universal coverage. Microinsurance units are part of this picture, and have great potential, particularly among the 19 million people in the informal sector. These people are excluded by PhilHealth's premium prices and by their geographic inaccessibility to health care providers.

Our survey indicates potential coverage of about 100,000 people, paying low premiums (on average 3.5 times lower than PhilHealth's) in exchange for lower benefits. In those markets, microinsurers, acting as multiple insurers, will be PhilHealth's best partners in achieving universal coverage. Forms of cooperation, including support to the microinsurers and operational guidelines, will have to be developed (now being negotiated). At this stage, microinsurers' management skills and tools would need to be enhanced and standardized, and some measures of efficiency should be introduced to boost the benefits. Simultaneously, to attract members, the population should be sensitized to the advantages of prepayment. Incorporation into developing interlocal health zones may also be necessary. PhilHealth needs to make some serious moves to elaborate the links to CBHCOs, and their complementary roles, in addition to their existing operations. PHIC can be the visible hand coordinating the development of this insurance network.

The weaknesses of the CBHCOs need to be mitigated, and their strengths further enhanced. Social reinsurance provides one as yet untried but promising approach to stabilize these CBHCOs and make them more attractive for investment or mere participation. Although some CBHCOs need to demonstrate that they can enlarge their membership, 43 percent of the survey schemes already have more than 1,000 beneficiaries. Most of the schemes need considerable help (both technical and financial) to adjust to a more regulated, demanding, and rigorous environment. The schemes should be supported and enhanced to overcome weak management. Acceptable risk levels need to be carefully determined and maintained. Despite their managerial weaknesses, CBHCOs have demonstrated their capacity to survive in a difficult environment, their essential role in responding to economic and social demand, and their common-sense approach to problem solving. Low- to middle-income members are attracted by the small benefits they can get apart from or in addition to benefits they already get from PhilHealth. Dealing with individual schemes, although possible, would increase the administrative burden. Dealing with federations or second-tier associations of CBHCOs could lighten this load. However, organizing microinsurers to function in tandem or as federations, a desirable move for pooling purposes and for standardization of managerial practices, is not in PhilHealth's mandate. Nor is PhilHealth able or legally mandated to provide reinsurance.

The survey showed that few schemes have external financial support (representing only 4 percent of their total revenue), but that the social capital being mobilized is a significant resource. When expanding the membership and the benefit package, the best way to provide subsidies will have to be assessed, as poorly designed subsidy mechanisms weaken community organizations instead of strengthening them (chapter 2, figure 2.3). In the meantime, hidden subsidies in the form of technical assistance rather than money may prevent harm to CBHCOs.

Own reserves are an expensive and inefficient way of managing risk, especially for microinsurers strapped for cash in the first place. Liquidity risks can be managed more efficiently through a liquidity fund maintained by a third party for several CBHCOs.[13] Such a fund can also serve as a vehicle for inducing standardization and more rigorous management systems among microinsurers. Microinsurers will need the right incentives to accept this idea.

As a product or service offered to CBHCOs, social reinsurance is highly conceptual, intangible, and new to prospective buyers of reinsurance. While some schemes have shown a tentative interest in reinsurance, its full impact will be better understood once a few microinsurers are covered by it under a pilot project. A reinsurance body and PhilHealth may also be reluctant to extend the investment to microinsurers that are perceived as high risk and unmanageable. CBHCO leaders and managers have to be educated on risk management so they can appreciate the value of reinsurance. Expanding management's horizons in this way must be attended to from the initial phases of the introduction of *Social Re*.

NOTES

1. The HDI consists of three components defining human development: long life, educational level, and the standard of living. Longevity is measured by life expectancy. The level of education is measured by a combination of adult literacy rate and the average number of years of schooling. Standard of living is measured by real per-capita GDP corrected for local prices.

2. U5MR = deaths under five years/1,000 live births.

3. Technical guidance is provided free of charge to the LGUs for administrative, managerial, and clinical issues. Social health insurance matters are left to the Regional Health Insurance Offices of the PHIC.

4. District hospitals have bed occupancy rates of 50 percent or less.

5.   PhilHealth is the name given to the Philippine Health Insurance Corporation (PHIC), mandated to implement the National Health Insurance Program.

6.   The *program utilization rate* is the number of claims paid divided by the number of members.

7.   The average size of the household is 5.04 members (PSY 1999, p. 1-28 and 2-13, tables 1.7 and 2.3).

8.   Minimum wages are set at PHP 250 a day. A bill was recently proposed by Senator J. Flavier to increase the minimum wage by 50 percent.

9.   The schemes were ranked according to five criteria: the scheme had to still be in operation; its ownership was to be balanced to ensure a representative mix of community and LGU schemes; the original scheme pattern was preferred to replications; the health care delivery proposed by the scheme was to be balanced between various systems; and priority was given to larger membership bases.

10. Eighty-one percent of the health care providers are reimbursed on a fee-for-service basis.

11. Support value in this survey was based on the reported total amount of claims and the total amount paid out by each CBHCO scheme. *Support value* equals the total amount of claims paid out divided by the total amount claimed. It is the percentage of the total health cost defrayed by the scheme.

12. This scheme is highly subsidized by an LGU; excluding it from the sample lowers the overall subsidy from 61 to 4 percent.

13. As demonstrated in the NATCCO liquidity funds (Bautista, Yap, and Soriano 1999).

REFERENCES

Bautista, M.C., M.E. Yap, and E. Soriano. 1999. "Local Governments' Health Financing Initiatives: Evaluation, Synthesis, and Prospects for the NHIP in the Philippines." Small Applied Research 7. Bethesda, Md.: Abt Associates Inc., Partnerships for Health Reform.

Development Academy of the Philippines. 1994a. *Family Income and Expenditure Survey*. Manila: DAP.

_____. 1994b. *Regional Distribution of Physicians and DOH Personnel (1990)*. Manila: DAP.

Flavier, J.D. 1998. "Technical Assistance Report to the World Bank." Washington, D.C.: World Bank. Unpublished.

GTZ (German Technical Corporation). 2000. "LEAPS in Health." Appraisal Report. Unpublished.

JSI (John Snow, Inc., Research and Training Institute). 2000. "Information sheet/flyer." Manila: JSI.

NSCB (National Statistical Coordination Board). 2001. "1991–1999 Philippine National Health Accounts." Manila. May.

PHIC (Philippine Health Insurance Corporation). 2001. "PhilHealth Operations Report." Corporate Planning Department. Manila. Unpublished. March.

PSY (Philippine Statistical Yearbook). 1999. National Statistical Coordination Board, Manila. October.

SHINE–GTZ (Social Health Insurance Networking and Empowerment–German Technical Corporation) 2001. "Data on Local Health Insurance Schemes Survey." Manila. Unpublished. May.

UNDP (United Nations Development Programme). 1999. "The Human Development Report." Office Calculations. www.undp.org

World Bank. 2000. "Country Data: Country at a Glance Tables." http://www.worldbank.org/data/countrydata/countrydata.html

CHAPTER 18

Epidemiological Data on Health Risks in the Philippines

Jeannie Haggerty and Tracey Reid

E*pidemiology* is the study of the distribution and determinants of disease in populations. The analysis of illness patterns by characteristics of person, space, and time gives clues about health needs that will affect both the population's demand for medical services and the type of medical services that are needed. In turn, illness patterns will give insight about the adequacy of the medical services. Epidemiological analysis, therefore, is part of the assistance that the *Social Re* program can offer microinsurance units to assess the frequency of use of certain medical services where local utilization patterns are unknown or unreliable, and to help in the definition of the benefit package.

THE CONTRIBUTION OF EPIDEMIOLOGY

The goal of medical care is to provide effective treatment for disruptions in health so that negative sequelae—disability and death—can be prevented. The analysis of disability and death can identify where medical care can be most usefully directed within the constraint of a limited benefit package. The focus is on illnesses for which clinical care is clearly indicated and cost-effective.

For medical services to be effective, access to accurate diagnosis and to efficacious interventions must be timely. Health insurance reduces the immediate financial barriers to seeking timely care. But to appropriately establish the insurance premium and plan services, the insurance scheme must have a reasonable estimate of the demand for health care and the intensity of care that will be needed. To attract consumers, a benefit package has to cover services that matter to the constituency—services that are perceived to be beneficial not only for rare and catastrophic events but also for more commonly occurring illnesses where timely treatment makes the difference between health and disability. Microinsurance then will benefit from an epidemiological analysis to identify the type and severity of common illnesses as well as the rate of occurrences of rare and

For her helpful comments on a draft of this chapter, the authors thank Joyce Pickering, M.D., M.Sc., Assistant Professor, Departments of Medicine and Epidemiology and Biostatistics, McGill University, Montreal, Quebec, Canada.

catastrophic events among its potential members. This information is equally useful to the reinsurer for assessing the financial viability of the microinsurance unit. Finally, epidemiological analysis can contribute to decisions about whether a condition is insurable or uninsurable (chapter 6, this volume).

The role of epidemiology in planning health insurance is to:

- Identify the major health needs in the constituency to be served.

- Set priorities for the services to be covered in the benefit package on the basis of health needs.

- Estimate the rate of occurrence of health events to be covered as well as average costs for care.

In this chapter, we outline the epidemiological approach to developing an expectation about the frequency of diseases that are amenable to medical care and most likely to be requested in a health insurance plan. This includes a brief description of the type and quality of data available to gain insights into the demographic, mortality, and morbidity (illness) profile of the country as a whole as well as reasonable expectations for illness patterns and occurrences in the locality where a scheme will be developed. We use the Philippines as an illustrative example to talk about the data sources and to make epidemiological interpretations of the data that would be useful to an insurance scheme as well as to the reinsurer. We use both national-level information and utilization data from two microinsurance units.

The Philippines

The World Bank has classified the Philippines as a "lower-middle-income economy" and "moderately indebted" developing country. Agriculture, forestry, fishing, manufacturing, and service industries drive the economy. Poverty is high in the Philippines, with 37.5 percent of the population living below the national poverty line in 1999 (World Bank 2000; chapter 17, this volume).

As a result of endemic diseases, the tropical climate, the increasing population, and industrialization, adverse environmental conditions are now common in the Philippines. Extensive deforestation, disposal of solid wastes (including toxic waste) in open dumpsites, and pollution of the air, water, and soil contribute to unsafe living conditions and increase the risk of vector-borne, vermin, parasite, and bacteria-related diseases (NDHS 1998).

Government spending on health care is low, with 3.5 percent of gross national product (GNP) spent on health care by government and private sectors in 1997 (DOH 1999a, p. 12). Access to health care is unevenly distributed among the population, given the financial barriers to health services. The per-capita expenditure on health care in 1997 was 100 international dollars, giving the Philippines a rank of 124 out of the 191 members of the World Health Organization (2000). The greatest burden of health care spending is on individual residents, who account for 46 percent of the money spent on health care (DOH 1999a, p.13).

Although the Department of Health (DOH) and the local government units employ many health personnel, access to health services is still limited because of the clustering of medical personnel in urban centers. In 1997, the government employed 7,359 physicians, 9,719 nurses, 1,961 dentists, and 15,888 midwives. Existing health care facilities in 1997 included 1,816 hospitals (644 public hospitals and 1,172 private, with a bed capacity of 81,905), 2,405 rural health units, and 13,556 barangay health stations (DOH 1999a, pp. 13-14).

The Two Microinsurance Units

The two microinsurance units are located in the provinces of La Union and Tarlac.

Province of La Union. The ORT Health Plus Scheme is based in the province of La Union, in the Ilocos region (Region 1) on the Northwest side of the island of Luzon. The province consists of 19 municipalities, 576 barangays, and one city—San Fernando City—the region's center with a population of 102,082. The province has a population of 657,945, with a population density of 441 per kilometer, an average household size of 5.15 people, and an average annual growth rate of 1.83 percent during the past decade (NSO 2000).

Health facilities located in the province of La Union include 7 government hospitals (total bed capacity of 415, 2 tertiary, 4 district secondary, and 1 medicare primary hospital) and 12 licensed private hospitals (bed capacity of 3,232: 2 tertiary and 10 primary hospitals). Four of the private hospitals are located in San Fernando City.

Province of Tarlac. The constituency of the Tarlac Health Maintenance Plan reside in the province of Tarlac in the Central Luzon region (Region 3). This landlocked, first-class province is one of the six comprising the Central Luzon region. Located in the middle of Luzon, the province of Tarlac consists of 17 municipalities, one city (Tarlac City, the provincial capital, population 262,481) and 510 barangays (Department of Interior and Local Government 1999). The province has a population of 1,068,783, population density of 350 people per square kilometer, 4.96 people per household on average, and an average annual population growth rate in the past decade of 2.2 percent (NSO 2000).

The province of Tarlac has 5 government hospitals (390 beds in 1 tertiary center, 2 secondary district, 1 secondary military, and 1 medicare primary hospital) and 16 private hospitals (447 beds in 3 tertiary, 5 secondary, and 8 primary hospitals (DOH 1999b).

Expectations of Similarity between Local and National Levels

Data at the national and regional level are readily available on the Internet, via reliable Philippine and international organizations. However, it is difficult to obtain detailed information at a provincial level. Inferences about the epidemiological profile of the constituency for a microinsurance scheme from existing sources of data will be based on regional data. Information will need to be collected first-hand for more precise information about smaller units (for example, a municipality or a barangay; see chapter 17, this volume).

Although statistics such as population density, average household size, and average annual growth rate vary only slightly between the two provinces and the rest of the country, the epidemiological profile of these two regions/provinces will be similar to the national picture, as both provinces are located on Luzon, where 56 percent of the total Philippine population lives. However, national statistics are probably driven more by the national capital region than by any other area because it is the most populous area. Thus, national data, the most readily available data, will be driven by the country's largest urban center.

FIRST IMPRESSIONS: DEMOGRAPHICS

Demographic data are the information that is most readily available. Most countries regularly conduct a census to count the population. Sociodemographic data are also collected from vital statistics registries (births, deaths, and marriages). This information, used for many purposes, including taxation bases and political processes, is relatively accurate.

Information on registration certificates usually includes a breakdown by sex, age, and region and, when combined with denominator information from periodic censuses, these data are used to calculate the important demographic indicators (for example, infant mortality, fertility rates, maternal mortality ratios, and crude birth and death rates).

The age-sex composition of a population is particularly relevant for planning preventive care, which is indicated principally by age, sex, and predictable life-cycle events rather than by the onset of symptoms. The type and intensity of curative services also vary by age and sex. For instance, illnesses among children aged less than five years are common, tend to be acute in nature, and can usually be resolved easily at the ambulatory level. Timely access to care is critical because health can deteriorate rapidly when care is delayed. At the other end of the age spectrum, the elderly population (over 60 years of age in many developing countries) manifests high morbidity from chronic conditions and multiple illnesses, but the use of ambulatory services declines and is replaced with more expensive hospital care. During the middle years, ages 15 to 45, there is a wide discrepancy in health care use between women and men, with high rates of accidents and injuries in men, and care related to childbearing in women.

Demographic Profile of the Philippines

A useful snapshot of the demographic composition of a country is the population pyramid, illustrated in figure 18.1 for the Philippines. Here we observe the wide base and narrow top that is typical of high fertility countries. Although the average number of births per woman (fertility rate) has decreased, the current rate of

FIGURE 18.1   Philippines: Population Pyramid, 1998

Age group

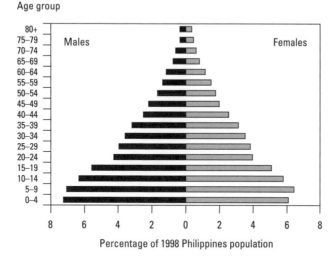

Percentage of 1998 Philippines population

Sources: DOH 1999a; NDHS 1998.

3.7 (NDHS 1998) still remains higher than the average of 2.1 for the entire East Asia and Pacific region. Approximately 38 percent of the population is less than15 years of age. Because of the declining birth rate and better survival at all ages, the median age of the population is increasing, as is the proportion of older people. There will be an increasing requirement for medical services to meet the needs of an aging population, but the needs for maternal and child services will continue to predominate, particularly in rural areas where the fertility rate is 4.7 children per woman compared with 3 children per woman in urban areas (NDHS 1998).

The term *demographic transition* refers to the phenomenon in which countries pass from a demographic equilibrium of high birth rates and high death rates to an equilibrium of low birth rates and low death rates. The former is typical of agrarian societies, and the latter are observed currently in industrial countries. During the demographic transition from one state of equilibrium to another, death rates drop before birth rates, resulting in a rapid increase in the absolute number of people at all ages. In the Philippines, crude birth rates have fallen since 1970, as have crude death rates, but they are not in equilibrium (table 18.1) and the total population is still growing (GDN 1999). However, the annual growth rate is declining and is projected to be 1.6 percent in 2015 (World Bank 2001), and for the first time there are more children aged 1 to 4 years than aged 5 to 9. While maternal and child health will continue as a dominant concern for the next few decades, the median age of the population will increase more rapidly, and care for

TABLE 18.1   Philippines: Key Demographic Trends, 1970–99

Indicator	1970	1980	1985	1990	1999
Population, total	37,890,000	48,317,000	54,668,000	60,687,000	74,259,000
Annual population growth (percent)	3.0	2.1	2.2	2.2	1.9
Urban population (percent of total population)	33.0	37.5	43.0	48.8	57.4
Total fertility rate (births per woman)	5.1	4.8	4.5	4.1	3.5
Crude birth rate (per 1,000 people)	39	35	33	31	27
Crude death rate (per 1,000 people)	10	9	8	7	6

Source: GDN 1999.

accidents and chronic disease will be of increasing concern to a constituency interested in purchasing health insurance.

PROFILING HEALTH NEEDS: THE EPIDEMIOLOGICAL SNAPSHOT

Three types of data will be used to complete an epidemiological profile: mortality data, where causes of death reflect both past and current exposures to health risks; morbidity data, where the presence of nonfatal illnesses reflects the current disease trends; and information on the prevalence of risk factors, which forms an impression about future trends in disease.

Examining the relative proportions of communicable (including maternal and perinatal causes) and noncontagious diseases and injuries gives an impression of the major illness trends in the country. To stage a country with respect to the epidemiological transition (see next page), we focus on contagious and noncontagious diseases. The issue of injuries will be examined separately.

Mortality

Mortality data follow demographic data in terms of availability, validity, and precision. Countries vary greatly in terms of the detail and accuracy of mortality data. Industrial countries have instituted standardized processes for reporting information on death certificates, and consequently age- and sex-specific death rates are relatively accurate and readily available. For very low-income countries such as Bolivia and Uganda, without standardized collection methods, mortality rates are estimated from sentinel health care institutions or even community surveys using verbal autopsies.

Information on sex and age for broad groups of diseases is relatively accurate, but considerable error can crop up in coding specific causes of death. Error may arise from failure to diagnose illnesses accurately, difficulty in determining the underlying cause of death when there are multiple diseases, lack of care taken by certifying physicians, or cultural and political pressures that limit the identification of causes such as suicide or AIDS. Note in table 18.2, for instance, how the number of deaths from and cases of AIDS change from one source to another. However, the number of deaths from diseases such as typhoid fever and malignant neoplasm is stable across all sources.

Mortality data by age and sex for the Philippines were freely available from the WHO Statistical Information System for 1996 (WHO 1996). Death from "signs, symptoms and other ill-defined conditions" and "senility" accounted for 5 percent of deaths, indicating lack of accuracy in coding. But for most disease categories, mortality rates and trends from various sources were comparable, suggesting that the epidemiological inferences about large mortality tendencies can be considered to be robust.

The epidemiological transition. The prevailing rates and causes of death can be used to stage a population within the epidemiological transition.[1] The first stage is referred to as the *age of pestilence and famine.* This is typical of agrarian societies where recurring epidemics of infectious disease such as typhoid, tuberculosis, cholera, measles, and meningitis are superimposed on high endemic rates of less dramatic infections such as gastrointestinal infections and pneumonia. The picture is of a high mortality rate in both children and adults, with cyclic troughs and peaks in death rates corresponding to different epidemics. The low life expectancy at birth reflects a high mortality in children aged less than five years, but the population remains susceptible to infectious diseases through adulthood. Mortality is high and morbidity is low given the high lethality of diseases.

During the stage of pestilence, the occurrence (or incidence) of disease is very high; illnesses are acute and rapidly progress to death. The most important interventions to improve the health situation are larger than those offered by clinical medical services: improvements in water and sanitation, mass vaccinations, spraying, and vector control. Nonetheless, medical services will be required to diagnose accurately and respond rapidly to these acute conditions with appropriate treatment. Timeliness is of the essence in preventing subsequent complications or death. A preponderance of these illnesses, if diagnosed early, can be treated cost-effectively in ambulatory services. Consequently, a microinsurance scheme

TABLE 18.2   Philippines: Deaths from and Cases of AIDS, 1996

Cases	Deaths	Source
22	19	National Statistics Coordination Board Department of Health, Manila http://www.nscb.gov.ph/secstat
53	30	National Epidemiology Center, Department of Health, Manila http://www.doh.gov.ph/NEC
n.a.	None	WHO Statistical Information Systems, Statistical Information, Mortality data http://www.who.int/whosis/statistics

n.a. Not applicable.

within this epidemiological profile should provide its members with ready access to health services. This means low financial and geographic barriers to ambulatory services and ready availability or transportation to specialized services. Prevention of future occurrences of disease needs to be a principal concern for the insurance scheme as well as for the insured populations. This implies that the scheme must work in close coordination with public health initiatives such as mass vaccinations and vector control or that it covers these basic preventive services where public health coverage is inadequate.

The second stage in the epidemiological transition is the *age of receding epidemics*. Epidemics become less frequent and, although contagious diseases continue to occur frequently, the survival rates are better. Life expectancy increases dramatically as a larger proportion of the population survives childhood. More survivors will die of other causes, resulting in an increased prevalence of chronic and degenerative disease. Implications for medical care in countries in this second stage will be discussed in detail later in this chapter.

The third stage is the *age of degenerative and man-made diseases*. Epidemics and communicable diseases are no longer a threat to mortality, and a large proportion of the population survives into adulthood where they succumb to accumulated risks that lead to chronic diseases or the "diseases of affluence": cardiovascular conditions, diabetes, and certain types of cancer.

A further stage in this transition has been called the age of *delayed degenerative diseases*. The aging population lives longer with these diseases and a substantial proportion has more than one condition. In the United States, 41 percent of the population has a diagnosed chronic condition, and of these 40 percent have at least two (Bierman and Clancy 1999). Medicare data show that 65 percent of individuals aged 65 years and over have two or more chronic conditions, and that the mean per-capita health expenditures increase almost exponentially—not additively—with each additional chronic condition (Starfield 2001).

In the third stage, a major concern for medical services becomes the prevention and treatment of acute exacerbation and complications of these degenerative and chronic conditions. A major concern for an insurance scheme will be to identify the care that is cost-effective for its benefit package. This care will likely include early detection for disease at a stage where it is most amenable to treatment, providing guidelines for frequency and content of follow-up visits for detected conditions, and providing guidelines for treatment protocols of common conditions. The health scheme will require assistance in technology assessment, guideline development, and provider profiling.

Epidemiological staging of the Philippines. The trend of the top five leading causes of mortality in the Philippines from 1975 to 1995 illustrates the epidemiological transition in this country. In 1975, pneumonia and tuberculosis (contagious disease) were the leading causes of mortality, while over time the degenerative diseases of the heart and vascular system became more prominent. The transition in mortality is illustrated in table 18.3.

TABLE 18.3   Philippines: Trend of Five Leading Causes of Mortality, 1975–95

Rank	1975	1980	1985	1990	1995
1	Pneumonias	Pneumonias	Pneumonias	Heart diseases	Heart diseases
2	Tuberculosis	Heart diseases	Heart diseases	Pneumonias	Diseases of the vascular system
3	Heart diseases	Tuberculosis	Tuberculosis	Diseases of the vascular system	Pneumonias
4	Diseases of the vascular system	Diseases of the vascular system	Diseases of the vascular system	Tuberculosis	Malignant neoplasms
5	Malignant neoplasms	Malignant neoplasms	Malignant neoplasms	Malignant neoplasms	Tuberculosis

Source: DOH 1999a.

The Philippines is in the age of receding epidemics. High rates of contagious disease coexist with high rates of degenerative and chronic diseases. Different regions within the country are at different points along the transition from infectious to degenerative diseases. As the distance from the capital region of Manila increases, so too does the frequency of childhood respiratory infection, diarrhea, and fever. In contrast, the occurrence of cancer becomes more frequent in closer proximity to the capital region. Regardless of region, rural areas show a more infectious profile than do urban areas. As a general rule, poor and rural populations have a higher infectious disease profile, and the urban wealthy have more of a degenerative disease profile. The susceptibility of the poor to infectious diseases includes those in urban areas where internal urban migration exceeds the infrastructure of housing and sanitation. Internal migration has seen an increase in the urban population from 33 percent of the total population in 1970 to 57.7 percent in 1999 (GDN 1999).

The applicability of these national data to local microinsurance can be surmised by examining the survey database of the Social Health Insurance Networking and Empowerment (SHINE) project that analyzes data from 35 community-based microinsurance units in the Philippines. The Philippines' six leading causes of mortality countrywide were also the six leading causes for mortality in the surveyed health care organizations. Even the order of causes was largely similar: heart disease, pneumonia, vascular diseases, tuberculosis, malignant neoplasm, and accidents (in decreasing order). However, the ranking of diseases within each health care organization differed from organization to organization and included more diseases than those listed here. Thus, the mortality picture will change in local contexts, but much of the profile will be predictable by extrapolating from national data.

The "double burden" of infectious and degenerative disease puts a strain on the health care system. Although different populations within the country will share more of one burden than the other, a health plan cannot simply provide infectious disease care in rural areas, and degenerative disease care in urban areas. Much of the population faces both assaults. For instance, adults who were low-birth-weight babies have a much higher rate of diabetes mellitus and cardiovascular disease as adults than do normal-weight babies. In the Philippines, cardiovascular disease is highest in the more urban regions and in the Visayas archipelago in the center of the country. In the cities, it is thought to be attributable mostly to lifestyle factors such as diet, smoking, and a sedentary lifestyle, whereas in the Visayas regions previous infections from rheumatic fever heighten susceptibility to heart disease.

This predisposition may partially account for the observation that mortality from degenerative diseases occurs at a younger age in the Philippines than it does in an industrial country such as Canada. The median age of death (age by which 50 percent of deaths have occurred) is approximately 10 years younger in the Philippines than in Canada for diabetes mellitus and diseases of the circulatory system, and almost 15 years earlier for all malignant neoplasms (WHO 1996). The delay in Canada is also attributable to earlier and more advanced treatment of diagnosed conditions—an expected result of better health insurance and access to care.

Avoidable mortality. The effectiveness of the health care system in responding to health needs can be gauged by assessing avoidable mortality. These are deaths from conditions for which there is effective treatment and where most of deaths could be avoided by timely treatment. These sentinel health events are often used to indicate the responsiveness of the health care system or problems of access by the population (Rutstein and others 1976). Avoidable mortality or morbidity may result from failure to prevent the initial occurrence of an illness, as in the case of vaccine-preventable conditions such as measles, tetanus, or diphtheria. Such mortality generally points to a failure of the public health system. In the Philippines, despite reported immunization coverage of between 70 and 90 percent, measles break out regularly and more than 80 percent of the cases have not been vaccinated (NESSS 2001).

Avoidable mortality may also reflect failure to access health services in a timely manner or receive appropriate care. Examples of these include all maternal deaths, appendicitis, hypertension, asthma, typhoid fever, diarrhea, and most pneumonias. All but appendicitis figure among the major causes of mortality in the Philippines. The maternal mortality ratio was 180/100,000 live births in 1995. Although this represents a small decrease from the previous decades, it is still much higher than in other Asian countries with a similar economic development (Malaysia: 20/100,000 live births). Most health insurance schemes in the Philippines cover deliveries in medical facilities only for first births and for pregnancies classified as high risk, but the high maternal mortality suggests that the benefit package should include more mechanisms for rapid response to obstetrical emergencies.

Avoidable mortality may also result from delayed detection of underlying conditions. For instance, the mortality rate from kidney conditions (nephritis and nephrosis) is very high in the Philippines (10/100,000) and is among the top 15 leading causes of death. These deaths principally result from failure to detect chronic glomerulonephritis, diabetes mellitus, and hypertension at early stages. Before dying of kidney failure, many people will have lived with end-stage kidney disease, and less than 15 percent of them will have received dialysis to prolong their lives. An insurance scheme may or may not decide to cover dialysis, but for long-term viability it would be prudent to ensure that the scheme provides case-finding for chronic glomerulonephritis, diabetes, and hypertension.[2]

Morbidity

Morbidity data generally come from utilization statistics kept by health facilities. The diagnostic information is usually accurate because qualified health professionals make the diagnoses. Hospital discharge data are the most commonly used source of morbidity data, followed by reasons for ambulatory care visits. Hospital morbidity is based on discharge information, and most patients leave the hospital with a diagnosis. Hospital data generally show the tip of the iceberg in terms of disease, but inferring the rates and probabilities of use to the whole population may be biased because hospital services are more easily accessed by the urban wealthy and also reflect provider-practice styles. Nonetheless, hospital data are a relatively accurate source of information for serious diseases that require surgical interventions or intensive therapy. Information from ambulatory care centers is usually less biased by issues of access, but the information often pertains to symptoms or general conditions rather than to specific diagnostic labels.

Another important source of morbidity information is notifiable diseases.[3] National as well as international agencies usually organize reporting, which, although possibly incomplete at any one time, provides a valuable insight into the context of illness in a country. The *WHO Weekly Epidemiologic Record* publishes weekly statistics on reported cases of diseases subject to international health regulation: cholera, yellow fever, and plague. These show cholera outbreaks in the Philippines in both 2000 and 2001, but no cases in the regions where our sample microinsurance schemes operate. Influenza and dengue fever outbreaks have also been reported for the Philippines. Although not all regions are equally susceptible, the frequent outbreaks of contagious diseases suggest that health services and the insurance (and reinsurance) schemes need to be prepared to respond to epidemics.

In addition to the internationally notifiable diseases, countries often select to monitor the occurrence of specific diseases with epidemic potential. These data are usually collected from sentinel health institutions, and excess occurrences of diseases are investigated. For instance, in the Philippines, the National Epidemic Sentinel Surveillance System (NESSS) relies heavily on admissions to the San Lazaro Hospital in Manila. The hospital issues weekly reports on admissions for dengue fever, diphtheria, hepatitis A, hepatitis B, leptospirosis, malaria, meningitis, measles, tetanus, rabies, and typhoid fever. NESSS has been able to track, for instance, the increasing epidemic of dengue fever, showing that most cases occur from September through November in urban concentrations. The system even identified the localities where cases tended to cluster (NESSS 2001).

Often the most valid way to measure the prevalence of illness is through a population survey. Community surveys identify the prevalence of symptoms, limitations in function, illness days, and risk factors such as overweight and smoking that may be related to ill health. Although these surveys do not provide precise diagnostic information, they are closely related to manifestations of diseases and people's decisions to seek medical care for them.

A rich source of community prevalence of illness and the propensity to use medical services is the demographic health surveys (DHS). These are country-level household surveys of issues related to family planning, child survival, and some health service issues. They are carried out periodically in most developing countries following a methodology that permits comparisons between countries. They are a good source of information on maternal and child health. DHS data offer the advantage of allowing access to the raw data for analyses of the subcomponent that may be most similar to the local context of interest. The use of health services is assessed only for diarrhea, respiratory infections, immunization, and family planning. Despite this limitation, the information gives an insight into the propensity to use health care services for common conditions.

In general, the DHS surveys indicate a high propensity to use health services for childhood illnesses in the Philippines. For instance, the 1993 survey showed that the two-week prevalence of nonspecific fever in children less than five years of age was 24 percent in Ilocos, where the ORT scheme is located, and 19 percent in Central Luzon, where the Tarlac scheme is located (NSO and MI 1994). More than half of the children were taken to a health facility for diagnosis and treatment. Likewise, the prevalence of diarrhea was 13.6 percent in Ilocos and 6.5 percent in Central Luzon, and 35 percent of these children were taken to health facilities in both areas. By comparison, only 15 percent of children in Uganda with the same condition were taken to health facilities.

Morbidity profile of the Philippines. The DOH in the Philippines publishes the top 10 causes of morbidity every year. These data are generated by the Field Health Service Information System, which consolidates information from health facility records all the way from community midwives through to the tertiary care hospitals. Data from private clinics and hospitals are not included, but the information does provide an insight into the illness patterns that might be expected in the target population for microinsurance schemes. In keeping with the expectation of a country in the age of receding epidemics, where the mortality from infectious diseases is decreasing but the incidence remains high, infectious diseases comprised 8 of the top 10 causes of illness requiring medical care in 1999 (table 18.4.)

The top six diseases have remained stable over the past few years, although their relative position changes from year to year. Diseases lower in the list reflect periodic epidemics of measles, typhoid fever, and chicken pox. The pattern of diseases seen in health facilities suggests that children are the highest users of the health care system, and that use decreases with age. This pattern is expected to change over the

TABLE 18.4   Philippines: Ten Leading Causes of Morbidity, 1999

Cause	Rate per 100,000 population	Class of disease
Diarrheas	1,190	Contagious
Bronchitis/bronchiolitis	939	Contagious
Pneumonias	908	Contagious
Influenza	674	Contagious
Hypertension	273	Degenerative
Tuberculosis, respiratory	190	Contagious
Malaria	89	Contagious
Heart diseases	83	Degenerative
Chicken pox	47	Contagious
Typhoid and paratyphoid fever	23	Contagious

Source: DOH 1999c.

next decade or two as the proportion of young children in the population decreases relative to the proportion of older people. We would expect to see heart and circulatory diseases as well as diabetes emerge as leading causes of illness care. This trend will occur earlier in regions that are farther in the epidemiological transitions: the national capital region, followed by Central Luzon, then Ilocos.

Morbidity profile of the case insurance schemes. The two insurance schemes on which we have limited utilization data are the Tarlac Health Maintenance Plan in the province of Tarlac, Central Luzon region, and the ORT Health Plus Scheme, based in the province of La Union in the Ilocos region. Membership in both schemes is by household, with monthly premiums based on the number of dependents per member in the ORT scheme and a standard yearly premium per member (regardless of number of dependents) in the Tarlac plan. Membership in the Tarlac plan is immediately terminated if premiums have not been paid by the due date, whereas membership in the ORT scheme is cancelled for failure to pay the monthly premium for two consecutive months. Reinstatement in the both plans is possible, but waiting periods are imposed before coverage resumes.

The ORT Health Plus Scheme includes 13 clinics and the regional tertiary hospital (Ilocos Training and Regional Medical Centre) in the city of San Fernando. The satellite clinics provide primary care and are staffed by a volunteer health worker. Five nurses and three physicians visit each of the 13 clinics twice a week. The nurses and physicians who work in outpatient services are salaried while inpatient hospital services (for example, professional fees and medications) are covered by a standard monthly capitation fee for each ORT member.

Insurable benefits for ORT scheme members include primary health care consultations, immunizations, and other preventive care, prenatal visits and well-baby care, essential medications prescribed by an ORT provider, diagnostic tests, and outpatient and inpatient services provided at the Ilocos Training and Regional Medical Centre. Certain services, such as dialysis, open-heart surgery, and dental care, are not included in the benefit package. Since individual consultations do not generate a claim in the ORT plan, and diagnostic information is recorded only for hospitalizations, our capacity to make inferences about the illness profile and utilization rates was very limited.

The Tarlac health plan insures outpatient consultation, diagnostic services, minor surgery, and inpatient fees (for example, medication, room and board, diagnostic tests, and physicians' fees). Each benefit has an annual monetary ceiling per family. Certain services and diseases or injuries are excluded from the benefit package, including outpatient medications, health care received from a provider outside the Tarlac plan (except in emergencies), deliveries after the first born, and treatment of congenital or neonatal abnormalities, sexually transmitted diseases, AIDS, psychiatric illness, and injuries resulting from the abuse of alcohol or drugs, suicide, war, or service in the military or police forces.

Services to members of the Tarlac Health Maintenance Plan are provided by reimbursing services of physicians and health care facilities that are accredited by the plan. All private and public physicians, hospitals, and diagnostic centers based in the province of Tarlac and licensed by DOH or the Professional Regulations Committee are eligible for application to render services in the Tarlac plan. Currently, the Tarlac plan includes 14 hospitals (4 primary, 6 secondary, and 4 tertiary), 1 diagnostic center, and 130 physicians (90 of them based in Tarlac City and 40 based in nine municipalities). Of these 130 physicians, 16 are general practitioners, and the rest practice specialty medicine. Providers are paid on a fee-for-service basis. Analysis of the illness profile and utilization rates was possible because of the fee-for-service payment mechanism and the fact that the plan has been recording diagnoses for both outpatient and inpatient claims in the last four months of the data available to us.

Based on the epidemiological profile at a regional level, we hypothesized that the Tarlac membership would experience a slightly higher proportion of degenerative diseases than the country as a whole but would still be subject to high rates of contagious diseases. Of the leading causes of morbidity in the Philippines we expected that malaria would be rare because Tarlac is not in the malaria-endemic region. The expectation of higher rates of degenerative disease is based on the Central Luzon region's being a Class 1 Region, with a high per-capita income and the vast majority of members living in or near the urban area of Tarlac City. Plan members appear to be employed principally in small enterprise, but some are farmers, and others, such as maids and general laborers, work in informal-sector occupations. Table 18.5 shows the top 13 diagnoses in service claims over a four-month period from September to December 1999. Together they comprise 85 percent of the reasons for visits where a diagnosis was coded.[4] Contagious diseases accounted for 54 percent, and degenerative diseases for 31 percent of the claims. Infectious diseases, although still more common than chronic degenerative diseases, played a

TABLE 18.5   Tarlac Health Maintenance Plan, Philippines: 13 Leading Causes of Morbidity, Outpatients and Inpatients, September to December 1999

Cause	Number (percent) of claims	Number (percent) seen as outpatients	Estimated yearly rate per 1,000[a]	Mean (SD) outpatient cost	Mean (SD) inpatient cost	Number (percent) of outpatient claims > 40 pesos[b]	Mean (SD) outpatient cost if > 40 pesos[b]
Acute respiratory infection, bronchitis	82 (20.9)	69 (84.1)	57.3	46.2 (28.2)	1,141.7 (716.1)	5 (7.2)	126.0 (70.6)
Diabetes mellitus	39 (9.7)	28 (71.8)	27.2	63.9 (35.4)	1,093.9 (594.2)	13 (46.4)	91.5 (35.8)
Hypertension	31 (7.7)	21 (67.7)	21.6	50.5 (30.7)	1,053.4 (697.4)	3 (14.3)	113.3 (50.3)
Urinary tract infection	30 (7.5)	20 (66.7)	20.9	50.5 (29.1)	1,355.3 (795.9)	4 (20.0)	100.0 (34.6)
Heart diseases	28 (7.0)	14 (50.0)	19.5	82.9 (55.4)	1,020.9 (565.8)	7 (50.0)	125.7 (48.6)
Tonsillitis, pharyngitis	28 (7.0)	25 (89.3)	19.5	40.8 (4.0)	1,028.8 (435.0)	1 (4.0)	60.0 (—)
Diarrhea, gastroenteritis	26 (6.5)	11 (42.3)	18.1	52.5 (48.3)	1,067.1 (618.1)	1 (9.1)	197.6 (—)
Pneumonia	20 (5.0)	7 (35.0)	13.9	40.0 (0.0)	1,361.9 (942.8)	0 (0.0)	— (—)
Tuberculosis, respiratory	13 (3.2)	11 (84.6)	9.1	52.7 (24.1)	1,124.3 (620.0)	3 (27.3)	86.7 (23.1)
Vertigo	13 (3.2)	10 (76.9)	9.1	59.0 (46.8)	508.7 (94.6)	3 (30.0)	103.3 (75.1)
Asthma	12 (3.0)	6 (50.0)	8.4	40.0 (0.0)	1,115.8 (420.9)	0 (0.0)	— (—)
Typhoid fever	12 (3.0)	4 (33.3)	8.4	699.4[c] (1306.0)	1,124.5 (604.5)	2 (50.0)	1358.9[c] (1836.9)
Nephrosis, nephritis	10 (2.5)	6 (60.0)	7.0	35.0 (5.5)	1,000.3 (730.0)	0 (0.0)	— (—)

— Not available.

Note: Diagnoses were recorded for 401/563 (71 percent) of claims. Percentages are calculated using 401 as the denominator.

a. Estimates of rate per 1,000 calculated as follows: (number of cases in 4 months X 3) ÷ 4,295 members in the plan.

b. These are consultations that generated ancillary costs over and above the PHP 40 professional fee for outpatient consultation.

c. This figure includes a reimbursement of PHP 2,657 for services received outside the plan. Its classification as an outpatient consultation may be the result of a coding error.

Source: Claims for services, September to December 1999, Tarlac Health Maintenance Plan.

lesser role in the morbidity patterns among Tarlac beneficiaries than among the Philippine population as a whole. Diabetes, hypertension, and heart disease, all chronic degenerative diseases, were included among the top five diagnoses recorded on the Tarlac reimbursement claims. However, the absolute rates of occurrence of these illnesses are substantially higher than morbidity rates recorded for the Philippines as a whole. In the absence of more information about how national rates were calculated, however, it is difficult to interpret why this occurs.

Table 18.5 also shows the mean outpatient and inpatient costs for these diseases. Notice the remarkable similarity of costs for mean outpatient and inpatient across diagnoses. The table also shows the impact of the changing epidemiological profile on costs of care. The degenerative conditions have much higher average costs associated with consultations than do the infectious diseases.

The probability in Tarlac of an outpatient consultation was 0.25, and of hospitalization 0.07, for a total 0.32 probability of health care use in Tarlac.[5] Comparable figures are not available for outpatient consultations in the ORT scheme, because providers are paid on a salary rather than fee-for-service basis. Claims are available only for ancillary services in outpatient visits (laboratory tests, X rays, electrocardiograms, special examinations). If we assume that 37 percent of outpatient visits in ORT generated an ancillary cost—as they did in the Tarlac scheme— the probability of outpatient visits in ORT is 0.67.[6] This figure is highly uncertain, but even if the proportion of ancillary services were as high as 60 percent in ORT, the probability of outpatient visits would still be much higher than in Tarlac. It may be that the ORT members are closer to services or more trusting of providers.

For hospitalizations, the figures are more reliable, and here we notice striking differences in the pattern of hospitalizations between the two schemes. The probability of hospitalization in Tarlac in 1999 was three times that for ORT (0.07 vs. 0.02), even when obstetrical cases were excluded. In contrast, the length of stay for ORT hospitalizations was almost double the 2.9-day mean stay in Tarlac. This funding suggests that the threshold for hospitalization is lower in Tarlac and that hospitalizations occur for less serious conditions. Such situations are more likely the result of differences in provider discretion than of differences in burden of disease in the membership, as seen in the subsequent analysis of avoidable hospitalizations.

Avoidable hospitalizations. Avoidable hospitalizations are admissions for conditions that can usually be managed with timely and effective treatment in an outpatient setting. Hospitalization for conditions such as asthma, diabetes, hypertension, and pneumonia are often interpreted to result from a lack of access to primary care or failure to diagnose and treat appropriately at the ambulatory care level (Bindman and others 1995). Indeed, the rates of hospitalization for avoidable morbidity are much higher in the Tarlac scheme than in the ORT scheme. Patient or provider barriers to outpatient services may be too high in Tarlac. It is also possible, however, that the differences can be attributed to physician-practice style. One indication of discretionary physician behavior is the occurrence of admissions for nonspecific conditions such as vertigo and edema: Physicians admit patients to hospitals to make diagnoses instead of treating diseases diagnosed in the outpatient setting. This provider behavior is probably attributable to differences in the definitions of the benefit package or provider-payment mechanisms between the two schemes. There may be a hidden incentive to hospitalize in Tarlac or a disincentive in the ORT scheme. It would be worthwhile to evaluate whether the benefit package for ambulatory services in Tarlac could be modified to avoid costly hospitalizations.

It seems likely, on the other hand, that outpatient visits in ORT are associated with a higher use of laboratory tests. The ORT scheme has a strikingly higher rate of tests that are usually used for early detection of disease (urinalysis, pap smears, and electrocardiograms). This higher rate may reflect a more preventive orientation and a strong primary care system, but it may also reflect a professional payment scheme that favors laboratory testing.

The limitation of this morbidity information is that it is based on health service utilization data. The propensity to use health services reflects not only the occurrence of illness but also the characteristics of the users, the providers, and the payment method for services. The propensity to seek medical services for a new health problem (patient-initiated care) will vary with the population's cultural and sociodemographic characteristics. In the results of the SHINE survey, key informants from the health care organizations indicated that, in the constituencies of all the organizations, people resorted to home remedies before consulting medical providers, and going to see traditional healers was ranked higher as an illness response than going to private medical providers. Once a patient is in the system, however, the characteristics of the providers or the payment method for services will have a large influence on higher-level services that patients receive. Even within the limitations of utilization data, epidemiological analysis can help to monitor patient- and provider-induced moral hazard within the insurance scheme.

Accidents and Injuries

The issue of accidents and injuries deserves special attention because they are the types of health events that fall within the classic insurance paradigm of insurable events. The epidemiological transition focuses more on the relative burden of contagious versus degenerative diseases, but a rapid industrialization and urbanization process is often accompanied by an increase in intentional and unintentional injuries. These are often consequences of increased economic activity, population mobility, and social problems. Prevention of injuries is largely a matter of public policy to enhance road and occupational safety and reduce social tension. Medical services still have an important role to play not only in treatment but also in the detection of factors that increase the risk of accidents and injuries. Risk factors in which medical services play an important role are the detection of problem drinking, depression, and family violence.

As with noncontagious diseases, accidents are becoming increasingly prominent as a leading cause of death in the Philippines. The annual death rate from accidents increased 20 percent between 1991 and 1994 to 21.5 deaths per 100,000 people. Intentional injuries (homicide and suicide) make up slightly more of the deaths than unintentional injuries (motor vehicle accidents, drowning, head injuries, fractures). For the country as a whole, the morbidity from accidents and injuries in 1994 was 308/100,000; it was 405/100,000 in Central Luzon, and 150/100,000 in Ilocos (DOH 1999a, p. 116). Injuries accounted for two hospitalizations in a four-month period among members of the Tarlac Health Plan, and in three hospitalizations over a one-year period in the ORT scheme. In the SHINE survey, accidents were the sixth leading cause of mortality.

PROFILING FUTURE HEALTH NEEDS: HEALTH RISK FACTORS

In addition to having information on the mortality and morbidity in the country, information on the prevalence of important risk factors helps predict the types of illness patterns that will emerge over the next decades.

Risk Factors for Contagious Diseases

The risk factors for contagious diseases are the presence of infectious agents, the quality of water and sanitation facilities, the immunization coverage, and safe sex practices. Since maternal and perinatal conditions are included in this classification, risk factors extend to family planning coverage and access to services. Interventions to reduce exposure to these risk factors are part of public health services, public policy, and development.

As noted, the fatality rate from contagious diseases is declining in the Philippines, but these conditions will continue to be a major source of morbidity for at least the next decade, especially among children, the poor, and residents of the southern parts of the country. Tuberculosis and dengue are endemic in urban areas, and malaria and schistosomiasis are still endemic in the southern and rural parts of the country. Information from epidemiological surveillance programs suggests that, in addition to a high baseline occurrence of contagious diseases, outbreaks of conditions such as malaria, dengue, and cholera occur regularly within the country. Although these epidemics may not occur frequently in a given locality, health insurance and reinsurance schemes will need to account for this probability.

Likewise, although fertility is falling in the Philippines, maternal mortality has not been dropping at the same rate. This disparity suggests that obstetrical emergencies will remain an important concern for health services into the next decade.

Risk Factors for Noncontagious Diseases

The risk factors of greatest concern to the emergence of degenerative and chronic diseases are lifestyle choices and exposure to pollutants. Smoking and obesity are lifestyle choices of particular interest. Problem drinking and depression affect the risk of accidents and injuries, but little information is available on either issue.

Cigarette smoking is the single most important modifiable risk factor for future illness. Smoking accounts for more than 80 percent of all occurrences of cancer, 70 percent of chronic obstructive lung disease, and 35 percent of deaths from heart disease. Children exposed to second-hand smoke are more than twice as likely to have respiratory infections and ear infections.

National surveys in the Philippines show that in 1998 the prevalence of smokers was 59 percent of individuals aged 55 and above, 52 percent of individuals aged 40 to 54 years, and 39 percent of individuals aged 20 to 39 years (DOH 1999a, p. 205). The vast majority of smokers are males. Although the age trend of lower prevalence in younger age groups is encouraging, the DHS survey showed that 60 percent of all households include members who smoke. Smoking-related diseases will account for high rates of death and illness, especially among middle-aged and older males, and infectious diseases will be exacerbated among children in smokers' households.

PREDICTING HEALTH CARE DEMAND AT THE LOCAL LEVEL

The ultimate aim of epidemiological analysis within the framework of micro-insurance is to estimate the demand for health care in the local context in which the insurance scheme will be established. The epidemiological profile provided up to this point will provide a general framework for the local estimation.

Various ways of estimating the demand for health care have been developed, most of them involving regression modeling of population and provider characteristics on the probability and mean level of health care use. These methods have been developed principally in industrial countries (Hakkinen 1991; Anderson and Newman 1973; Tataryn, Roos, and Black 1995), and some preliminary research will have to be carried out to determine how applicable the coefficients and variables are for developing countries. The variables most often used in this type of modeling are listed in table 18.6. The sets of variables are listed in decreasing order of data availability.

In countries such as the Philippines, where there is relatively good availability of information, many of the variables can be obtained from existing data sources. To test the regression model and to determine the epidemiological profile of disease, however, utilization information will almost certainly have to be obtained from a local source. Understanding of local heath needs and health care utilization patterns, both current and future, will only be refined by collecting data first-hand in the community to be served. The information to be collected pertains to both health needs and the tendency to use health services.

Local Surveys

The first step in a local survey is to define the constituency and develop an exhaustive list of all people or households who can be included (*sampling frame*).

TABLE 18.6   Variables Commonly Used for Regression Modeling of Health Care Demand

Information to be collected	Potential sources of data
1. Sociodemographic information • Age-gender structure (produce a population pyramid by 15-year age group) • Age-gender structure of household • Average household size • Gender and educational achievement of household head • Unemployment rates • Population density (overcrowding index)	Census Bureau or extrapolation from demographic health surveys
2. Environmental health factors • Infrastructure of houses (building materials, cooking facilities) • Sanitation and garbage disposal facilities • Access to potable water • High-risk occupations	Department of Health, municipal offices, Census Bureau
3. Access to health services • Number of providers per 1,000 population • Number of hospital beds per capita • Distance to health care centers (time and space)	Department of Health, demographic health surveys
4. Illness and disability • Presence of illness in last two or four weeks • Presence of chronic illnesses (use local nomenclatures) • Extent of activity limitations in household members • Presence of major health event in last year	Community surveys, extrapolations from demographic health surveys, estimations from utilization statistics
5. Health service utilization • Response to illness in last four weeks • Use of formal versus informal care • Intensity of care received (consultations, diagnostic services, prescriptions, other therapy) • Reasons for not seeking medical care	Community surveys, estimations from utilization statistics
6. Health risks • Smoking • Problem drinking • Obesity • Undernutrition (especially children, and women in childbearing years)	Community surveys

Where the constituency is in a geographically defined area, circumscribing and identifying the constituency is relatively straightforward, with the use of local vital registries or voting lists. Otherwise, it can be very challenging.

Once identified, the constituency can be sampled rigorously and systematically to ensure that it represents the constituency. The recommended sampling unit for these types of surveys is the household, because information can be gleaned on the health behavior of more than one person and the household is the membership unit in most health insurance plans. One key informant can provide adequate information for the household. A sample of 200 households will generally provide adequately precise estimates and is operationally feasible for a small organization.

The analysis will focus on identifying and understanding the factors affecting health care utilization. Illness, health care utilization patterns, and risk factors will be broken down by age, gender, and other available categories to estimate the potential demand for health services covered by the benefit package. The combination of the expected probability of health care use, the average intensity of use, and the average cost of services on the basis of data collected from local health care providers provides information for the parameters used in calculating the insurance premium.

CONCLUSIONS

This chapter illustrates how the epidemiological analysis of demographic, mortality, morbidity, and risk information at a national level can provide clues to the major health needs in a country and, to a certain extent, within the local context for microinsurance schemes. In the context of a specific scheme, however, this analysis will help identify information gaps that may have to be filled with original data collected locally.

This chapter also demonstrates how the epidemiological analysis of available data was used to provide clues to the risk profile for microinsurance schemes in the Philippines. The Philippines is a country in both demographic and epidemiological transition, both of which have implications for health services. As the Philippines is still characterized by high fertility rates, maternal and child services will continue to predominate among its people's health concerns. Within the epidemiological transition, the country faces a double burden of a high occurrence of infectious diseases and an increasing prevalence of chronic and degenerative diseases. The continued endemic nature of infectious diseases, as well as the high prevalence of risk factors, suggest that the health service offered by microinsurance units would have to accommodate both.

What does the epidemiological analysis tell us about the priority of services that should be offered within the benefit package? What does the epidemiological analysis suggest are the services that will be perceived by the insureds as meeting their major health needs? To address the problem of commonly occurring diseases, there is a continuing need for first-contact ambulatory services that are responsive (ready access) and able to resolve most problems (effective). Although mortality from pregnancy is relatively rare, it has enormous social consequences and is largely preventable through ready access to good emergency obstetrical care. Finally, the epidemiological profile suggests the potential for an outbreak of contagious disease, which will affect both the insurance scheme and the reinsurer.

The insurance membership will also be increasingly concerned about the onset of chronic diseases that compromise quality of life and drain health care resources. The long-term nature of health expenditures for these conditions will also concern the insurance scheme. The insurer will have to make difficult choices about treatments to include in the benefit package, as effective but expensive alternatives continue to emerge. The insurer will need access to health technology–assessment services to be able to weigh alternatives in terms of cost-effectiveness. The membership may have to consider obtaining upgrades in coverage to receive treatments excluded from the basic package.

Although preventive care does not fall within the services considered insurable, prevention has to be an important part of service coverage to avert more expensive health services later. This is particularly true for early detection of asymptomatic conditions in which early intervention improves health outcomes: detection of diabetes, hypertension, and breast and cervical cancer. Clinicians also need to be proactive in addressing risk factors such as smoking, problem drinking, obesity, depression, and domestic violence.

Our analysis of information from two microinsurance units has shown that utilization patterns can differ markedly from one plan to another. Such utilization is more likely to be affected by differences in the members' propensity to use outpatient services and the type and intensity of services generated by providers than by large differences in the prevalence and incidence of disease in the two populations. There are undoubtedly differences in the type of illness burden between the two contexts—we expected a higher burden from degenerative diseases and accidents in Tarlac. But the most striking differences are probably influenced by the availability of services, the form of provider payment, the relationship of the members to the unit, and the definition of the benefit package.

Careful definition of the benefit package can ensure that barriers are lowest for acute conditions for which timeliness is critical. For chronic conditions, the benefit package can also ensure that care is appropriately limited to cost-effective treatments. Limiting benefits to effective care can protect patients against excess use of interventions of dubious effectiveness. The definition of the benefit package need not be viewed only as a means of limiting services but also as a means of protecting the health of all members and enhancing the equity of access to health services.

NOTES

1. *Epidemiological transition* is the term used to describe the major epidemiological trends observed during the past two centuries (Omran 1971).

2. *Case-finding* refers to the performance of routine diagnostic examinations on apparently healthy persons to detect illness prior to the development of symptoms so that presymptomatic conditions can be treated to prevent the occurrence of more serious diseases.

3. *Notifiable diseases* are those subject to national or international quarantine or public health measures.

4. Of the 563 claims, diagnoses were recorded for 401 (71 percent); inferences about morbidity are based on the latter.

5. Tarlac: 305 hospitalizations plus 1,127 outpatient visits by 4,295 individuals.

6. ORT: 51 hospitalizations plus 535 ancillary outpatient claims by 2,167 individuals. (Assuming that ancillary services occur in 37 percent of outpatient consultations, then there were 1,446 consultations. For the denominator, we assume that the membership in 2000 is approximately similar to that for 1999.)

REFERENCES

Anderson, R., and J.F. Newman. 1973. "Societal and Individual Determinants of Medical Care Utilization in the United States." *Milbank Memorial Quarterly* 51:95–124.

Bierman, A.S., and C.M. Clancy. 1999. "Women's Health, Chronic Disease and Disease Management: New Words and Old Music?" *Women's Health Issues* 9(1):2–17.

Bindman, A.B., K. Grumbach, D.H. Osmond, M. Komaromy, K. Vranizan, N. Lurie, J. Billings, and A.L. Stewart. 1995. "Preventable Hospitalizations and Access to Health Care." *Journal of the American Medical Association* 274(4):305–11.

DOH (Department of Health). 1999a. National Objectives for Health: Philippines 1999–2004. Custodio, G.G.V, Ed. Manila: DOH, Office of the Secretary. http://doh.gov.ph/noh/.

_____. 1999b. "Health Facilities." http://www.doh.gov.ph/hosp/hospitalist.htm.

_____. 1999c. *Field Health Service Information System Annual Report.* Manila: DOH. Table 9-4.

Department of Interior and Local Government. 1999. "Number of Regions/Provinces/Cities/Municipalities/Barangays." http://www.dilg.gov.ph/lgusum.html.

Hakkinen, U. 1991. "The Production of Health and the Demand for Health Care in Finland." *Social Science in Medicine* 33(3):225–37.

GDN (Global Development Network). 1999. "Data Query of the World Bank's Global Development Finance (GDF) and World Development Indicators (WDI) Database." http://www.gdnet.org/GDN-Query.htm.

NDHS (National Demographic and Health Survey). 1998. Manila: Department of Health, National Statistics Office and Macro International, Inc.

NESSS (National Epidemic Sentinel Surveillance System). 2001. "NESSS-SLH Reports, Admissions at San Lazaro Hospital, 2001, Surveillance Update." Manila: Department of Health, National Epidemiology Centre. http://www.doh.gov.ph/NEC_wpage/Download/Dload_slh.htm.

NSO (National Statistics Office). 2000. "Census 2000 Final Counts Summary: Total Population, Number of Households, Average Household Size, Population Growth Rate and Population Density by Region, Province and Highly Urbanized City: as of May 1, 2000." Department of Health, NSO. http://www.census.gov.ph/census2000/.

NSO and MI (National Statistics Office and Macro International). 1994. *Demographic and Health Survey 1993.* Manila: NSO, Department of Health, and Calverton, Md.: Macro International, Inc.

Omran, A.R., 1971. "The Epidemiological Transition. A Theory of the Epidemiology of Population Change." *Milbank Memorial Fund Quarterly* 49(4):509–38.

Rutstein, D.D., W. Berenberg, T.C. Chalmers, C.G. Child, A.P. Fishman, E.B. Perrin, and Working Group on Preventable and Manageable Diseases. 1976 "Measuring the Quality of Medical Care." *New England Journal of Medicine* 294:582–88.

Starfield, B. 2001. "The Value of Primary Care." Plenary Presentation, North American Primary Care Research Group, Twenty-eighth Annual Meeting, Amelia Island, FL, November 14–17, 2001.

Tataryn, D.J., N.P. Roos, and D. Black. 1995. "Utilization of Physician Resources for Ambulatory Care." *Medical Care* 33:DS84–DS99.

WHO (World Health Organization). 1996. Geneva: WHO Statistical Information System. "Statistical Information. Mortality Data. Numbers of Deaths and Death Rates." http://www-nt.who.int/whosis/statistics/.

_____. 2000. Epidemiologic Fact Sheet on HIV/AIDS and Sexually Transmitted Infections in the Philippines: 2000 Update. http://www.who.int/emc-hiv/fact_sheets/pdfs/philippines.pdf.

World Bank. 2000. "Country Data: Country at a Glance Tables." http://www.worldbank.org/data/countrydata/countrydata.html.

_____. 2001. *World Development Indicators.* http://www.worldbank.org/data/wdi2001/.

CHAPTER 19

Attitudes toward Solidarity, Risk, and Insurance in the Rural Philippines

Elmer S. Soriano, M.D., David M. Dror, Erwin Alampay, and Yolanda Bayugo

Every managerial act rests on assumptions, generalizations, and hypotheses—that is to say on theory. Our assumptions are frequently implicit, sometimes quite unconscious, often conflicting; nevertheless, they determine our predictions that if we do A, B will occur. Theory and practice are inseparable.

—Douglas McGregor 1960

A sustainable health reinsurance system can be fashioned for the informal sector by mobilizing social and economic forces operating within individual communities. The economic analysis in part 1 of this book draws conclusions from success stories in industrial countries and failures in low- and medium-income countries. This analysis leads to the premise that decentralized development of microinsurance units, operating in a market segment left out by for-profit health insurance firms and by national schemes, can be stabilized financially through their affiliation with a reinsurance facility—*Social Re*[1] (part 1, this volume; Dror and Duru 2000, pp. 30–40; Dror 2001).

Dror, Preker, and Jakab, in chapter 2 of this book, explain how the sociological dimension would theoretically affect the performance of a microinsurer. Findings of the Institute of Medicine reaffirm the active interplay of biology, psychology, behavior, and society in determining people's health attitudes. The institute further reports that, although people's attitudes and actions can readily be altered, these changes need support and reinforcement over time to guarantee better health. Attitudinal and behavioral changes are best prolonged through interventions at multiple levels, from the individual to society at large (Institute of Medicine 2001, pp. 1-1–1-8).

Efforts are required to address the psychosocial factors that influence health status, including, for example, proposing measures such as microinsurance to persuade individuals to accept a healthy way of life and permanently modify their health behavior. Microinsurance schemes provide individuals, households, and

The authors gratefully recognize useful comments by Soledad A. Hernando, Ph.D., Asian Institute of Management, Makati City, the Philippines, and John W. Peabody, M.D., Ph.D., Institute for Global Health, San Francisco, who reviewed this chapter.

communities mechanisms for financing their health through group risk-pooling mechanisms, leading to a sustained improvement in their access to health services.

Higher up on the social scale, well-evaluated interventions at the organizational level should be encouraged, giving credit to organizations' vital role in influencing individual behavior. Still farther up the scale, community involvement in health-promotion strategies should not be overlooked, because some disease-related factors that are beyond an individual's capacity to modify can be significantly minimized through community efforts. Community empowerment, social support, and other values that protect members from stress are strengthened through community-level interventions. Finally, interventions at the societal level recognize the role of collective organizations influencing individuals' everyday existence (Institute of Medicine 2001, pp. 1-1–1-8).

Underlying assumptions are that members' affiliation with microinsurers is voluntary (individuals can join, stay enrolled, or withdraw at will) and that microinsurers will voluntarily join *Social Re*. A clue is therefore needed about the considerations that shape individual and collective choices. According to one opinion, "The underlying economic motivation for joining a microinsurance unit is assumed to be a desire to seek reciprocity in sustaining risk-sharing arrangements among essentially self-interested individuals" (Dror and Jacquier 1999, p. 79). This assumption implies that joining a microinsurance unit (and *Social Re*) is a predictable, rational economic choice by self-interested individuals to maximize total utility *(optimal choice theory)*, and an act of reciprocity, in which giving and getting are somehow linked. According to the utility motive, people will join if they can benefit from joining. However, considering that many people will pay a health insurance premium without getting any cash benefits (if they stay healthy), is it really clear what each individual would consider as his or her exact utility from being insured? As Herrnstein points out, because utility cannot be directly observed, it must be inferred from behavior, from the choices individuals make. Thus, utility is synonymous with the modern concept of reinforcement in behavioral psychology (Herrnstein 1997, p. 226). Dror and Jacquier mention a second motive for joining a microinsurance unit: people's desire to improve their health by controlling their living and working conditions. This control is linked to a deep-rooted human need to seek voluntary and repeated interaction with others in daily life (Dror and Jacquier 1999, p. 80). These interactions may provide material reciprocity or they may reflect altruistic, nonmaterial interactions. The three authors mentioned above suggest that, to understand how microinsurers can attract and retain their clients, they have to know what shapes their clients' behavior in their specific operating context. The same reasoning applies to a microinsurer's decision to affiliate with *Social Re*.

Since *Social Re* will be piloted in the Philippines, this examination will be done with reference to that country and culture. The rest of this chapter will provide an overview of the social and institutional structure of Philippine rural and informal society and the attitudes toward solidarity, risk, and insurance that influence choices and help shape the role of microinsurance. This role is quite different from what could be conjured from classical economic theory on utility, as will be shown. This analysis leads to the conclusion that in the rural Philippines, the introduction of insurance and reinsurance hinges as much, perhaps more, on the structure of society than on the profile of risks and the existence of a market for insurance.

A BRIEF OVERVIEW OF PHILIPPINE SOCIAL HISTORY

Most Filipinos trace their roots to the Malay people; others are descendents of the Chinese, Indians, Arabs, Spaniards, and Americans. The location of the Philippines, an archipelago of more than 7,000 islands in Southeast Asia, explains some of these lineages. History, colonization, and cultural influences explain the rest. Seventy-six million people, scattered over half of the islands, live with great diversity in language (several dozens are known to be in use), in degree of development, and in prevalent habits. Cultural and political diversity was not always welcome, as attested by the country's history.

Precolonial Culture

Before the 16th century, the big islands of Luzon, Mindanao, and Samar were dotted with many independent villages, each a closed, self-contained political, socioeconomic, and ecological system. Each had its own way of regulating village life, mobilizing village resources, enforcing rules, and dispensing justice. Religion and mysticism largely determined village laws and norms. The system of governance varied, as did religions and beliefs.

Society at the village level was loosely stratified into three classes—the nobility, commoners, and *alipin* (household and farm help), with mobility across classes permitted. Despite some evidence of intervillage alliances and an awareness of commonality among the different ethnolinguistic groups, national consciousness and culture were absent.[2]

The Spanish Colonial Experience: Introduction of Central Institutions

The Spaniards, arriving in the middle of the 16th century, established central authority over a vast territory that had never before been bound together as one political entity. The Spanish system of governance, operating out of Manila, was designed to subdue the native inhabitants and maintain control over the territory through the combined interventions of administrative, military, and religious personnel. The Roman Catholic Church reinforced the legitimacy of the Spanish government and was equally influential in the natives' political-economic life. The Spanish governor-general was the undisputed chief executive, legislator, chief justice, and commander-in-chief of the Spanish armed forces over all the Philippine Islands. The territory was divided into geopolitical units, with regional new towns (centrally planned from Manila) serving as centers *(hamlets)* for indoctrination of the natives in the Christian religion and for administrative control. In the three centuries of Spanish rule, the people of Luzon and Visayas adapted their indigenous ways to the culture of their new colonial masters, sometimes viewed as "superior" and more "refined." A collective amnesia of precolonial cultures prevailed among the Philippine lowlanders. Villages (or submunicipal groupings) retained their Spanish appellation: *barangay(s)*.

The American Influence: Economic Forces Gain Political Power

When the Americans arrived in the late 19th century, they retained the key components of the Spanish organization across the country. The Americans established a bicameral legislature, modeled after their own system of democracy. The newly found democratic space allowed landed local elites to access political power, thus combining their political and economic strength into semifeudal structures.

Patronage Politics and New Entrants into the Political Space

Philippine political and economic elites drew their position largely from ownership of vast tracts of land their families had accumulated during the Spanish and American eras. Land ownership was concentrated in few hands, with 14 percent of all landholders owning 64 percent of cultivated lands (Putzel 1992). A reciprocal yet unequal patron-client relationship evolved between landlords and their tenants.[3] Tenants bore the risk of failed crops or damage from natural calamities (for example, typhoons). In the absence of any form of financial risk transfer, landlords were the only fallback to provide some protection and help. As a reciprocal measure of loyalty, tenants' debts of gratitude to landlords (like their other debts) were paid by the labor of tenants' sons in the landlords' fields and their daughters' service as domestics in the masters' households, for little or no pay.

To this day, the old power elites dominate national and provincial elections, based on regional representation and patronage politics. Local politics is gradually changing, as well-educated, local professionals acquire some power in the provinces, municipalities, and barangays through their personal authority or entrepreneurial activities.

SALIENT CULTURAL TRAITS

Anthropologists observed that, despite a large variety of ethnolinguistic origins, some features of Philippine beliefs and practices associated with community life are commonly shared.

Jocano (1990) points to the predominance of the kin group and the peer group as bases for collective consciousness. The kin group is composed of near and distant relatives who are known to an individual. It assists the individual or group in times of need, especially when the nuclear family cannot do so. Kin groups range from a few dozen to more than a hundred in a rural community.

Membership in a peer group, loosely organized among equals, enhances an individual's social prestige and acceptance in the community. From peer groups, individuals derive psychological and economic support outside the family and kin group. Peer groups range from three individuals to a few dozen.

Gambling has been identified as a popular practice, dating to pre-Hispanic times. Trimillos (1992) explains that current rural religious practices reflect Catholic practices attributable to the Spanish, mixed with singing, storytelling, and gambling typical of pre-Hispanic Southeast Asian traditions.

Kapwa Psychology and the Corresponding Behaviors

Interpersonal relationships among Filipinos are guided by the notion of the "shared inner self," the assumption that what is good for one person is also good for others and that, conversely, what is detrimental to one person is detrimental to others. This is known in Filipino (the national language) as *kapwa*. A person who is kapwa with another will not act or make any decision that would offend the other person's dignity because he appreciates the other person's being as completely as if it were an extension of his own self (Enriquez 1978). Kapwa may be practiced at varying levels of depths and modes of social interaction. The first five levels apply in relationships with individuals outside the kin or peer group and can be translated as meaning that the prescribed behavior should be sensitivity, conformity, and reciprocity.[4] More intimate relationships, especially those within the family, kin group, or peer group, would command a higher commitment to the welfare of the other.[5]

PERSPECTIVES ON ORGANIZATIONAL BEHAVIOR IN MICROINSURANCE UNITS

The description of the social structure in the rural Philippines invites a query on the powers at play when people are free to make their own choices about insurance, for example, regarding affiliation with microinsurers.

Weber's Bureaucratization Theory versus Social Capital

The description of the formal hierarchy leads to the conclusion that political power is vertical and top-down. The president heads the central government, which enjoys the strongest formal legitimacy, followed by the provincial government with a provincial governor at its head, down to the municipality level, and ending at the barangay level. Within this structure, order is maintained through formal rules (the interest groups alluded to above wield influence mainly by interpreting formal rules to accommodate sectarian interests). Society's goals are defined and achieved through specialization, formalization, and bureaucratization. Specialists, reporting upward, are assigned functions in an organization and are compensated for their contribution to the organizational objectives defined at the higher level. Most people who live at the low end of the hierarchy perceive this structure as remote from their reality and, in fact, it has not changed essentially since the Spanish period. The keen sense of distance and anonymity accompanying this hierarchical power structure at the grass-roots level translates into distrust of people higher up in this chain. Consequently, grass-roots populations often prefer to limit their interaction with authorities to encounters to obtain immediate and specific material aid instead of engaging in interactive and empowering involvement in decisions and priority setting. This structure, by and large, conforms to Weber's theory of bureaucratization (Silos 1991).

The formal top-down power structure does not deliver universal access to health care and has been unforthcoming in providing support to communities that tried to elaborate alternative solutions (Flavier, Soriano, and Nicolay, chapter 17, this volume). This state of affairs has added distance to a relationship between the informal and the formal sectors that has been characterized by mutual reserve and sometimes distrust. Bearing in mind the mounting empirical evidence that confidence, honest dialogue, even income distribution, social mobility, family relations, religion, and the like are indicators of economic growth, the distance between the informal and the formal sectors has more than ethnological significance (La Porta and others 1997, p. 5; Knack and Keefer 1997; Hjerppe 1998, p. 5; Rothstein 1998, p. 5; Temple and Johnson 1998; Hjerppe and Kajanoja 2000). Low trust can mean lower capacity to reverse the excluded population's unfavorable situation. This consequence of distrust can be reinforced, or abated, by trust within the community.

The few investigations into the internal dynamics of Philippine rural communities recognize that the glue binding people in these social networks and institutions is their acceptance of the prevailing social values and an attitude of trust (Albano 2000). Repeated face-to-face interactions increase mutual respect for group reputation, trust, and acceptance of norms of cooperation and mutual reciprocity. For instance, one microinsurer (Medical Mission Group Hospital and Health Services Cooperative) reported that the increased social cohesion allowed reductions in monitoring and enforcement costs. Another source reported that community-based health organizations generated high social capital—85 percent of their workers were volunteers—a resource contribution that allows these schemes to stretch their limited funds (chapter 17, this volume).

Trust and social capital have a direct impact not only on the degree of grass-roots social organization and operating costs but also on health status. A study from a remote region in Finland compared the health status of Finnish speakers and Swedish speakers. The two groups had the same health benefits from the formal system and were much alike in their classical demographic, social, and economic variables. But significant differences in variables describing social capital appeared to explain why the Swedish-speaking minority was healthier than the Finnish-speaking group (Hyyppä and Mäki 2000, p. 5). The conditional variable was trust, rather than a difference in economic or other quantifiable variable or in access to care. Thus, where affiliation is voluntary and highly influenced by trust, there would seem to be more reason to believe that health outcomes are linked to social capital. This conclusion provides further strong support for the hypothesis that microinsurers enjoying high social capital are more likely to achieve better results in enhancing both outreach and health outcomes in the excluded catchment population.

The Institute of Medicine (2001, p. 4-19) adds that the impact of social capital on health, as manifested in increased convenience to local services and facilities through united social action, and in supplying more direct social support, increases self-esteem and mutual respect. Even politically, policies that protect the individual's interests are followed in countries that have a strong collective philosophy.

If mutual reciprocity is an expression of social capital, might it be measured by the rate of membership retention? Committed participation in reciprocal arrangements would reduce defection on the grounds that a person has paid for a long time without receiving anything. Yet, all community schemes in the Philippines have large dropout rates. Such dropout rates suggest that Filipinos view membership as participation in a reciprocal arrangement in which gifts are exchanged. They do not view it as an insurance arrangement in which—in the long term—some lucky persons avoid risk and always pay without getting anything in return and some unlucky persons fall ill or sustain losses and repeatedly get more out than they put in. In fact, with the prospect of future repayments, members are more willing to pay than they would be without a return on their payments. Moreover, even if the time of repayment is unknown and the return gift is not of identical value to the original contribution, reciprocity would be considered balanced (Platteau 1997, pp. 767–78). Because of the informal nature of the arrangement, mutual reciprocity requires great trust, strengthened by intimate knowledge of community members, thus reducing the risks of free riding and adverse selection associated with information asymmetry. At the same time, the assumption cannot be rejected that these communities operate a solidarity scheme, founded on dissociation from the idea of risk pooling and possible income redistribution among the members—a transfer that will never be repaid. Members of such schemes in the Philippines reported satisfaction with health services and solidarity with the community as the two top reasons for retaining membership, suggesting that renewal was based on monetary and nonmonetary reasons simultaneously (chapter 17, this volume).

In light of this situation, is the underlying principle of insurance acceptable at all in the Philippine cultural context of kapwa? Kapwa may discourage individuals from acting only upon their personal utility but, in reality, can kapwa exist between one person who is repeatedly lucky and another who is consistently unlucky? Constant good or bad luck might be interpreted to signify supernatural interventions (which break down trust among peers) instead of being viewed simply as fluctuations, explained by normal statistical rules that apply equally to all members. The solution will depend on perceptions of the root cause of misfortune. Supernatural signals call for magical corrections, whereas statistical fluctuations call for measures to narrow distributions and spread the resultant cost among all players. To explore the approach to insurance further, the next section looks at the relevance of economic thinking to individual choice in this context.

Utility Theory versus Regret and Prospect Theory

The utility (or optimal choice) theory assumes that consumers make choices with the sole objective of maximizing gains. Insurance models based on this (prevalent) assumption view the estimated probability of encountering a contingency, and its average cost, as indicators of individual willingness to pay insurance premiums to remove the risk. This theory implies knowledge of the gain (that is, comparing the cost of the premium with the probability and cost of the risk), but is there sufficient proof that people in the rural Philippines have that knowledge? A different economic theory on utility, the regret theory, holds that people want to replicate good feelings and lessen feelings of regret. When deciding whether or not to buy insurance, people usually act at the beginning of a period but assess their choice at the end, based on the outcome. The pleasure or displeasure associated with a result therefore depends not only on the result itself but also on the alternatives. If, in retrospect, an individual appears to have made the right decision, it is associated with rejoicing, while the wrong decision is associated with feelings of regret (Loomes and Sugden 1982, p. 778). Shafir, Simonson, and Tversky (1993) take this argument a step further, by claiming that decisions are reached by focusing on reasons for a selection instead of on the economics of a problem. Hence, they conclude that, often, perceived utility will not be solely or even mainly the result of pure economic gain or loss.

In their prospect theory, Kahneman and Tversky (2000) suggest a descriptive, value-based analysis of reasons individuals behave differently from what utility theory predicts when making risky choices. They also try to explain why individuals' responses to variations of probability are not linear, as utility theory would predict. Kahneman and Tversky have shown that gains and losses cannot simply be translated into discrete expressions of assets or liabilities; perception of risk influences the way decisions are fashioned or framed; and the experienced utility (the actual experience of an outcome) is a major criterion for evaluating decisions about the intensity of anticipated pleasure or pain.

Within this same concept, health behavior theory, as presented by the Institute of Medicine (2001, p. 5-4), explains why people do not persist in performing activities that inhibit or identify an illness early on. The model illustrates the role of apparent vulnerability, an individual's awareness of risk of acquiring a certain condition and its gravity, and the extent to which an individual ascribes harmful costs when illness is established, in supplying the driving force to reduce or eliminate concerns. People's actions are influenced by their perceptions of what reduces a health hazard as well as by the likely harmful results of those actions.

Organizations, both formal and informal, play a role in shaping the social and physical conditions that influence people's choices. Their influence depends on individual "membership" as worker, patron, client, or patient. A health-conscious organizational culture would most probably implement rules and activities and focus on concerns that would encourage its members' well-being. Such endeavors would signify the organization's culture of health awareness (Institute of Medicine 2001 pp. 6-1–6-2).

Bearing in mind the attributes of Philippine society, particularly the predominant role of reciprocal interactions with peers and kin and the authority of village elites over external influences, social choice among rural Filipinos seems to be context dependent. Thus, for microinsurers, a scheme's acceptance will depend less on its objective characteristics than on whether village dignitaries promote it; whether it addresses locally recognizable problems (instead of introducing protection against unknown and unappreciated risks); and whether it offers reciprocity to all players instead of instituting a game of winners and losers. Under these circumstances, can informal risk-sharing and pooling arrangements function at all in the Philippines?

EVIDENCE FROM PHILIPPINE RURAL MICROINSURERS

To answer this question, the prevalent attitudes of several microinsurers were studied, through interviews of management, staff, and members; program document reviews; and on-site inspections of the project offices. The microinsurers visited include Bagong Silang Multi-Purpose Cooperative (BSMPC),[6] Angono Credit and Development Cooperative (ACDECO),[7] the Barangay Health Workers Aid Organization (BAHAO),[8] Medical Mission Group Hospital and Health Services Cooperative (MMG),[9] Peso-for-Health,[10] and ORT Health Plus Scheme (OHPS).[11]

The first item of interest was whether the microinsurers are run under informal or formal rules. As a short reminder, the traditional system bases compliance or controls on the application of implicit and customary rules for social relationships. In the Philippines, subjectivity, personalism,[12] familism,[13] and reciprocity are key themes that guide social relationships (Jocano 1990). When the microinsurance system leaves ambiguity or a policy gap, members intuitively assume that the customary conventions for social relationships are the default guidelines and behave accordingly. The ambiguity of customary conventions is often reduced as the organization writes down, or codifies, its conventions as formal policies to be enforced by the institution.

The limited field study suggests three prototypes for the way traditional risk-pooling systems and modern insurance systems are used in the installation of a microinsurance system:

- An organization implements the community's traditional solidarity and risk-pooling mechanisms. The scheme implemented within the context of the organization retains its traditional form, with limited written policies and relying on social conventions (for example, ACDECO).

- An organization implements microinsurance modeled after modern insurance systems by applying, from inception, the microinsurer's written systems, policies, and procedures (for example, BSMPC as originally conceptualized).

- Traditional systems of solidarity and risk sharing are applied within the microinsurance unit but with a conscious and progressive effort to codify the conventions. The microinsurance that evolves begins to resemble the impersonal and bureaucratic systems of the modern insurance system.

In microinsurance run by public authorities (both local government units and the National Health Insurance Program, NHIP), one problem is finding the right pitch to market the plan to targeted families. For instance, the government offered benefits to alleviate hardship among specific groups (for example, the elderly or indigents), but some families rejected these special privileges, partly because they did not want the "stigma" of being called old or being identified as the poorest in the community. In ACDECO, where the insurance program, run by informal rules, was labeled "the manager's," some members decided against participation because of the label and its possible implications in terms of formalization of the scheme's rules.

Microinsurers run by cooperatives have emphasized insurance principles (risk reduction through resource pooling, and the larger the pool the better). These microinsurers have also promoted a sense of ownership among their members. Since affiliation is voluntary, members were concerned about having to pay an additional contribution without the assurance of balanced reciprocity.

An interesting example was BSMPC. When marketed as formal insurance, the project was rejected, but the group reacted favorably when it was marketed as a form of "caring for each other" (*damayan*).[14]

Microinsurers such as the BSMPC and BAHAO use more personal dynamics in their operations. Thus, informal communication such as *pakiusapan* is routinely practiced.[15] Traditional microinsurers gained members' acceptance by emphasizing the principles of solidarity and sharing. In sociological terms, this is reminiscent of "Theory Y."[16] Groups that operate a microfinance institution have already accumulated similar experiences. For instance, a borrower who does not pay his or her debts on time receives bimonthly visits from a collector to trigger *hiya* (fear of losing face), thus forcing the debtor to pay without resort to legal procedures.

Several of the microinsurers studied (ACDECO, BSMPC, BAHAO), especially the member-managed schemes, have modified their policies, hence their norms, over the past 12 months. Viewed in terms of sociological and insurance theory discussed earlier, a slow but steady evolution seems to be occurring from balanced reciprocity, based on informality and members' sense of ownership through strong social capital, to formal insurance, with impersonal rules, an implicit notion of winners and losers, and therefore little or no accommodation for personal hardships.

Silos (2001, pp. 2–25) proposes another possible outcome based on the "emergent" theory of Asian organizations. He explains how Asian organizations have been able to install formal codified systems while maintaining traditional values as part of the organizational culture without sacrificing organizational effectiveness. He further explains how integrating values and formal systems within the organization enhances organizational performance. In this scenario, formal insurance systems can theoretically be applied without sacrificing social capital, sense of ownership, and the solidarity ethic within the microinsurance unit.

SPIRAL EVOLUTION OF MICROINSURERS

The microinsurer's norms and values (as expressed in written or unwritten policies) undergo processes of preservation, elimination, and innovation (table 19.1). The review of existing norms may be set in motion when questions arise about their continued relevance and responsiveness to members' needs. A norm that outlasts its usefulness becomes obsolete or irrelevant (ACDECO). But any conflict between new and old norms generates confusion and tension, which may disrupt the microinsurance system. Unless the microinsurer's leaders have appropriate insurance-management skills and knowledge, revision of the system may result in design flaws in the new norms and policies (MMG). However, if members perceive the new norms as an extension of the existing norms and an expression of existing values, the new norms may be easily integrated into the system (BSMPC). Members' rejection of newly announced norms may result in dysfunctional behavior or withdrawal from active participation in the scheme

TABLE 19.1 Microinsurers' Spiral Learning Process

Step	Process	Gains	Risks
1. Current norm	Updating, stabilization	Stabilization, finding equilibrium, clarity for members	Obsolescence
2. Challenge of old	Reviewing existing norms vis-à-vis emerging local realities and member needs	Openness to new relevance	Political tension
3. Revision of norms	Reengineering of microinsurer design, systems, policies, and norms	Acquisition of new learning, skills, sophistication	Design flaws, incompatibility, new policy gaps
4. Communication and implementation of new norm	Decision point for members —recommitment	Learning for members as well as improved system performance	Rejection

(BAHAO). The new norms, if accepted, become the basis for behavior, and members recommit and conform to them.

SECTORAL CULTURES AND RISK

The microinsurers studied have retained some characteristics that can be traced to their origin as state, business, or civil society organizations (respectively, Peso-for-Health, ACDECO, and OHPS). Both Peso-for-Health and BAHAO were state-launched free programs that eventually started to collect contributions to supplement tax financing. Peso-for-Health used the provincial health office as its extended management system, thus giving the scheme a subsidy covering most or all of its administrative cost. OHPS was started by a nongovernmental organization (NGO) that was financed through grants and technical assistance from foreign donors but that had to resort to various revenue-generating schemes because of grant insufficiency. ACDECO is primarily a business endeavor, owned by its 2,500 members. Although conscious about break-even and cost recoveries, its main concern remains its members' welfare.

The sectoral distinction seems to be losing some of its edge in the rural Philippines. With low effective demand for privately provided services, businesses tend to engage in social causes; low revenues through taxation push government agencies to charge user fees; and drying up of donations for NGOs have accelerated entrepreneurial ventures of civil society organizations (Alampay 1999).

STAKEHOLDER INTEREST AND RISK

Microinsurers can also be looked at according to their corporate character. Three distinct microinsurance options are present in the rural Philippines: consumer-driven (ACDECO, BSMPC), provider-driven (MMG), and fund manager–driven (Peso-for-Health). The three models differ in the degree of voice the members can exercise and their impact on decisions.

Consumer-driven microinsurers give priority to solidarity and members' welfare. Unlike other schemes where members pay the projected premium, BSMPC collects contributions only for hospitalization. Members agree on the contribution amount and the other fund guidelines. All members seem comfortable with this form of reciprocity, which is at odds with the notion of insurance but perfectly in line with the balanced-reciprocity theory. The practical difference between these two economic theories would depend on the frequency of risk events that call for contributions under the reciprocity model. The higher the frequency, the more similar is the outcome of applying one or the other.

Consumer-driven microinsurers that have evolved from other economic activities (for example, microfinance) have experience with profitability as a key to sustainability. ACDECO is a good example of a group whose common denominator is its savings and lending operations. Its efficient and sophisticated financial services have influenced its approach to operating a microinsurance unit. The other aspect of multifunctional schemes is that the balanced reciprocity of participating in microinsurance may be perceived as being gained through benefits from other services that provide protection against other risks. Alternatively, revenues from other operations may be used to subsidize social services (for example, ACDECO), or a limited and less costly activity that can reduce health risk exposure (for example, health educational programs run by BAHAO resulted in improved health behaviors by members, which reduced health expenditures).

MMG, a cooperative of health service providers, is a provider-driven microinsurer. Its members consider MMG a third party and do not feel a sense of ownership over the funds or a sense of solidarity with other insureds. The dominant logic for enrolling in a microinsurance scheme is to derive maximum utility from its members' premium payments.

Peso-for-Health has been considered fund manager–driven, since its managers have the authority to decide on the rules of the scheme. (Since it operates out of a hospital, however, it could be viewed as a provider-driven scheme.) Conceived as a way of enhancing outreach as well as income from a very poor population, this project generated new income for the hospital and, for clients, a more attractive payment scheme than user fees. The scheme can offer benefits at extremely low cost (5 or 10 pesos per family per month), partly because hospital personnel handle the plan's administration, and the hospital absorbs the full cost.

Figure 19.1 depicts the different levels of consciousness of the individual (top half) and of the group (bottom half). The sociocultural realm on the left and the economic realm on the right reflect the scale of group consciousness as sociocultural needs and economic needs are addressed. The collective here is the kin group or peer group, less formalized than an organization.

The heavy line delimiting the organizational and supraorganizational levels reflects the psychological barrier that Philippine organizations have to transcend to pursue interorganizational (supraorganizational) interests collectively. This supraorganizational level is theoretically especially difficult to attain because of the small-scale kin and peer-group consciousness that predominate in Philippine social relationships.

In the figure, BSMPC and ACDECO operate in most quadrants because they are member-driven: their members are conscious of organizational interests and pursue them both as members and as an organization. ACDECO is in the supraorganizational level (lower left quadrant), because it has begun to engage in supraorganizational pursuits through a national confederation of cooperatives.

Member-driven BAHAO's profile is similar to BSMPC's and ACDECO's but closer to the collective level because it has not yet developed the more sophisticated organizational system.

The members in Peso-for-Health and OHPS function mainly as individual clients and consumers, hence their location in the individual level in Quadrant B. Logic or participation in these two schemes closely approximates that described

FIGURE 19.1   Stages and Alternatives in Development of Consciousness in Microinsurance Units

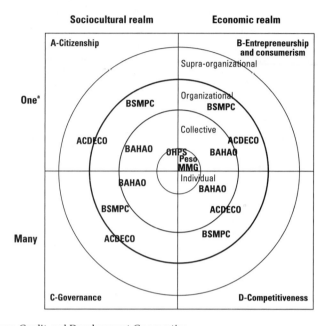

ACDECO Angono Credit and Development Cooperative.
BAHAO Barangay Health Workers Aid Organization.
BSMPC Bagong Silang Multi-Purpose Cooperative.
MMG Medical Mission Group Hospital and Health Services Cooperative.
OHPS ORT Health Plus Scheme.
Peso Peso-for-Health.
a. *One* person would relate as "I," as distinct from more than one person *(many)*, which could be "we" or "they."
Source: Adapted from K. Wilber 2000.

by utility theory. MMG is also in this quadrant because its large membership (32,000 individuals) dilutes the individual sense of solidarity and ownership.

CONCLUSIONS

The social and institutional structure of Philippine rural and informal society explains why a single-insurer model is impractical without central government funding for universal access to health care. In the absence of such top-down engagement, single communities at the barangay and subbarangay level use such traditional mechanisms for dealing with risk as kapwa and damayan, based on balanced reciprocity.

The small group size, a handicap in terms of insurance calculations, is an asset in terms of social capital. Repeated social interactions among group members reduce classical market failures, such as free riding and moral hazard, linked to insurer asymmetric information. Small size also increases trust among group members who know each other, a proven asset for improving both health outcomes and scheme management efficiency.

In deciding whether or not to join a microinsurance scheme, individuals in the rural Philippines are likely to be influenced by the views of the group, their own past exposure to risk (rather than abstract risk assessment), and their expectation of reciprocity in return for payment of the contribution. This fundamental attitude toward risk is enhanced by traditional cultural traits such as kapwa. Neither the microinsurer's decisionmaking style (member-driven, provider-driven, or fund manager–driven), nor its ownership (public, NGO, or private) seems to affect these criteria significantly. Nor is there any evidence to support the assumption that optimal or rational choice theory can explain an individual's decision to affiliate and retain membership in a microinsurance scheme. Individuals cannot exercise informed choice without knowing their risk probabilities or their expected cost. At the same time, the prevalence of betting and gambling suggests that people play winner-loser games when they know the cost of a loss in advance and can afford it, even when they do not know the probability. This social custom suggests that if the cost of the insurance premium is perceived as affordable and the risk is better defined, people can be persuaded to buy insurance.

Members are more likely to join a microinsurance scheme if they can participate in other economic activities within the same group. The availability of multiple activities increases the likelihood that a member will obtain the desired return (reciprocity) for contributions paid. People are also more likely to join if their past experience with risk has been negative.

In the process of changing social attitudes to accommodate insurance activity, the roles of group consensus and the village elite are decisive. Communities that have had experience with microfinance give more attention to solvency, profitability, efficiency, and good management than do communities unfamiliar with these ideas. The rules underlying risk transfer are more difficult to modify, however, and in their redesign will have to accommodate mechanisms favoring reciprocation. One such option might be to link the introduction of *Social Re* with benefit enhancement, offering benefits with high externalities but significant short-term effects. Such a policy can also create acceptance by discounting the reinsurer's premium cost.

Last, there is no evidence that reinsurance would be harder to introduce than first-line insurance. Since the prime motivation is group influence and reciprocity rather than individual risk avoidance, the reinsurance facility could be introduced by targeting communities that have experience with financial accounting and mediation (mainly through functioning microfinance institutions). Such communities will have developed both a concern for profitability and modalities for cross-subsidization across their different economic activities (for example, by subsidizing health insurance premiums from earnings on their savings).

NOTES

1. *Social Re* is the name of the first pilot reinsurance operation for community-financed health schemes. Part 4 of this book provides more details on the preparations for such a pilot and the conditions under which it could be operated.

2. Prior to the Spanish colonization, no predominant cultural group had emerged in the Philippines as the political and economic elite. In this, the Philippines was unlike its Asian neighbors, Imperial China, Thailand (the Chakri dynasty), or Indonesia (the Sri Vijaya and Madjapahit empires).

3. Some Western writers have described the dynamics of rural politics by reference to the "cacique politics" framework of analysis in the South American countries (McCoy and de Jesus 1998).

4. Transaction/civility *(pakikitungo);* interaction with *(pakikisalamuha);* joining/participation with *(pakikilahok);* in conformity with/in accord with *(pakikibagay);* and being/going along with *(pakikisama).*

5. Being one with *(pakikiisa);* getting involved *(pakikisangkot);* being in rapport/understanding/acceptance of *(pakikipagpalagayan/pakikipagpalagayang-loob).*

6. BSMPC is a 40-member farmers' cooperative founded in 1996. It purchases farm inputs in bulk and lends them to its members. Its microinsurance unit was started in 1999 and is based in Nueva Ecija.

7. ACDECO is a community-based cooperative founded in 1966. Its microinsurance unit was started in 1988 and now has 2,500 members. Its activities include lending and deposit taking and running other coop enterprises such as a printing press, a grocery, and a bottled-water store. It is located in Rizal Province.

8. BAHAO is a 100-member association of village health workers, mostly women, organized in 1998. Besides its microinsurance activities, it runs income-generating projects such as medicinal soap-making and iodized salt production. It is located in Cavite Province.

9. MMG, a cooperative of health professionals, runs a coop-owned hospital and a coop-microinsurance unit. Since its founding in 1991, it has established more than a dozen branches all over the country. MMG started its microinsurance unit in 1991, which by 2001 had some 32,000 members. MMG is located in Davao City.

10. Peso for Health is a government-initiated program attached to the district hospital. Its microinsurance unit, located in Negros Oriental Province, has some 3,000 members.

11. OHPS, an NGO-driven microinsurance unit, started in 1990 with 6,250 members. OHPS, located in La Union Province, also runs early child development programs.

12. *Personalism* is an individual's special concern for the welfare of another.

13. *Familism* is the habit of emphasizing the interests of the family or kin group.

14. Damayan also refers to a traditional solidarity mechanism where community members contribute cash to a deceased neighbor's surviving dependents.

15. *Pakiusapan* means talking issues over discretely and personally before resorting to coercion or litigation.

16. Douglas McGregor (1960) provides two sets of sociological assumptions underlying rulemaking at work: *Theory X* presents people/workers as lazy, relatively unintelligent, and prone to avoiding work if they can. Under those assumptions, managers must install rigid control systems and use rewards, punishments, and coercion to meet productivity targets. *Theory Y* presupposes that workers naturally enjoy work and, if given an opportunity, they will be productive, since doing their jobs well gives them a sense of fulfillment. The manager's role in this scenario is to provide an environment that fosters cooperation and nurtures workers' enthusiasm. Insurance schemes often assume Theory X and thus use control mechanisms, incentives, and disincentives to reduce moral hazard and adverse selection.

REFERENCES

Alampay, E. 1999. *Organizations in Development: The Changing Nature of Service Provision in the Philippines*. ISS Working Paper Series No. 299.

Albano, J. 2000. "Social Capital and Health." *Conjuncture* 12(2):7–9.

Dror, D. 2001. "Reinsurance of Health Insurance for the Informal Sector." *Bulletin of the World Health Organization* 79(7):672–78.

Dror, D., and G. Duru. 2000. "Financing Micro-Insurance: Perspective and Prospective." Keynote address at Seventh International Conference on System Science in Health Care, organized by ISSCHC and Semmelweis University, Budapest, May 29–June 2, 2000. In A. Javor, W. van Eimeren, and G. Duru, eds., *International Society for System Science in Health Care, Proceedings*. Vol. 1. Budapest: ISSCHC, 2000.

Dror, D., and C. Jacquier. 1999. "Micro-insurance: Extending Health Insurance to the Excluded." *International Social Security Review* 52(1):71–97.

Enriquez, V. 1978. "From Colonial Liberation Psychology." *Philippine Social Science and Humanities Review* 42(1–4):73–95.

Herrnstein, R. 1997. "Rational Choice Theory: Necessary but Not Sufficient." Chapter 11 in H. Rachlin and D. Laibson, eds., *The Matching Law: Papers in Psychology and Economics*. Cambridge, Mass.: Harvard University Press.

Hjerppe, R. 1998. Cited in R. Hjerppe and J. Kajanoja, "Social Capital: The Missing Link in the Performance Measurement." Paper prepared for delivery at the Year 2000 International Research Conference on Social Security, September 25–27, 2000, Helsinki.

Hjerppe, R., and J. Kajanoja. 2000. "Social Capital: The Missing Link in the Performance Measurement." Paper prepared for delivery at the Year 2000 International Research Conference on Social Security, September 25–27, 2000, Helsinki.

Hyyppä, M., and Juhani Mäki. 2000. Cited in R. Hjerppe and J. Kajanoja, "Social Capital: The Missing Link in the Performance Measurement." Paper prepared for delivery at the Year 2000 International Research Conference on Social Security, September 25–27, 2000, Helsinki.

Institute of Medicine, Committee on Health and Behavior Research, Practice, and Policy, Board on Neuroscience and Behavioral Health. 2001. *Health and Behavior: The Interplay of Biological, Behavioral, and Societal Influences.* National Academy of Sciences. Washington, D.C.: National Academy Press.

Jocano, F. 1990. *Management by Culture: Fine-tuning Management to Filipino Culture.* Manila: Punlad Research House.

Kahneman, D., and A. Tversky, eds. 2000. *Choices, Values, and Frames.* Cambridge: Cambridge University Press.

Knack, S., and P. Keefer. 1997. "Does Social Capital Have an Economic Payoff? A Cross-Country Investigation." *Quarterly Journal of Economics* 112(4):1251–88.

La Porta, R., F. Lopez-De Silanes, A. Shleifer, and R. Vishny. 1997. "Trust in Large Organizations." *American Economic Review* 87(2):333–38. Cited in R. Hjerppe and J. Kajanoja, "Social Capital: The Missing Link in the Performance Measurement." Paper prepared for delivery at the Year 2000 International Research Conference on Social Security, September 25–27, 2000, Helsinki.

Loomes, G., and R. Sugden. 1982. "Regret Theory: An Alternative Theory of Rational Choice Under Uncertainty." *Economic Journal* 368:805–24. Quoted in J-P. Platteau. 1997. "Mutual Insurance as an Elusive Concept in Traditional Rural Communities." *Journal of Development Studies* 33(6):764–96.

McCoy, Alfred, and Ed de Jesus, eds. 1998. *Philippine Social History.* Manila: Ateneo de Manila University Press.

McGregor, D. 1960. *The Human Side of Enterprise.* New York: McGraw-Hill.

Platteau, J-P. 1997. "Mutual Insurance as an Elusive Concept in Traditional Rural Communities." *Journal of Development Studies* 33(6):764–96.

Putzel, J. 1992. *A Captive Land: The Politics of Agrarian Reform in the Philippines.* Manila: Ateneo de Manila University Press.

Rothstein, B. 1998 (in Finnish). Cited in R. Hjerppe and J. Kajanoja, "Social Capital: The Missing Link in the Performance Measurement." Paper prepared for delivery at the Year 2000 International Research Conference on Social Security, September 25–27, 2000, Helsinki.

Shafir, E., I. Simonson, and A. Tversky. 1993. "Reason-Based Choice." *Cognition* 49:11–36.

Silos, L. 1991. *Oikos: The Two Faces of Organization.* Makati, the Philippines: Asian Institute of Management.

_____. 2001. *The Asian Organization.* Makati, the Philippines: Asian Institute of Management.

Temple, J., and P. Johnson. 1998. "Social Capability and Economic Growth." *Quarterly Journal of Economics* 113(3):965–90.

Tracy, P., and M. Tracy. 2000: "A Conceptual Framework of Social Capital and Civil Society: The Re-emergence of John Dewey." Paper prepared for delivery at the Year 2000 International Research Conference on Social Security, Helsinki, September 25–27, 2000.

Trimillos, R. 1992. "The Lenten Practice of Pasyon as Southeast Asian Theater—A Structural Analysis of Performance, Practice and Protocol." School for Hawaiian, Asian and Pacific Studies, University of Hawaii, Honolulu. http://wuarchive.wustl.edu/doc/coombspapers/coombsarchives/political-and-social-change/philippine-studies/confr-1992/abstr-poetry-epic-tradition.tx

Wilber, K. 2000. *Integral Psychology.* Boston, Mass.: Shambahala Publications.

CHAPTER 20

Structuring Demand and Supply in Community Health in Philippine Insurance

Avi Kupferman and Aviva Ron

M ost of this chapter comes from recent, first-hand experience setting up community health insurance schemes in developing countries. The experience encompasses feasibility studies, design, implementation, and monitoring over a lengthy period as well as adaptation of the core design to the needs of new communities. The most recent experience relates to the ORT Health Plus Scheme (OHPS), developed in the Philippines since 1994 by the ORT (Ron and Kupferman 1996; Flavier, Soriano, and Nicolay, chapter 17, this volume).

Before attempting to evaluate the scope of reinsurance in developing countries, we have to define the parameters for community health insurance schemes or microinsurance. Chapter 2 of this book covers the overall concept of microinsurance, but several areas should be stressed. First, the context covered is social insurance, in which financial sustainability is a goal but not the major criterion for success. The real test of community health insurance schemes is in their ability to bring their members sustained access to health care, to protect them against the hazards of health expenditure, and ultimately to improve their health. Many of these schemes required external funds and technical assistance for their initial development, as noted in the literature (Bennett, Creese and Monasch 1998; van Ginneken 1999). Their success should therefore also be reflected in their weaning from outside assistance, both financial and administrative.

A second area needing clarification, and related to the viability of a scheme, is the ability to accumulate reserve funds. Like any other scheme involving the collection and holding of money for largely unpredictable contingencies, the ability to earn interest on surplus funds may become overly attractive. In nonprofit community health insurance schemes, the ability to extend benefits and coverage is considered more important than the interest a fund can earn on reserves derived from any surplus of revenues over the expenditures.

Third, the beneficiary populations of such schemes now are mainly low-income groups in urban and rural areas. These populations typically work in the

The authors acknowledge, with thanks, helpful comments on a draft of this chapter from Guido Carrin, Health Economist, World Health Organization, Geneva, and Dyna Arhin, Lecturer, London School of Hygiene and Tropical Health.

informal labor sector or are self-employed workers, excluded from social security schemes. Their incomes may be low and unstable, but they generally do not perceive themselves as indigent nor do they want to seek health care as charity patients with the attached stigma.

The fourth area needing clarification concerns ways of measuring coverage and compliance, itself important in any contributory social protection scheme. As noted in the literature, the coverage of community health insurance schemes is generally low (van Ginneken 1999; Carrin, Desmet, and Basaza 2001, pp. 125–49). However, coverage has to be measured in the context of the target population, not the population at large. Community health insurance schemes are usually voluntary unless the organization or cooperative operating the schemes requires membership as a condition of affiliation. To measure coverage, both actual numerator and target denominator have to be defined. In some schemes, the numerator may be the number of registered "members"—individuals or households, without listing every family member or household dependent. This would reduce the proportion of coverage. Other schemes may record all registered members at any time, giving little attention to their current entitlement in terms of continued and current payment of contributions.

On the denominator side in measuring health insurance coverage, there is a tendency to count the entire population. The appropriate denominator would be the target population covered by the organization. To define the total eligible population, it has to be known whether health insurance coverage is extended only to "members" of the sponsoring organization or whether it is open to other groups. If a health care provider operates the scheme, it may be open to the entire population in a feasible catchment area. For these reasons, the percentage of coverage is appropriate only when both numerator and denominator are defined or, as an alternative, follow the growth trends in absolute numbers over time.

To summarize, the parameters can be briefly termed the real goals of community health insurance, the ability to extend benefits and coverage rather than accumulate reserves, the dignity of the beneficiary population, and the appropriate measurement of scheme growth.

Structuring demand and supply is the terminology used from here on. It is the term used in this book to describe the process of identifying and prioritizing needs for community health insurance or microinsurance units. The process of structuring demand and supply is linked to several factors, each with implications for both financial and operational viability and health outcomes.

ENVIRONMENT CONDUCIVE TO MICROINSURANCE DEVELOPMENT

Over the last two decades of the 20th century, most governments cut spending on social services and stopped delivering health care free of charge at point of use to all but their poorest citizens.

Limited Government Resources

Without external funding, free health care is limited to what governments can afford from their own resources. The amount and scope of free care may also be determined by governments' ability to mobilize external resources for health services. However, even when up to 80 percent of total spending on health care comes from external sources, the range of services included as essential care may be limited. Personal health care may be limited to preventive services such as immunization and basic maternal and child health care covering only vulnerable periods in the life cycle. Preventive health services required for public health may become seriously underfunded (for example, safe food and water, and sanitation). In parallel, public health facilities show signs of marked deterioration in infrastructure and capacity to deal with the usual burden of health care, let alone additional demands caused by disasters or the morbidity changes linked to demographic shifts. Poor planning and basic inefficiency may cause some waste in the public system, but rigid systems of resource allocation often do facilitate the shifting of resources to areas of greatest need.

This reduction in government capacity to deliver health care is often accompanied by dissatisfaction among public health workers with very low and sometimes irregular remuneration as well as little hope of improvement in either pay or working conditions. Since these health workers are civil servants, they justifiably perceive that better regular remuneration can come about only through major change in civil service conditions and therefore appreciate the advantages and disadvantages of such reform. Even major health care reforms have done little to improve salaried health workers' remuneration. Seeing little hope of better incomes through their public jobs in the short term, health workers may try to engage in private practice, often at the expense of their government job working hours. When possibilities for private practice are limited, they are more likely to seek additional income by requesting "under-the-table" payments from patients.

Repercussions of Health Care Reform

Some components of health care reform in developing countries have stimulated interest in social health insurance in general, and microinsurance in particular. These components are decentralization, transfer of financial autonomy to public health providers, and privatization of health care.

Decentralization. In large countries that spend little on health care, decentralization has exacerbated inadequate public health funding in relatively poor and economically underdeveloped provinces. In some countries, decentralization may also have been implemented without adequate preparation for the administrative and financial tasks involved in a decentralized health system.

Transfer of financial autonomy. The transfer of financial autonomy to public health care providers may have disrupted the balance between the available free-of-charge public health care and the low-income population with low utilization patterns and perhaps low expectations of public health care. Public providers' new pressures to acquire revenue cause this disruption. They soon realize that generating demand among people poorly informed about health care is the simplest and fastest way to prosper. Out-of-pocket user charges quickly shift from nominal registration fees to substantial charges for a broader range of services. Weaknesses in the decentralization process, combined with increasing user charges linked to public provider financial autonomy, can rapidly put an unbearable load on household health expenditure.

Some exemptions from user chargers may be arranged for poor, disadvantaged, and vulnerable individuals. But the exemptions do not always work well, particularly in poor areas, as decentralized funding may also mean that the mechanisms for distributing funds and grant-justified exemptions are not well developed or bound by legislation. User charges, as well as exemption mechanisms, are especially problematic in remote rural areas where the limited availability of both public and private resources leads to difficulties in understanding and accepting such new measures. People are reluctant to pay for services when they do not see any improvement in quality and supply. Exemption mechanisms, particularly those requiring some form of means testing, may not be well accepted in small communities (Arhin 1995).

Apart from the economic burden, user charges may also change health care–seeking behavior. Out-of-pocket user charges at the time of illness, when earnings may be reduced, can lead to irrational behavior such as delays in seeking care, poor decisions about which family member should have priority, and what services to purchase beyond the initial consultation with a doctor or nurse (Ron 1999).

Gaps in Social Protection

The extent of social protection in a country's health care will be a crucial factor in this scenario. The development of social health insurance, as part of a broad social security system or as a separate program for health care, is covered by Preker, Langenbrunner, and Jakab in chapter 1 of this book. Although universal health insurance coverage may be a stated goal of health care and social security reforms, it is usually implemented in stages, first covering salaried workers in large and medium-size enterprises, and then slowly extended to smaller enterprises. In many developing countries, the vast majority of the population will not fit into those groups, even when the schemes cover both public and private salaried employees and when family members or dependents are included as beneficiaries. Most of these people, particularly those with the lowest incomes, are informal-sector workers and their dependents.

For short-term social security benefits such as health insurance, few countries have enabled voluntary affiliation for the self-employed and informal sectors or even for salaried workers' dependents in countries where only individual workers are covered (Ron, Carrin, and Tien 1998). Most social security systems allow voluntary affiliation only for the full benefit package—including pension, disability, and other scheme benefits. Relatively new social security systems usually plead weak administrative capacity to explain this attitude. Admittedly, it is very difficult for fledgling social security systems to take on individuals with unstable incomes for a single benefit. Not only is the health care benefit the one most frequently used, but it is also complex in terms of the scope of benefits covered. Making a case for including these nonsalaried workers is also difficult, when most of them cannot pay the full contribution costs, which cannot be shared with employers.

Erosion of Traditional Support Systems

Savings and support from the community at large used to help families deal with the dual burden of sickness and its financial costs.

Savings. Once well rooted in the cultures of many developing countries, the concept of saving for contingencies such as health care for family members has eroded. Today, the capacity to save is minimal among the poor. For low- and middle-income earners, the rationale for saving has also changed. The current concept of savings focuses on small and slow saving for desired events. Examples are education for children, assets that may increase family income, or assets such as housing or appliances that will improve family comfort. In this approach, there is a large and usually informed element of choice regarding the product, time, and amount of savings needed. If hard-earned savings are used for health care, consumers have little choice regarding product and timing and little control over the amount charged. The patient and family are usually at a disadvantage regarding knowledge to determine the appropriateness of the services prescribed. Nor is there any guarantee of care quality or outcome. Ill health is not a desired event, and the fairness of relying on a population's past saving practices can indeed be questioned.

Solidarity issues. In parallel with the change in the concept of savings, radical shifts may have occurred in the ways different societies in developing countries deal with the need for financial or other support in times of ill health and personal crises. Independence from colonial rule or cultural revolutions often reduced the activities of charitable institutions and nongovernmental organizations (NGOs) providing health care, if they did not entirely eliminate the institutions themselves. Organizations now returning usually operate as private for-profit providers, with limited capacity to serve the indigent as "charity cases."

That leaves the majority of the population to confront new and increasing user chargers, underfunded public health systems, generally unsympathetic health workers, and scant attention from political sources. The acceptance of user fees is particularly problematic for the elderly, who come into old age with low-income capacity and, in most developing countries, the double burden of both acute communicable diseases and chronic diseases (Ron 1998). Despite mounting concern about poverty reduction from the international community and from national governments, the extent to which the financial burden for health care pushes families and individuals below the poverty line is not yet fully understood.

Other factors. The main point here is that it is insufficient to analyze the growth, or lack of growth, of social health insurance at the national or community level within the context of the core functions of health systems. Poor resource allocation and inefficient purchasing arrangements and service delivery also narrow all population sectors' access to health care. Also required is an understanding of the reasons social safety nets have not been developed prior to or in parallel with substantial health care reforms. The term "social safety net" covers both contributory social protection and social assistance (Chu and Gupta 1998a, pp. 7–23). If no safety nets are in place or their coverage is not extended through legislation and guarantees of government funds, there is a hole in social protection. Community health insurance schemes spring up in this void.

Filling the gap. Who takes the initiative to create health care and other community social-protection schemes? This is the next issue related to the gap in social protection. Microinsurance implies a contributory mechanism for the regularly scheduled accumulation of personal savings—instead of sporadic deposits when there is spare cash. Apart from solidarity issues among community members, the contributory initiative first has to be justified. The participants, whether residents of specific areas or members of a defined group, need to see clear advantages in assuming direct financial responsibility for their own health care. Most participants will be used to the government's bearing this responsibility and will not fully understand why government assistance has been so drastically curtailed as to place a heavy financial burden on them at the time of illness. If local community members contribute regularly to create a stable financing mechanism, they can legitimately expect government to recognize their efforts as a form of cost sharing. Government would then be expected to sustain at least its current level of funding and continue to guarantee and improve public health services delivery as well as personal health care for the most vulnerable individuals.

The environment described above chiefly reflects failures in governments' commitment to provide basic social services and in mechanisms for doing so. To repair the gaps in social protection, government has to play an active role in promoting community health care financing initiatives that can provide immediate solutions and ultimately form part of a national network to ensure universal coverage. However, before government can take this role, the initial development of community schemes is likely to come from the people, mainly through initiatives of civil society organizations and through voluntary mechanisms. Demand for such schemes is connected not only with the existence and strength of civil society organizations and their interest in obtaining basic social services through self-reliance but also with the potential consumers' basic characteristics (Amalric 2001).

DEMAND ISSUES LINKED TO THE TARGET POPULATION

Community or microinsurance schemes meet the needs of any population excluded from coverage or seeking alternatives when social insurance schemes for health care have not been developed at all. Such schemes are therefore not limited to the informal sector, but it is likely to constitute most of the target population. Who, then, and where are these prospective microinsurance subscribers?

Prospective Microinsurance Subscribers

The informal sector includes both economically active and economically inactive individuals and their dependents.

Economically active. The economically active include workers in agriculture, forestry, and fishing who may be engaged in both the primary and secondary aspects of their occupations as self-employed, family, or short-term contract workers without formal employer-employee relationships. Some occupations such as construction work are seasonal or casual work linked to market demand over which workers have little influence. Then there are market vendors, workers in small enterprises, and service providers such as tailors and barbers. Some occupational markets are more susceptible than others to repercussions from recession, or inflation. Some individuals may receive regular salaries as workers in small enterprises or households. All these workers have one thing in common: They are not registered as salaried workers—nor can they register as self-employed workers—under any social security scheme.

Despite two decades of economic growth, the informal sector may still be expanding instead of contracting. Transition economies moving from centrally planned to market economies are likely to have growing numbers of informal-sector workers as state enterprises close or are streamlined toward privatization (Chu and Gupta 1998b, pp. 94–113). Such economies may have incomplete registration of new and small private enterprises and their workers, particularly when many of them are family members. In the process, many workers may lose their previous social security arrangements. The globalization process also contributes to the growing number of unprotected workers by increasing the movement of labor between countries. The current lack of social protection for migrant workers contrasts sharply with past experience in Western Europe (Ron 1986). But it also reflects the preference of many migrant workers from developing countries for having employment, any employment, over social protection. Labor patterns are also changing in the host countries, where a growing proportion of the national labor force is willing to accept short-term contractual employment without social security benefits.

Economically inactive. Economically inactive individuals may make up a larger part of the target population than estimated. Without well-established national social security mechanisms to replace income for the old and disabled, more and more retired workers and surviving spouses are likely to join the ranks of the self-employed while also holding salaried positions. Although not every retiree fits the description of "very poor," some are still strapped for cash. They may own physical assets such as the house they live in, but using savings or cash from the sale of nonessential assets for their own health care may conflict with their desires to leave their children an inheritance.

Cultural and Societal Factors

Most of the target population described, including both active and retired workers, is generally not organized through labor or professional organizations. However, in many countries these populations may have well-developed civil society organizations or the community itself may be cohesive.

Civil society organizations. Civil society organizations may be strong grass-roots or community associations and cooperatives, based on various types of affiliation such as religion, occupation, shared interests or personal characteristics, or residence within defined neighborhoods. A starting point for creating microinsurance is therefore identifying such organizations and learning about their histories, structures, and affiliations with other civil society organizations and local governments. It is also essential to know their interest in and potential for meeting such a scheme's administrative requirements. "Interest" includes negative or conflicting motivations as in the case of a microcredit cooperative that sees a community health insurance fund as a source of short-term money for earning dividends.

The absence of community organizations does not rule out the creation of microinsurance for local populations. If the new microinsurer cannot handle its own administration, those functions can be taken on by, for example, a health care provider (Moens 1990). In that case, the civil society organization could facilitate community or membership participation in the microinsurance. Community identity through such organizations and local leadership is needed to develop microinsurers with a clear sense of ownership.

Identifying civil society organizations within a community is relatively easy, but their cultural and societal characteristics must also be recognized and understood. These factors will not necessarily prevent the establishment of a microinsurance unit, but understanding them will help in dealing with any obstacle that arises and might also allow any opposition to be redirected toward success. Relevant cultural and societal factors include community solidarity, familiarity with the insurance concept, approach to illness, and attitude toward Western medicine.

Community solidarity. The first factor concerns the nature and extent of a community's solidarity mechanisms. Limited access to health care is usually not the community's only disadvantage, and its residents may have established effective ways of dealing with crises requiring immediate cash. The more positive mechanisms are family support, spread among large clans instead of the small nuclear family. The limitations of this approach become apparent as family size decreases and health care costs increase. This point can be used to promote social insurance.

If solidarity mechanisms are based on deep-rooted religions and traditions with wide community support, reasons for changing may be less apparent and acceptable to the community. Community charitable institutions themselves may want to retain their status as protectors of the poor (Ron 1999). Such past practice may have created a "dole-out" mentality and the perception, among the poorest members of the population, that help will come if they wait long enough or if the illness is serious enough. Although the dole-out factor may not be widespread, it is more intractable than cultural solidarity mechanisms that can be used as a point of departure in creating microinsurance.

Unfamiliarity with the insurance concept. People may not be familiar with the concept of insurance against an uncertainty. This factor is especially likely in rural populations engaged in nonmechanized occupations, where insurance for motorized vehicles or appliances is uncommon. At best, households may be willing to prepay for goods or services but may not renew the payment if they obtained no benefits in the initial period of coverage. Some members will drop out for this reason but quickly request reentry when faced with bills for acute care. Renewing membership under such conditions may be seen as adverse selection to some extent. In the scheme's early development, this phenomenon should be expected and dealt with case by case in ways that discourage others from defecting during healthy periods. For example, reentry into membership may require payment of premiums for a period longer than the original qualifying period. Whatever shape preexisting solidarity takes, marketing voluntary insurance becomes complicated when community members are expected to understand and accept that people outside the immediate family and larger clan are using their payments.

The lack of experience with insurance becomes more daunting if, in the past, illness has not entailed much out-of-pocket expenditure for the necessary services. At the household level, it may be easier to sell insurance for a new utility (for example, a costly appliance or farm machine) than for health care.

Even after the idea of health care insurance is accepted, it may be rejected if communities perceive insurance as a commercial and highly profitable business and possibly exploitation in a new guise. A community's fear of outside exploitation alone would justify the development of the microinsurer as a community-owned venture and not an external initiative.

Traditional approach to illness. A third set of factors relates to the community's approach to illness and health care seeking. The target population groups typically use medical care infrequently and not just because it is inaccessible. Their knowledge and expectations of modern medical care are generally not high for reasons including a deep-rooted belief in and use of traditional or indigenous health care. Although traditional medicine may not be free, the charges may be flexible and payable in kind.

Reported utilization of modern or Western medicine in the microinsurance target population may be low for a combination of reasons, including limited knowledge, limited access to health care, and limited diagnostic capacity. Yet these people may have unmet health care needs such as prolonged neglect of chronic conditions. Enrollment in a health insurance scheme may not immediately change health care–seeking behavior, but initial contacts with health care providers are likely to result in the diagnosis of advanced stages of long-neglected conditions.

All these characteristics of the target population are important in identifying demand and potential for the development of microinsurance. The same factors are also crucial in designing the schemes that best meet the people's needs and suit their cultural and societal attributes.

DEMAND ISSUES LINKED TO SCHEME DESIGN

Once the target population and basic administrative structures have been identified, designing microinsurers for the specific community environment is the single most important step for sustainable implementation. Although community ownership is also an important factor in sustainability, good and simple design should grow out of adequate technical inputs, based on first-hand experiences and adapted through consensus to suit each new target population. Community ownership is not necessarily the foundation of design but should be an end result of the design process.

Design Tailored to Target Population

Good design has to be based on adequate analysis of factors relevant to the population, its health status and patterns of health behavior, and availability of health care resources. Often, because the information on these matters is limited in scope and reliability, detailed planning has to depend on reasonable assumptions. Good design can still be achieved with the understanding that risks will be involved. Although willingness to pay health insurance contributions is an important factor, data gained from studies to identify individuals in the target community are not the major determinants for initial implementation. In some populations, customary priorities in daily household spending may interfere with rational thinking regarding the amount the family would willingly set aside for health care through a prepayment scheme.

In the design process, simplicity and attractiveness of the scheme and ability to meet health care needs should outweigh immediate financial viability. The target population may initially be attracted if the contribution is considered affordable and fair and if the benefits are understood and guaranteed against changes, except by bodies representing the community. Simple procedures for registration and contribution collection, as well as clear statements regarding benefits and limitations, will promote and expand enrollment. However, people will remain in the voluntary scheme only if the benefits cover their most likely illnesses and conditions, as well as those involving high costs, and if no additional payments are required when they use either low- or high-cost services.

Microinsurers may end up with new members with acute and serious needs as soon as entitlement is established. The scheme therefore has to accept that serious illness may surface with the removal of financial and other treatment barriers and that the liability to provide the benefits stems from the contract created by prepayment. A qualifying period of payment before entitlement is a generally understandable means of preventing moral hazard.

Basically, the scheme has to show that insurance protects members from the hazards of paying for health care when ill through payments made all year, not just at the onset of illness, and that each insured individual is entitled to "no fault" benefits. For that reason, the package must include, not exclude, care for preexisting conditions, sexually transmitted infections, mental health, and injuries caused by accidents and violence. It is also important to include preventive services, particularly those with visible benefits for others who are not acutely ill. Preventive services, by enabling the early detection of disease, will also work in the interests of cost control (Ron 1993). In the case of mental health, limitations can be linked to acute care, while for chronic conditions, limitations on inpatient care can be based on time instead of maximum charge. Exclusions can be linked to services that are neither medically necessary nor available through the designated providers of the health care benefits.

The assumption here is that this population will eventually have fewer neglected health needs and that the design will promote health-care-seeking behavior that encourages early detection of disease through primary prevention. Early in implementation, contributions may not correspond to actual utilization and costs for lack of reliable estimating information. Over time, however, analysis of actual patient utilization and scheme operating costs may allow rate adjustments. The initial financial risk, which may seem enormous, can be dealt with through expenditure controls instead of benefit limitations.

Core Principles of Design

The design should therefore follow a set of core principles. The four principles given here, drawn from the experience of the initial OHPS, guided later adaptations in the Philippines:

- A family contribution, affordable by most of the target population, entitles all family members to health insurance benefits.

- Health care benefits will include ambulatory and inpatient care, with a strong primary care base, and prescription drugs.

- Administration of the scheme, including financial control with separate accounting, will be the responsibility of a defined community organization or a designated provider institution, and a designated community board will oversee and monitor the scheme's development.

- Health services will be provided through a capitation-payment contract with health care facilities serving a specific community or through a combination of direct provision of primary health care services and capitation-payment contract for hospital-based services.

These core principles do not limit the form or number of consultations or episodes or set cash limits on benefits. Nor are any copayments required at time of use. The principles are designed to protect and provide necessary health care for each family member. The design precludes payment methods that might encourage providers to generate demand. These arrangements protect the fund's financial viability, which also means that the need to adjust contribution rates can be controlled.

The third principle above, dealing with the microinsurer's administration, refers to two possibilities: a defined community organization or a designated provider institution. Other options might be linked to a microinsurer's initiators or sponsors. By law, whatever management structure is chosen, it must be a legal and duly registered entity with a community board and well-defined guidelines for overseeing, monitoring, and further developing the scheme.

The scheme therefore functions according to additional principles such as continuity of health care, with good primary care serving as the gatekeeper for hospital-based care. The contracted hospital provider will have a stake in controlling expenditure and retaining as much revenue as possible from the capitation payment. Underservicing by providers can be problematic, especially when the number of potential provider partners is limited in the particular locality. However, an appropriate information system, oriented toward quality control, should minimize underservicing. In this respect, community organizations must fulfill a crucial watchdog role.

SUPPLY FACTORS

Discussion so far has focused on the demand side of creating microinsurers. On the supply side, there are two requirements for civil society organizations such as cooperatives: They must exist and they must be willing to take on health-protection responsibilities by establishing formal prepayment schemes. This undertaking may encompass all the ramifications of involvement in both administration and health care delivery for nonprofit purposes.

Availability of Insurance, Resources, and Workers

The main supply-side issues concern the availability of insurance, health care resources, and health workers.

The first supply-side issue is related to the availability of health insurance. As noted, microinsurers' target populations may not be covered by social insurance, and they cannot afford private, for-profit health insurance. Even if they could afford it, many individuals' preexisting health conditions would bar them from private coverage.

The second supply-side factor concerns the availability of health care resources. It is generally believed that prepayment systems cannot be established unless the health care resources are in place. The approach taken here sees two options:

- Resources are available, but financial barriers limit access, a situation more relevant to urban areas with large, low-income populations than to rural populations. Removing the financial barriers is the microinsurer's main task in this instance.

- Resources themselves are extremely limited, a common situation in rural areas with widely scattered populations. In this case, the microinsurer's tasks include creating selected resources and persuading government or other health care providers to allocate complementary resources to these areas. The microinsurer would, for example, recruit primary health care workers, pay their salaries, and procure and distribute essential drugs. The microinsurer could also take on preventive activities such as providing safe water and sanitation, which would significantly reduce the burden of disease (Ron 1993).

The next supply issue relates to the qualifications of the health workers that can be recruited and the structures that can be coopted to provide the health care benefits. Microinsurers in the target population areas have to work with whatever staffing is available; they cannot bring in specialized, highly trained health workers from outside. However, locally available health workers will probably not have a good understanding of either community health or social health insurance. Microinsurance development will therefore require considerable capacity building in social and community health consciousness. Lay community members may also need training to perform specific tasks.

Under good leadership and a teamwork approach, and with heavy investments of time and effort, a trained and committed staff can be assembled to perform both administrative and health care functions. This situation led to low staff attrition and turnover rates at the first OHPS in La Union (Ron 1999). If the scheme itself takes on the delivery of primary health care, the health care team's commitment will grow through mutual professional respect as the members learn to work together. The entire staff's commitment will grow stronger as new members join the scheme and its representative governing bodies recognize good management practices.

Additional Supply Factors

Understanding of the prepayment/insurance/solidarity concepts will not alone launch successful community health care financing systems using these mechanisms. In the rural target communities, with their low and sometimes unstable-income families, it may be difficult to find the necessary administrative structures for efficient registration, premium collection, health care and human resource mobilization, and financial controls to run a viable health insurance scheme. Another supply element is needed to support the venture: mechanisms to regulate microinsurers' operations. The existence of, and high compliance with, regulations regarding civil society organizations and cooperatives, particularly regarding fund holding, accountability, and board composition, will facilitate the development of appropriate microinsurance regulations.

An appropriate regulatory environment also assists microinsurers' operations, particularly contract negotiations with providers and strict enforcement of their accountability requirements. Revenues from contributions are usually difficult to control in a community scheme, because sanctions are not easily imposed in this voluntary and grass-roots setting. The scheme's viability may therefore depend more on controlling expenditures in the first stages until the concepts of insurance and the links between compliance with contribution payment and entitlement are fully understood.

Within this process, health care providers have to be seen as partners in achieving access to care for the subscribers, usually newly insured. These providers stand to gain in at least two areas:

- In their ability to provide services appropriate to subscribers' needs within a framework of defined benefits. This framework may prescribe clinical behavior much different from clinicians' customary approach to treating poor patients as charity cases in both public and private hospitals.

- By receiving from a third party regular payments of revenues, set by contract, instead of having to collect fees from individuals who may or may not be satisfied with the treatment or its outcome.

To strengthen supply factors, the value of both the professional freedom and the revenue aspects should be promoted.

CONCLUSIONS

These opinions on community health insurance schemes come from first-hand experiences that provided both privileges and frustrations. The privileges included the close witnessing of social change and empowerment in access to basic social services and the emergence of a sense of pride in the realization of dignity instead of charity in accessing health care. In this process, the beneficiary population needs technical input, but the people themselves become the actors of development. This is a central principle in strategies for attaining social justice. It is a principle that emphasizes, as the source of social improvement, the creativity of local communities and of people, though living in poverty (Sen and Grown 1987).

Microinsurance cannot be forced on people. Microinsurance has to be developed in partnership with civil society organizations and, if not in full partnership with local government, following government policies. The process recognizes that successful schemes cannot be blindly replicated. Instead, after identifying the core elements, the model has to be adapted for each new group. Basic tools (for example, benefit definitions and membership database management) can be transferred, but each new microinsurer will always engender some innovation. The newly insured acquire ownership of the scheme through adaptation and innovation.

The impetus for the development of community health insurance may have come from the gap in access to health care and exclusion from existing social health protection mechanisms. The challenge now is to take the social transformation further, to universal coverage, but without compromising individual schemes' social and health care achievements. At the same time, the proliferation of such schemes is disquieting considering their wide range of contribution, benefit, and entitlement conditions, including the ability to transfer between schemes. To set minimum standards and create networks, government support becomes crucial.

The frustrations come from both civil society organizations and government. The growth of any voluntary scheme is usually slower than initially envisaged and slower than the usual pace of work of international development agencies. It takes time to appreciate that slower may be better in the long run, and to understand the local politics that hinder a scheme or help it succeed. Local government can be extremely helpful in providing support for extending coverage to new populations over which it has some leverage. Or it can delay growth by proposing alternatives that may not be better ideas but plans with vested interests or expressions of envy regarding the community-developed schemes' success. For the same reasons, as well as the old habit of neglecting the poor people usually covered by microinsurance, national governments may be slow to observe, analyze, and lend support to these new initiatives.

The donor community and international development agencies have been taking notice of microinsurance. Although assistance in technical inputs and seed money for new schemes may be crucial, even more important is limiting donor roles to allow microinsurers space to mature and develop sustainability. At the same time, communities have to learn to assume responsibility and accountability for their microinsurers.

The cooperative management responsible for the OHPS in La Union was glad to participate in a social reinsurance trial, and the same can be expected for the new OHPSs in the Philippines. The management was interested because of the approach to financial viability noted at the outset of this chapter: that financial viability should not be measured simply by the size of reserves and the return on investment. Financial viability includes a scheme's ability to solve sporadic financial overloads caused by specific health episodes or individual members' serious health crises. Random events in health and in cash availability among people with low and unstable incomes cause these situations, not constantly poor performance or mismanagement. The solutions may come from the mobilization of resources within the community, through earmarked community fund-raising activities, or from the private sector, as happened in OHPSs in the Philippines.

Resources cannot be mobilized in this way regularly or frequently. To do it all requires credibility based on the scheme's performance in terms of protection and on its administrative maturity. Since these factors take time to develop, social reinsurance could meet the unpredictable need for additional funds as new schemes are created with an umbrella of shared services and guarantees—with government backing.

Microinsurance for health care is what the term implies. It is insurance on a small scale, answering an immediate need for short-term benefits in the form of health services. Except for the few schemes that provide funeral benefits, microinsurers do not offer cash benefits to replace income in times of acute and continued need such as illness, invalidity, and old age, but they can provide solutions for immediate needs. Social reinsurance may be able to strengthen the schemes' financial base in the short to medium term. However, the ultimate goal should not be the creation of as many sustainable microinsurers as possible, covering all interested groups, even if these are connected through a national social reinsurance mechanism. The goal is to use microinsurance, created through peoples' initiatives with strong government support and guidance, to spread the understanding of the insurance concept, broaden access to health care, and promote health system development toward universal coverage. Universal coverage should provide broad social protection, not just health care, through appropriate burden sharing among households, employers, and government.

REFERENCES

Amalric, Franck. 2001. *From Food Aid to Community Empowerment: Food Security as a Political Project.* Report from the SID initiative "Food Security and Sustainable Livelihoods." Rome: Society for International Development.

Arhin, D. 1995. "Rural Health Insurance: A Viable Alternative to User Fees?" PHP Departmental Publication No. 19. London: London School of Hygiene and Tropical Medicine, Department of Public Health and Policy, Health Policy Unit.

Bennett, S., A. Creese, and R. Monasch. 1998. *Health Insurance Schemes for People Outside Formal Sector Employment.* WHO/ARA/CC/98.1. Geneva: World Health Organization.

Carrin, G., M. Desmet, and R. Basaza. 2001. "Social Health Insurance Development in Low-Income Developing Countries: New Roles for Government and Nonprofit Organizations in Africa and Asia." Chapter 10 in X. Scheil-Ablung, ed., *Building Social Security: The Challenge of Privatization.* Geneva: International Social Security Association.

Chu, K.Y., and S. Gupta. 1998a. "Social Safety Nets in Economic Reform." Chapter 2 in K. Chu and S. Gupta, *Social Safety Nets: Issues and Recent Experiences*. Washington, D.C.: International Monetary Fund.

_____. 1998b. "Social Protection in Transition Countries: Emerging Issues." Chapter 5 in K. Chu and S. Gupta, *Social Safety Nets: Issues and Recent Experiences*. Washington, D.C.: International Monetary Fund.

Moens, F. 1990. "Design, Implementation and Evaluation of a Community Financing Scheme for Hospital Care in Developing Countries: A Pre-paid Health Plan in the Bwamanda Health Zone, Zaire." *Social Sciences and Medicine* 30:1319–27.

Ron, A. 1986. "Sharing in the Financing of Health Care: Government, Insurance and the Patient." *Health Policy* 6:87–101.

_____. 1993. "Planning and Implementing Health Insurance in Developing Countries: Guidelines and Case Studies." *Macroeconomics, Health and Development*, No. 7. Geneva: World Health Organization.

_____. 1998. *Social Security Financing Policies and Rapidly Aging Populations*. World Bank Discussion Paper No. 392. Washington, D.C.: World Bank.

_____. 1999. "NGOs in Community Health Insurance Schemes: Examples From Guatemala and the Philippines." *Social Sciences and Medicine* 48(7):939–50.

Ron, A., and A. Kupferman. 1996. "A Community Health Insurance Scheme in the Philippines: Extension of a Community-Based Integrated Project." *Macroeconomics, Health and Development*, No. 19. Geneva: World Health Organization.

Ron, A., G. Carrin, and Tran Van Tien. 1998. "Viet Nam: The Development of National Health Insurance." *International Social Security Review* 51(3):89–103.

Sen, G., and C. Grown. 1987. *Development, Crises and Alternative Visions, Third World Women's Perspectives*. New York: Monthly Review Press.

van Ginneken, W. 1999. "Social Security for the Informal Sector: A New Challenge for Developing Countries." *International Social Security Review* 52(1):49–69.

CHAPTER 21

Actuarial Assessment of the ORT Health Plus Scheme in the Philippines

Hiroshi Yamabana

T he ORT Health Plus Scheme (OHPS) was created in July 1994 by the ORT Multipurpose Cooperative in San Fernando, based on Republican Act No.6938, the Cooperative Code of the Philippines. At the outset of the scheme, Australian International Development Aid supported the OHPS financially and the International Labour Organization (ILO) provided technical assistance. The government of La Union Province pays some staff salaries.

COVERAGE

Scheme coverage is voluntary and open to all residents of La Union Province. ORT covered about 700 families with 2,500 family members in May 2001. More than 40 percent of scheme members are also covered by the Social Security System (SSS) managed by the Philippine Health Insurance Corporation. As the SSS does not cover most outpatient care and has ceilings on inpatient care, OHPS benefits supplement those of the SSS.

ORT membership expanded from 153 families at the end of 1994 to 700 families in May 2001, but the scheme has a high and rising dropout rate—30 percent in 1996 and more than 75 percent in 2000. Thus, the scheme faces an almost complete turnover of insured persons about every two years.

MEDICAL FACILITIES AND PERSONNEL

The 14 ORT day-care centers (satellites), the ORT Central Unit, and the OHPS Clinic at Ilocos Training and Regional Medical Centre (ITRMC) provide primary care and pharmaceuticals. One full-time and three part-time doctors, one full-time supervisory nurse, and four full-time nurses visit the satellites on a rotational basis. The

The author thanks Michael Cichon, Chief, Financial, Actuarial and Statistical Branch, International Labour Office, for his helpful comments on this chapter.

scheme has a capitation contract with the ITRMC, mainly for inpatient care. The OHPS clinic at ITRMC serves as a gatekeeper for care at ITRMC.

BENEFITS

The main benefits are primary health care, drugs, ancillary services, and hospital care.

Doctors or nurses provide primary health care free of charge at the 14 satellites, the ORT central unit, and the OHPS clinic.

Essential drugs, prescribed by an OHPS doctor or nurse from an approved drug list, are free of charge for scheme members. Over-the-counter drugs, those not appearing on the list or nonprescribed drugs, are sold at preferential prices (the wholesale price plus some profit margin). On average the markup is around 20 percent for members and 50 percent for nonmembers, resulting in average profit margins of around 30 percent.

Outpatient services (specialist consultations, laboratory tests, and X rays) and inpatient services (room and board, doctors' services, drugs, X rays, and laboratory tests) are provided at the ITRMC free of charge on referral from the OHPS. Inpatient care is covered for up to 45 days per stay.

Some services are not covered: dental care, optometrist care, cosmetic surgeries, organ transplants, open-heart surgeries, and dialysis. Other primary health care benefits are provided after a one-month contributing period. Inpatient benefits are provided after two months' contributions. Maternity benefits are provided after 12 months, and patients must see the OHPS physicians at least six times prior to delivery. Benefits are suspended after nonpayment of two consecutive monthly contributions.

FINANCING

Income

Most of the scheme's financing comes from flat-rate contributions from families and single persons. Single persons pay PHP 70 a month; standard families (two to six people) pay PHP 120, and large families (seven or more members) pay PHP 150. Until February 1999, non-SSS members paid PHP 25, 70, or 95 each while non-SSS members paid PHP 50, 100, or 130 each since the SSS provided no inpatient care coverage for its members. The contribution rate was raised to present levels and applied to both SSS and non-SSS members in March 1999. Contributions are payable monthly, quarterly, or semi-annually, after an initial payment of three monthly contributions upon registration.

The provincial government subsidizes the scheme by paying some administrative and medical staff salaries. These staff members also perform other duties so the exact value of this subsidy is difficult to quantify.

Expenditure

The main categories of expenditure are net expenditure on medicines (wholesale purchases of pharmaceutical supplies minus income obtained by selling medicines), salaries for doctors and nurses, and the capitation payment to the ITRMC.

The annual capitation fee per family member of active contributors, regardless of age, gender, chronic condition, need for surgery, care, or inpatient admission, was PHP 100 for a non-SSS member and PHP 30 for an SSS member until March 1999. The PHP 30 covered only outpatient services provided by the ITRMC, while inpatient care for SSS members was provided not by the scheme but by the SSS. The capitation fee for SSS members was increased to the same level of PHP 100 in April 1999 when the cost of inpatient care for SSS members exceeding the SSS ceiling was also borne by the scheme. The capitation fee was again increased in July 2000, to PHP 120. Theoretically, the capitation contract, which determines the capitation fee as well as benefit packages from June to May of each year, is negotiated annually between the OHPS and the ITRMC.

ECONOMIC AND DEMOGRAPHIC CONTEXT

Region I, the Ilocos region, is composed of four provinces (Ilocos Norte, Ilocos Sur, La Union, and Pangasinan), five cities, 120 municipalities, and 3,250 barangays.

In May 2001 the population of the region was 4,174,000, with 554,000 living in La Union, the location of the scheme. The average household size is five people. The annual rate of population growth in 2000 was estimated at about 2 percent. Average life expectancy at birth was 66.2 years for males and 71.3 years for females, and the total fertility rate was 3.5 on average during the period 1995–2000.

In 2000, real gross regional domestic product (GRDP) increased by 6.7 percent, and real per-capita GRDP by 4.8 percent. The average annual increase in real GRDP and per-capita GRDP in the nine years from 1990 to 1999 was 3.6 percent and 0.7 percent, respectively. Agriculture accounted for 43 percent of GRDP, industry for 16 percent, and services for 41 percent in 2000. The regional inflation rate was 10.3 percent in 1998, 8.1 percent in 1999, and 6 to 7 percent in the first quarter of 2001.

In 1999, the total population above 15 years of age was 2,684,000. The labor force numbered 1,761,000; 1,608,000 persons were employed, and 153,000 were unemployed. In January 2001, the labor force participation rate was 64.8 percent; the unemployment rate was 10.8 percent. In October 1999, 44 percent of workers were wage and salary earners, 40 percent were self-employed, and 16 percent were unpaid family workers. Agricultural workers accounted for 46 percent, production workers for 21 percent, service and sales workers for 23 percent, and the rest were professional, administrative, or clerical workers.

According to a survey conducted in 1997, the Ilocos region had an average annual family income of PHP 102,597 and an average annual family expenditure of PHP 83,307. However, the average annual family income and expenditure in the rural areas were PHP 85,483 and 70,541, respectively. On the assumption that most of the OHPS members live in rural areas, the average contribution of PHP110 per month represented about 1.5 percent of household income. Attention should be given to the regressive nature of flat-sum contributions, especially since around 25 percent of the residents of the region's rural area have an annual income of less than PHP 40,000.

FINANCIAL AND ACTUARIAL ASSESSMENT OF THE SCHEME

Because of data deficiency, only a crude financial estimate of the scheme is carried out for 2001–03. The scheme started operating in 1994, and available data allow neither long-term nor in-depth observation. Consequently, this analysis should be considered limited with respect to its accuracy.

The data situation did not allow any actuarial estimates of the effects of random fluctuations of utilizations or unit cost on the scheme finance. Thus, the analysis should be viewed as a demonstration of the way increasing utilization or unit cost would undermine the scheme finance in the absence of reforms that would lead to either increases in income or containment of expenditure. However, fluctuations in utilization or unit cost would not have significant financial impacts in the short term (two- to three-year projection period) as long as the scheme continues to provide medications from the essential drug list, outpatient benefits provided by doctors and nurses employed directly by the scheme, and inpatient benefits based on the capitation contract with a public hospital.

If the scheme would like to include more expensive benefits with higher fluctuations either in unit cost or utilization (for example, HIV treatment) and these treatments could not be covered by the capitation contract with providers, assessing financial impacts of fluctuation would become essential in order to find ways of stabilizing scheme finance.

Methodology of the Estimate

The scheme theoretically runs on a pay-as-you-go basis without relying on either reserves or investment income. Short-term crude estimates are based on available historical data of the scheme's cash flow and utilization. Income and expenditure are estimated separately for main items, such as the contribution income, medical expenditure, salaries for doctors and nurses, and capitation payment to the ITRMC.

Contribution income. Estimated contribution income is based on assumptions about the number of active contributors classified by family type. As the number of contributing families has become more stable except during promotional campaigns, the number of families and the average size of each type are assumed to be constant for the projection years, the same as the average of the period from January to May 2001.

The contribution per family is kept constant. In spite of considerable payments in advance and in arrears,[1] the *global compliance rate,* the ratio of actual contributions over potential contributions, was stable. The rate estimated at 84.3 percent between January and May 2001 is kept constant throughout the projection. Actual contributions are estimated as the product of potential contributions multiplied by this compliance rate.

Other income. Other income is assumed to remain a fixed percentage of contribution income. Excluding "unusual income" (for example, sponsorships or lottery), the ratio was historically around 1 percent and assumed to be 1.5 percent for 2001 and 1 percent for 2002–03.

Medical expenditure. Estimated medical expenditures encompass the cost of free medicines and over-the-counter drugs, profits from the sale of over-the-counter drugs, and wholesale purchase of medicines.

The estimated cost of supplying free medicines (mostly antibiotics) is based on assumptions about the average number of prescriptions per individual (frequency) and the average cost per prescription. The frequency is assumed to be a constant 0.89 for the projection period. The average cost per prescription in 2001 is assumed to be the average of the first five months, PHP 77. Three different assumptions were made for cost increases (0 percent, 10 percent, and 20 percent) in 2002–03 to establish the sensitivity of the results.

The estimated cost of over-the-counter drugs is based on the assumption of the percentage of the cost of free drugs over all medication costs (35.7 percent).

Potential profits from sales of over-the-counter drugs are calculated on those products' assumed margins. The rate of profit margins over the cost, average profits divided by the average cost of over-the-counter drugs, is assumed conservatively as 22.3 percent. By adding the cost and the potential profits of over-the-counter drugs, potential charges of over-the-counter drugs are estimated. The actual income from drug sales is calculated by multiplying potential charges arising from sales by an assumed collection rate.

Wholesale purchase of medicines is estimated by multiplying the cost of both free and over-the-counter medicines by an assumed ratio of purchase amount over the cost of medicines.

Finally, net expenditure on medicines is estimated by subtracting income from medicine sales (amount actually collected by the scheme) from the scheme's wholesale purchase of medicines.

Salaries. Estimated salaries for 2001 are based on payments between January and May 2001, taking into account the "thirteenth month" payment at Christmas. The projections do not assume an increase in the number of staff as the scheme still has the capacity to cover more patients.

Doctors working part-time for the scheme with other professional income and nurses working in the scheme mainly to gain experience have not claimed major salary increases. However, it is unrealistic to assume this situation will last indefinitely, particularly in the Philippine's inflationary economy. Therefore, to test the sensitivity of the projections, three different assumptions are made about salary increases (0 percent, 10 percent, and 20 percent) in 2002–03.

Hospital fees. Estimated hospital fees are based on the assumed capitation fee per individual and the number of individuals in the scheme. For 2001, the capitation amount will not be changed, as the hospital is asking the scheme to accept a ceiling on high-cost inpatient treatments instead of increasing the capitation fee. Taking into account the increased inpatient cases and average hospital days, the capitation fees for 2002 (June 2002 to May 2003) and 2003 (June 2003 to May 2004) are assumed to increase by 0 percent, 10 percent, and 20 percent—again to test the sensitivity of results.

Other expenditure. Other scheme expenditure is assumed to be a fixed percentage (7 percent) of contribution income.

Results of the Projection

Taking into account the nature of unavoidable increases in unit costs of medicines and treatments because of general or medical inflation or salary increases of medical staff, the individual contribution must be increased at least to cover those expenditure increases as long as the scheme's benefit package is maintained. On top of the minimum increase, technological improvements might increase the unit cost more, and utilization will normally increase over time.

Based on the assumptions outlined above, it is estimated that the fund will run a deficit in 2001 that can be covered from its technical reserves. However, the reserves will be depleted in 2002 without any increases in medical costs, staff salaries, and capitation amount, as assumed. Thus, an increase in contributions seems to be inevitable. To achieve a three-year financial equilibrium:

- A 10 percent increase would be required in the average contribution in 2002 if pharmaceutical costs, staff salaries, or capitation amount remain static.

- A 25 percent increase would be necessary in the case of a 10 percent rise in pharmaceutical costs, staff salaries, or capitation fees.

- A 40 percent increase would be required in the case of a 20 percent rise in these costs (see figure 21.1).

An increase in the membership will ameliorate the scheme's financial situation only with regard to fixed costs (for example, staff salaries). However, it will have no impact on medical costs or capitation fees because they will increase in parallel with the membership.

An increase in "compliance" (contribution collection rate) will improve the scheme's financial situation. Although the present "global" compliance rate of nearly 85 percent is high, considering the voluntary nature of scheme participation, the reasons for delinquency should be examined so an attempt could be made to further improve compliance.

An increase in contributions might affect the membership. Therefore, to achieve consensus among members before putting the contribution increase into effect, members must be provided with crucial information about, for example, the financial situation and the utilization of the scheme.

The present schedule is extremely biased toward large families whose per capita cost is PHP 21.4 a month versus PHP 70 for a single person. Some adjustment to the schedule might be acceptable.

The alternative to contribution rate increases may be adjustments in the benefit schedule. To keep the financial balance of the scheme, long-term

FIGURE 21.1   Income/Expenditure Balance and Reserves

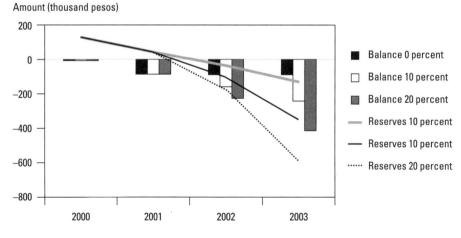

Source: Based on ORT data.

cost-containment measures could be considered. Introducing copayments would have a containing effect on utilization as well as on cost, notwithstanding debate on their appropriateness because of their regressive nature and, especially for the poor, their possible suppressive effects on necessary treatments. Raising profits on over-the-counter drugs would be another way of increasing revenue. Limiting the supply of essential drugs (mainly antibiotics) by changing providers' prescribing practices could also be beneficial. Tightening gate-keeping and reducing inpatient care service packages would lead to a slower increase in the capitation fee. However, just as in the case of increasing contributions rates, the elasticity of membership with regard to the offered benefits package has to be tested carefully. If the benefit package becomes too restrictive, the incentives to join the scheme might weaken considerably.

Standard Financial Procedures and Data Requirement

This analysis can only be of a preliminary nature mainly because of data constraints regarding disaggregation, consistency, lack of information (for example, on over-the-counter medicines), and the scheme's short history.

The present database should be expanded to permit more detailed analysis of the scheme. The age and gender structure of participants and patients should be clarified annually. Analysis of utilization by age and gender would provide a basis for further analysis on cost increases from aging.[2] The scheme should also have access to information on the finance and utilization of the hospital to aid capitation fee negotiations. In addition, a formal consistent accounting methodology should be established with a balance sheet that clearly delineates the scheme's assets and liabilities.

Based on these accounts and the information on utilization, annual budgeting and mid-term financial planning exercises are recommended to plan future reforms on the contribution and benefit sides.

CONCLUSIONS

The ORT scheme faces an imminent structural and systemic financial deficit. While it appears likely that the deficit emerging in 2001 can be absorbed by the technical reserve, an increase of at least 10 percent in the contribution rate or an equivalent reduction of expenditure would be necessary to maintain the scheme in financial equilibrium for at least three years.

The deficit is the result of the systemically increasing gap between expenditure and income, which is unrelated to random fluctuations in expenditure levels. This systemic gap has to be closed by a set of stringent measures before the scheme can seek protection through reinsurance against random fluctuations in expenditure or other income shortfalls. Simple mid-term financial projections should be repeated to see the normal path of the scheme's financial development.

NOTES

1. Payments in arrears exceeded 40 percent in 2000.

2. Utilization data should cover the frequency of inpatient and outpatient cases, the average hospital stay for inpatient cases, the frequency of prescriptions of free medicines and over-the-counter medicines, and the average cost per hospital day.

CHAPTER 22

Assessment of Piloting Social Reinsurance in the Philippines

Frank G. Feeley, Donato J. Gasparro, and Katherine Snowden

SOCIAL RE: THE CONCEPT, THE QUESTIONS, THE ASSUMPTIONS

Most microinsurance units have evolved in settings of severe economic constraint, political instability, and unsatisfactory governance, where community involvement is a first step toward improved financial protection against the cost of illness and improved access to priority health services (Preker and others 2001). Microinsurers do not always reach the poorest members of society, but they can offer social protection to a large group not currently served by formal social health insurance programs in many developing countries.

The sources of these schemes' vulnerability and insolvency have been discussed by Dror (chapter 5, this volume; Dror 2001). Reinsurance can address at least two major causes—shortage of reserve capital and the small size of the risk pool—but so far microinsurers have not had access to reinsurance. Commercial reinsurers see no profit in a market that is characterized by low premiums, badly identified risks, and widely variable management capacity of the primary insurers, the microinsurers. That is why reinsurance companies have never designed a product for this market.

But suppose microinsurers could obtain reinsurance through an organization with a social commitment? Such a program—*Social Re*—would provide coverage for microinsurers' unanticipated losses in return for a reinsurance premium paid from the microinsurers' contribution income.

Simulations show convincingly that microinsurers' danger of insolvency is reduced if risks are pooled through *Social Re* (Bonnevay and others, chapter 7, this volume). Assessing the plan to test *Social Re* requires reflection on the following:

- How large is the market for *Social Re* coverage in the Philippines, where the first pilot is being considered, because so many microinsurers already do business there? And what are the factors that will enable *Social Re* to tap this market?

For their useful comments on an earlier draft, the authors thank David Wilson and the International Labour Organisation Social Protection Assessment Group chaired by Dominique Peccoud. Attorney Manuel L. Ortega of Manila answered questions on the existing regulatory regime in the Philippines with professional clarity. The authors also acknowledge, with thanks, the useful comments by Christian Mumenthaler, Financial Analyst and Project Manager with the Finance Department, Swiss Reinsurance Company, Zurich, Switzerland.

- What is the best structure for *Social Re* to operate effectively, and how much will this cost? What is a plausible business plan for the start-up of *Social Re*?

- What are the financial and investment requirements? What are the projections for *Social Re* to break even on its reinsurance operations?

- What are the key issues and decisions in implementing *Social Re*?

- What are the key risks and uncertainties?

Our responses to these questions are based on the following assumptions. The benefit packages offered by microinsurers in the Philippines vary widely (Flavier, Soriano, and Nicolay, chapter 17, this volume). Reinsurance coverage would have to adapt to this variability in benefits and also premiums and could do so by using the model developed by Bonnevay and others (chapter 7, this volume). The model stipulates that *Social Re* would compensate a microinsurer for an annual loss (incurred claims) exceeding the assumed (long-term) average loss.

Based on statistical assumptions backed by simulations, the reinsurance premium is estimated at half the standard deviation of each microinsurer's mean benefit cost (when the pool size is optimal). Expressed as a percentage of that mean in the simulated scenarios (chapter 7), the premium can vary anywhere from 25 percent to 7 percent of the microinsurer's basic contribution income. An average value of 15 percent of the expected contribution income, used here, can serve as a point of departure. Defining the appropriate premium more precisely for each microinsurer will require more data than are available at this time.

Given the uncertainty about the reinsurer's actual losses, the analysis considers pure loss ratios of 75 percent, 100 percent, and 125 percent (the ratio of incurred claims to collected premium). The model (chapter 7) predicts a loss ratio of about 80 percent, when the premium is calculated correctly.

METHOD OF ANALYSIS

The pilot program in the Philippines was analyzed for several market scenarios, organizational structures, and additional requirements over a sufficiently long time span to evaluate the *Social Re* project.

Timeline

The period of analysis of operations is three years, identical to the planned pilot. This period should be long enough to test the Philippine market, but judging by simulations run under the conceptualization phase (chapter 7, this volume), it might be too short for *Social Re* to become fully self-supporting,[1] especially if it encounters bad years at the outset. At the end of the three-year pilot period, *Social Re* is projected to have 20 reinsured microinsurers, with an estimated total enrollment of about 240,000 individuals. Although still only 1 percent of the target population, this would be a large enough book of business to assess the *Social Re* concept's viability. By the end of this period, *Social Re* would have refined its systems and policy language and should be helping to bring new microinsurers into existence. It would have experience that can be transferred to *Social Re* start-ups in other countries or regions. In our analysis, success is defined as creating a viable organization with all necessary systems and enrolling 20 microinsurers with a loss ratio on the reinsurance written no greater than 125 percent.

Modeling Scenarios

To estimate the possible range of operating income, we have developed several market scenarios. For each scenario, we project the premium income and operating costs. To this, we add investment income from reserves. Then we can calculate:

- The first-year investment required

- The annual operating loss or gain for the reinsurance operation

- The costs of affiliated activities (the Project Office and technical assistance to microinsurers).

Later, any subsidies (for example, directed at benefit enhancements or at increasing enrollment) can be included in the model.

These results give the total funding required for the three-year *Social Re* experiment. The analysis is repeated for several market scenarios. The model can readily be adjusted to test the effects of:

- Different market scenarios

- Different assumptions about staffing levels and unit costs

- Different loss ratios

- Different levels of support for the Project Office, technical assistance, and microinsurance benefit enhancements.

Additional Scenarios

This model can be further modified to reflect:

- A change in the basic reinsurance structure (including a shift to coverage of excess costs of a specific benefit type, or single catastrophic claims, rather than for aggregate costs)

- Possible retrocession from *Social Re* to commercial reinsurers, assumed to be nil initially

- Different capitalization requirements, based on different licensing rules.

In addition, the model will allow for additional country operations if *Social Re* grows beyond the Philippines.

Structure

Social Re would have to perform several functions, supported by three organizational components: the Project Office (the holding company headquarters), the Philippines reinsurance operation, and technical assistance to microinsurers.

Project Office. Social Re is being created from scratch. It is a unique nonprofit organization aiming to achieve social goals that also meet the test of business viability. The new organization will inherit the knowledge gained from the conceptual phase, but it will not have the advantage of investors familiar with hands-on insurance operations or of being formed as a subsidiary of an existing insurance organization. A Project Office will have to oversee the creation of the new entity in the Philippines. At some point, this office may have to act as a holding company that would start other Social Re operations in other countries.

Reinsurance operation. The costs of *Social Re* operations were estimated using informants who know the insurance industry in the Philippines, as well as a multinational organization maintaining a Manila office. The cost structure is discussed more fully below, and assumptions about salaries and unit costs are shown in Annex 22A. Any cost factor can be changed as more accurate information becomes available.

Technical assistance. The technical-assistance function will be vital in improving microinsurers' management and increasing the number of families they cover. In the longer run, the operation should meet its operating costs. Therefore, sufficient accounting, auditing, claims monitoring, actuarial, and data-processing functions are needed in the staffing table.

Marketing. The marketing function spills into technical assistance, which will have to attract these services for microinsurers.

Government relations. Additionally, *Social Re* will need a strong government-relations function to coordinate its activities with PhilHealth, the government's social health insurance program. These functions go beyond those of a small commercial reinsurance organization, but they are indispensable to convince Philippine officials that *Social Re* is soundly run and can integrate into the policy for reaching the informal economy.

ASSESSING THE MARKET IN THE PHILIPPINES

Our assessment of the market for *Social Re* in the Philippines relied on the following sources:

- Data from the German Technical Corporation–Social Health Insurance Networking and Empowerment (GTZ/SHINE) program to support Philippine microinsurers, and the survey of microinsurer activity presented in chapter 19 of this volume

- Interviews conducted on our behalf by contacts in Manila, as well as comments from Sister Dulce Velasco, a leader in the Philippine community health movement

From these sources we conclude that:

- The total number of Filipinos currently participating in community health plans is estimated at 500,000 to 1,000,000. The number of Filipinos in the informal sector of the economy, with incomes above the poverty line, is estimated at 30 percent, about 20 million. Thus, *Social Re* has a large potential for outreach.

- The Philippines has a large cooperative movement that can serve as the springboard for the formation of new microinsurers. Interviews indicate that many cooperatives are interested in forming microinsurance units, and would welcome technical assistance from *Social Re*. Existing microinsurers have indicated in writing their interest in working with a *Social Re* experiment.

- Philippine microinsurers vary widely in sponsorship, size, and benefit package. The typical microinsurer has between 1,000 and 4,000 policyholders. Average family size is about 4, so the well-established microinsurer might cover 18,000 to 24,000 persons. However, many microinsurers are still very small.

- The estimated average premium mentioned in chapter 17 was about PHP 350 per family per year. However, the two plans studied in detail had annual premiums higher than PHP 1,000. Average claims costs in the sample were about PHP 1,671. Benefit ceilings reported in the survey averaged about PHP 11,500 annually.

STRUCTURING THE PILOT

Organization and Functions

The corporate office will evolve from the Project Office (initially in Geneva). Functions of the Project Office include:

- Developing the concept of *Social Re*

- Establishing a relationship with international agencies and foundations and raising funds to support the pilot program

- Establishing the *Social Re* presence in the Philippines and, pending the results of the pilot, in other countries

- Establishing a Board of Directors for *Social Re* and Advisory Panels, as needed

- Monitoring and evaluating operations in the Philippines

- Maintaining centralized accounts and reporting to donors or investors

- Selecting and supervising the top managers of the Philippine operation.

The regional office in Manila would be the operating reinsurer for Philippine microinsurers. Its functions would include:

- Establishing and maintaining a database of information on microinsurer operations that can be used to better quantify risks (that is, actuarial data), help microinsurers manage their programs, and evaluate needs for and uses of health care services in the informal sector

- Processing reinsurance claims from microinsurers

- Establishing and maintaining financial accounts and accounting procedures

- Periodically reviewing microinsurers' claims and financial records

- Marketing *Social Re*'s reinsurance to microinsurers

- Being responsible for complying with any local regulatory and licensing requirements

- Securing the approval and support of local agencies.

An office will have to be set up in Manila, and the expenses related to it (rent, equipment and supplies, printing, and communications) are included under start-up costs. Other expenses include travel costs (for trips by Manila staff to the microinsurers and for senior management travel between the Project Office in Geneva and Manila); fees, such as bank charges; and a 15 percent contingency allowance (applied to operating expenses, but not to losses).

Staffing Considerations

The Chief Executive Officer should be a person who understands the technical implications of reinsurance as well as the dynamics underlying each microinsurer. These dynamics include cultural differences, health care delivery systems, regional economics, and political influences. He or she will have overall responsibility for Manila-based operations and will report to the Chairperson of *Social Re*. Initially, the Chief Financial Officer and the Chief Information Officer roles could be combined, as both deal with supervisory responsibility for developing information and administrative systems and contracts to support the Manila reinsurance operations.

The Government Relations Manager will coordinate *Social Re*'s activities with those of PhilHealth on the national level and will also work with local government units to ensure support for the microinsurers.

The role of the Principal Underwriter is critical. Working with an independent actuary, he or she will evaluate premium adequacy and will decide which microinsurers to cover. This person must understand health care risks and recognize the economic, social, and cultural issues that influence access to and delivery of health care. In addition, the Principal Underwriter should communicate well with clinical personnel who know the local health care market. The Claims Manager will be responsible for the traditional functions of a claims department: confirming that the claims are covered by the terms of the reinsurance agreement, determining that the microinsurer followed agreed-on claims-management protocols, and verifying supporting documentation to confirm that it covers the claim payments requested. These functions will require both in-office claim reviews and on-site audits at the microinsurance unit. In the case of *Social Re*, the Manila Claims Manager will need to work closely with the microinsurers and their support staff to understand the implications of claims data and help the microinsurer plan and design changes in the health care scheme. In addition, the Claims Manager will work with microinsurers to give early warning of trends or epidemics that may be developing. Initially, one qualified person might be able to combine the activities of Principal Underwriter and Claims Manager.

Somewhat separate from the usual staffing for an insurance operation is the inclusion of technically qualified microinsurer support staff to work closely with microinsurers, both actual *Social Re* clients and prospective clients. *Social Re* in the Philippines will start with a staff of three individuals for microinsurer support. They will market the *Social Re* coverage and provide the microinsurers with technical assistance. Funds are also budgeted to cover training of microinsurer staff and to provide the microinsurers with computers. The financial model identifies this support as a separate activity, as funding for technical assistance could come from donors or government.

This technical support function will provide a full range of management and technical consulting to the plans. The integration of this technical assistance with the reinsurance function is an important strength of *Social Re*, but the costs are separated to highlight the need for ongoing external support for this function. This will also have to include support to users in the use of the *Social Re Data Template*, which is the main source of statistical and accounting information available to the reinsurer from the microinsurers.

The business plan includes funding for key consultations. We have budgeted $50,000 for each of the first two years for the systems development consultant.

Also shown at the Project Office level is a lump sum of $15,000 for an epidemiological study to assist in rate and policy development. Data from microinsurers to support real actuarial analysis will be scarce. It will be necessary to extrapolate likely utilization rates from other health data in the Philippines, notably the data provided by the microinsurers themselves through the *Data Template* (appendix A, this volume). Since this is a unique cost imposed by the experimental nature of *Social Re*, the Project Office, not the ongoing reinsurance operation, should carry it.

Expected salary levels are shown in annex 22A.

IMPLEMENTATION PLAN

There will be three phases in the evolution of *Social Re*: start-up, infrastructure development, and ongoing operations (including microinsurer support services).

Start-Up

The Geneva staff in the Project Office would begin working on program design, identification and selection of microinsurers, hiring the core staff, and securing funding for the pilot. Additionally, in the start-up phase, staff must address key legal and organizational issues and comply with other legal and regulatory requirements. Six months have been budgeted for this phase, which must be completed before operations begin in Manila.

Manila staff would start working three months prior to regular operations to install an office in Manila and adapt it for operations. Manila staff would be actively involved in the selection of participating microinsurers. During this period, start-up expenses will include one-time investments as well as normal operating expenses such as salaries and office expenses.

Infrastructure Development

The infrastructure development phase will complete the process of building administrative services for operations, begin marketing, and develop microinsurer support services. Administrative services include underwriting and actuarial support, claims administration, auditing, and operational administration, including support to microinsurers. Several subsidiary activities will have to be put in place, for example, contract development, finance and accounting, billing and collection, escrow account management, policy administration, rate filings (if required), and legal/general counsel. Financial analysis and reports should include periodic updating and adjustment of the business model developed for this assessment, the balance sheet, profit and loss, cash flow, sources and uses of funds, loss-ratio analysis, reserves, and working capital requirements as well as statistics on premium, insureds, and claims.

Underwriting and actuarial support. Specific underwriting guidelines will be needed to provide a standardized approach for evaluating each prospective microinsurer, taking into account heterogeneity in benefit packages and sociodemographic parameters of the membership.

Claims administration. Claims adjudication rules will have to be developed and may be customized for some microinsurers.

Auditing. Underwriting and claims must be continuously audited to confirm that procedures and policies are being followed, to identify any variations that imply that procedures or policy should be changed, and to identify any changes in risk exposure or claim frequency that differ from those assumed in the underwriting and actuarial projections.

Operational administration. Every reinsurance operation needs good systems to track all the business running through it. Reporting should be at least monthly, because senior managers need this information to set or adjust the company's direction.

Microinsurer Support Services

One of the most valuable roles that *Social Re* will play in the stabilization of these community-based risks is to provide consultative support to microinsurers. *Social Re* can provide technical insurance expertise and managerial services of four types: underwriting and actuarial, claims, provider contracting, and eligibility confirmation and procedures.

Underwriting and actuarial consulting to microinsurers. *Social Re* will work with the microinsurers to help set objectives and to identify and review the benefits that can be offered, taking into account members' needs and priorities, the existing supply of health care services and likely cost, the appropriate contribution level, and the maximum premium microinsurer members can afford.

Building claims-processing capacity. *Social Re* will help microinsurers set up a system to collect claims data, identify trends in claims experience, evaluate claims, and set reserves and changes in benefits. *Social Re* may offer advice on case management or other techniques for managing the cost of large claims.

Provider contracting. *Social Re* can help microinsurers by providing advice on selecting and qualifying medical service providers, setting rates, and confirming that providers meet standards of financial and professional integrity.

Eligibility confirmation. *Social Re* can share with microinsurers the most effective techniques for confirming eligibility, including (if needed) the use of photo identification cards and systems to enable providers to verify eligibility.

Ongoing Operations

Once its systems and personnel are in place, *Social Re* must focus on analyzing, monitoring, and reporting on its business operations. The purpose is to assess risk profiles and financial performance and identify trends requiring policy adaptation. *Social Re* will also need to address specialized insurance functions such as actuarial surplus analysis and regulatory reporting.

THE FINANCIAL MODEL

In the financial model of *Social Re*, revenues and expenses are consolidated for three levels of operation—local, regional, and central.

Local (or Microinsurer) Level

The variables that drive the microinsurer's contribution to *Social Re* and the *Social Re* claims expense are the number of microinsurers participating; the number of insureds covered by each microinsurer; the plan parameters (for example, the contribution charged by the microinsurer, benefits covered, and total benefit limit or cap per family); the average cost of claims and its variance or standard deviation;[2] structure of *Social Re* reinsurance coverage (for example, paying 100 percent of claims costs in excess of a specified level); and the loss ratio (actual losses [claims paid by *Social Re*] compared with premiums paid by microinsurers to *Social Re*). The loss-ratio parameter will yield the percentage of microinsurers' contribution revenue allocated to *Social Re*. The actual loss ratio is not known in advance, but its acceptable level determines the premium.

Regional Level

In the first three years, we assume the Manila office would incur all operating expenses, except the costs of the Project Office. These costs include personnel (both salaried and consultants), general office expenses, professional services for insurance activities (for example, underwriting and claims processing), and travel costs.

Technical assistance to provide assistance and training to microinsurers out of the Manila office is budgeted separately. Benefit enhancements are a separate cost line, which can be activated if such incentives are provided. Government fees and taxes are included as a line. These costs would depend on the legal structure of *Social Re* in the Philippines. At this point, we assume that *Social Re* will be chartered as a nonprofit corporation or international project, and thus will be exempt from premium taxes, corporate income taxes, or license fees.

Central (Project Office) Level

The plan includes salaries for a Chair of *Social Re* and an administrative assistant, plus a travel budget. We assume that office space and related expenses are provided as an in-kind donation by a supporting agency. Most of the financial work will be done in Manila, but the plan includes a modest budget for an annual corporate audit and for legal expenses associated with incorporation and start-up.

The *Social Re* program includes functions that fall outside those expected for normal insurance operations, notably the Project Office and the microinsurer support services. It seems appropriate to target foundations and other agencies to fund these costs. Because of start-up expenses and little investment income in the first year, these costs that are not covered by other income sources total about US$900,000 in year 1, fall to US$603,645 in year 2 and to US$560,797 in year 3 as more microinsurers join.

We assume that the *Social Re* Board will consist of members whose sponsoring agencies cover the delegate's travel and related expenses. No allowance is made for Board meetings.

Capitalization

If set up as a foreign-owned insurance or reinsurance company in the Philippines, *Social Re* must be capitalized at PHP 300 million (US$6 million) (Box 22.1). This capitalization is in excess of what would be required by insurance industry benchmarks in the early years of *Social Re*'s operation, where prudent insurance or reinsurance companies can usually operate with capital equal to 100 percent of retained annual premium, even with a new product such as that

---

BOX 22.1 REGULATORY CONSIDERATIONS

The Philippines has an active commercial health insurance industry, dynamic growth in community insurance plans, and relatively sophisticated insurance regulations (by developing-world standards). Terms, exclusions, and pricing of insurance policies are all subject to approval by the national Insurance Commission and must be justified by actuarial studies. The question is: Which regulations will apply to *Social Re*, and what form should the pilot take to minimize unnecessary regulatory burdens?

As currently proposed, *Social Re* will combine a number of other functions with its classic reinsurance role. It will provide technical assistance to community plans in activities including benefit design, pricing, eligibility verification, marketing and provider contracting, and payment. In addition, it may combine premium income with other sources of funds to spur the development of microinsurance plans. *Social Re* must be able to work constructively within the framework of the government's current health insurance initiative. It cannot afford the kind of controlled confrontation that characterizes the relationship between a regulated insurance entity and its regulator. For this reason, there may be a mutual advantage in its exemption from classical regulation.

Community health insurance schemes in the Philippines. Assuming that *Social Re* takes the form of a mutual or nonprofit organization in which any earnings are used to benefit the participating plans, which themselves appear to be exempt from licensing as insurance companies, a plausible case could be made for an exemption. Having some members of the *Social Re* Board—or at least the Philippine subsidiary of *Social Re*—drawn from the cooperative movement in the Philippines might strengthen this case. Also, if *Social Re* were a mutual reinsurer owned in part by the microinsurers that it reinsures, it would not need to use licensed agents and brokers.

If *Social Re* does not receive an exemption, it may be required to become the primary insurer. In such a case, the rules for capitalization are straightforward, whether the company is organized in the Philippines or as a foreign insurer

(Box continues on the following page.)

BOX 22.1 (continued)

operating a branch in the Philippines. If the company is 100 percent owned by Filipinos, it will require minimum capitalization—the excess of admitted assets over liabilities (including loss reserves)—of PHP 150 million, *plus* a margin of solvency set at 0.2 percent of the total value of insurance in force in the prior year. To illustrate, assume that *Social Re* offers reinsurance to 10 plans with 1,000 members each, for a total of 10,000 policies. The microinsurers pay the first PHP 10,000 of the insured medical costs, and the benefit limit is PHP 50,000. The required margin of solvency would be .002 times 10,000 policies times 40,000 (maximum *Social Re* obligation on any one policy), or PHP 800,000. If premiums cover projected losses, the initial capitalization would be PHP 150,800,000 and must grow by PHP 80 for every additional policy reinsured. At PHP 50 to US$1, this would require an initial investment of US$3,000,000. However, the assumption that premiums cover loss reserves is crucial. To the extent that *Social Re* deliberately underprices the coverage, or finds that losses exceed projections, it must immediately augment its capitalization by the amount of the shortfall.

Social Re need not be owned by Filipinos. An insurance or reinsurance company can be started in the Philippines with up to 100 percent foreign ownership, as long as a majority of the directors are Filipinos. For example, a Swiss-based trust or nonprofit corporation could own the company. Also, a foreign insurer can start a branch in the Philippines. In both cases, the capitalization requirements are higher than for a domestically owned company. As a branch of a foreign insurer, or as a Philippine company partially or wholly owned by non-Filipinos, a licensed insurance company must have capitalization of PHP 300 million, of which PHP 250 million must be paid up. In addition, it must meet the same margin of solvency requirements as the Filipino-owned insurer. Operating as a branch or subsidiary of a foreign corporation, *Social Re* would require capitalization of PHP 300,800,000 (US$6,016,000 at PHP 50 to US$1) in the scenario described in the preceding paragraph. The company would have the same requirement to supplement the margin of solvency as it grows the volume of insurance in force. It must also take the same steps to increase capitalization if surplus and the margin of solvency are eroded by inadequate premiums or unpredicted losses. Bank letters of credit based on securities held outside the Philippines do not qualify as an "admitted asset" in calculating required surplus, so the backers of *Social Re* must contribute about US$6,000,000 in cash or approved securities to start up a licensed insurance company.

Another alternative lies in the rule allowing Philippine insurance companies to purchase reinsurance from foreign reinsurers *not* licensed in the Philippines. *Social Re* might arrange *fronting*, where a Philippines-licensed company issues the policies to the community health plans, and *Social Re* (from its offshore location) issues a reinsurance policy. The rules require that the company purchasing the foreign reinsurance show that a Philippines-licensed reinsurer cannot match the terms offered. Furthermore, 25 percent of the total risk reinsured must be placed with Philippines-licensed companies. This set of rules permits foreign reinsurers to participate in risk-sharing arrangements with Philippines-licensed companies.

offered by *Social Re*. On this standard, in year 3 *Social Re* would need less than US$1,000,000 in capital.

However, to reassure the insurance regulators during the pilot stage and to facilitate transition to licensed operation at a later date, the capitalization is set at the higher level required of licensed foreign-owned insurers. The investment of US$6 million in reserve capital will not be required before the first reinsurance policies are written, near the end of year 1. In addition, *Social Re* must add a margin of solvency of 0.2 percent of the total value of insurance in force in the prior year. As the volume of insurance grows, additional capital is required to cover this margin of solvency. Additional capital would be needed if inadequate premiums or unpredicted losses erode the surplus. The model calculates the required capitalization based on these regulatory requirements. The value of insurance in force is the microinsurer's benefit limit per family less the expected (mean) claims cost per family times the number of policies reinsured. This formula expresses *Social Re*'s maximum exposure if all families reach their benefit ceiling.

Sources of Income

Social Re gets income from three general sources:

- Reinsurance premiums from microinsurers

- Grants and donations

- Investment income on its capital.

Because of the microinsurers' high price sensitivity and high membership turnover in the informal sector, the price *Social Re* charges its client microinsurers is initially intended to cover only the costs of the claims it will pay out (no more than 100 percent loss ratio). Eventually, the loss ratio would be less than 100 percent, allowing it to partially cover operating expenses through a reinsurance premium that includes a modest margin. A loss ratio above that level implies that *Social Re* would be subsidizing the reinsurance coverage provided.

Investment income is projected at 6 percent on *Social Re*'s equity (capitalization plus retained earnings, if any). We assume that this capital is not invested until the ninth month of the first year, thus earning only 25 percent of the expected annual interest in year 1.

The pilot of *Social Re* is initially planned for three years, but it should be noted that the plan could reach viability only after a longer period of about five to six years. In addition, during the first three years, grants and donations will have to cover the administrative, start-up, and other overhead costs, but over time this subsidy could be severed without endangering the reinsurance operation.

SCENARIOS TESTED

The model was tested with the following variables modified to produce different scenarios.

Exchange Rate

Amounts are stated in U.S. dollars, based on an exchange rate of PHP 50/US$1, assumed to be constant for the sake of simplification. These are real dollars, based on current 2001 price estimates.

Number of Participating Plans

The number of microinsurers that will buy *Social Re* coverage is uncertain. Around 65 microinsurers currently do business in the Philippines. Over time, a successful *Social Re* program would reach this number and encourage the creation of new microinsurers. For the analysis, we have assumed the following market penetration: end of year 1, 5 microinsurers; end of year 2, 12 microinsurers; end of year 3, 20 microinsurers—about a 30 percent market share of current microinsurers by the end of year 3.

Average Membership Size

The collected contribution to the microinsurance and reinsurance premiums are a direct function of membership size, so larger microinsurers will be more efficient customers. Because many microinsurers in the Philippines are still very small, we looked at this range of average size for participating plans. We used the assumption of 2,000 families for the baseline, with a steady growth in the total number of families to approximately 2,800 and a decrease in the average size of families from 4 to 3.8 over a period of three years.

Microinsurer Benefits and Contributions

A fixed annual contribution per family of PHP 1,200 (US$24) for a four-person family and PHP 950 (US$19) for a single person is assumed. This fee is what some of the microinsurers now operating charge (for example, ORT Health Plus, La Union).

Loss Ratios

Initial calculations were made with three different projected loss ratios: 75 percent, 100 percent, and 125 percent. However, simulations of the estimated minimal reinsurance premium, calculated by applying the reinsurance model (chapter 7), indicate that for an optimal size reinsurance fund the loss ratio is expected to be around 80 percent. In addition, the loss ratio will decrease further as the variance in benefit cost decreases, which is a function of membership size. Hence, loss ratios were assumed to be 75 percent at the baseline, with a slight drop in successive years to reflect the impact in the growing size of membership and of pooled microinsurance.

Reinsurance Premium

The model (chapter 7) forecasts that premiums of 50 percent of the expected standard deviation of the benefit expenditure would be adequate. Simulations show that 15 percent of contribution income can serve as a first approximation of this value. This value was assumed to be the constant percentage of contribution income payable as the reinsurance premium.

RESULTS

Net profit/loss from operations in years 1 to 3 is negative. About half the total net loss of about US$450,000 in year 1 is from reinsurance operations, and does not include the pilot overhead (technical assistance and Project Office). Total net loss in Year 2 drops to about US$120,000, and to about US$42,000 in year 3. Net profit from reinsurance operations can be reached in years 5 or 6, and even earlier if less additional capital than assumed is needed.

Manila expenses are fairly stable over the first three years and decline slightly in year 3 after systems development work has been completed. Personnel, travel, and communications costs for the Geneva Project Office remain stable for the entire period of the pilot.

Because fixed costs are relatively large compared with the costs for pure reinsurance operations during the first three years, the *Social Re* calculations seem relatively insensitive to alternative assumptions about microinsurer participation and characteristics.

Break-Even Analysis

It is unrealistic to expect *Social Re* to cover all its expenses through premium income or contributions from microinsurers. To address the entire set of issues or challenges facing microinsurers—inadequate financial reserves is one of them—a strong technical assistance program is included. The microinsurers do not have the income to pay for these services. In addition, there are project costs connected with testing and evaluating the Philippines program as a pilot and paving the way for possible expansion of the program to other countries. It is not appropriate to expect the Philippines pilot to support the costs associated with this larger effort. Therefore, we have limited the goal of *Social Re*'s financial sustainability to the reinsurance effort. In other words, can *Social Re* cover the Philippine insurance-related costs from investment and premium income?

Premium contributions from the microinsurers are split into two portions: the portion necessary to cover the claims incurred and the portion available to support *Social Re*'s insurance operating expenses. In a scenario with a 75 percent loss ratio some of the income can be used to cover operating costs; if the loss ratio were 100 percent, all the premium would be used to cover incurred claims and none would be available to cover operating expenses. The income earned on *Social Re*'s surplus is also applied to insurance operating expenses. In this scenario, premium and investment income is sufficient to cover claims incurred and the fixed and variable costs of insurance operations in Manila.

When costs are separated into fixed and variable costs, it becomes clear that most of the insurance-related costs are fixed. The variable insurance costs are, for instance, more staff for underwriting, claims, and accounting, and a modest incremental cost in audit fees with sufficient growth in the number of microinsurers served. We estimate the variable cost of taking on another microinsurer at about US$2,300 per year.

The costs of technical assistance are almost completely variable in nature. These costs include salaries and expenses for microinsurer support staff, who work closely with the microinsurers and spend a great deal of time on site, and the cost of annual training for microinsurer staff in Manila. We estimate the variable cost of providing technical assistance and training to an additional microinsurer at about US$4,100 per year.

In addition, there are variable start-up costs associated with adding a microinsurer. Bringing microinsurer staff to Manila for a week of initial training would cost about US$2,000. Another US$5,000 per microinsurer in the first year is needed for computers and related equipment. A third cost results from the Philippine government requirement of a contribution to surplus equal to 0.2 percent of the maximum exposure. Assuming a benefit limit of PHP 50,000 (US$1,000) per insured family, the additional surplus requirement would be US$2 per family, or US$8,000 for a microinsurer insuring 4,000 families.

To recap, the variable costs associated with serving an additional microinsurer with 4,000 households would be US$21,400 (composed of US$15,000 one-time cost for training, equipment, and surplus increment; US$2,300 per year for reinsurance-related costs; and US$4,100 per year for technical assistance). This incremental cost analysis suggests that, once *Social Re* is up and running, it could add microinsurers for an incremental investment of US$1.68 per family. An annual subsidy of US$1.02 per family would be required to continue technical assistance to microinsurers at the level offered during this demonstration phase. The reinsurance program would be self-supporting in covering its operating costs and loss payments. If the technical assistance is effective and the microinsurers set sound contribution levels and effective methods to secure a high compliance rate, the system will be self-sustaining with this US$1 per family annual subsidy—less than the cost of a single course of many prescription drugs.

Based on the assumptions in the model, *Social Re* would need to enroll between 20 and 30 microinsurers to break even on insurance-related costs. Figure 22.1 illustrates the funding needs of *Social Re* up to the point when it can break even on the reinsurance operation. As can be seen, the need for external injection of capital is concentrated mostly during the initial three years.

FIGURE 22.1   Funding Needs of *Social Re*

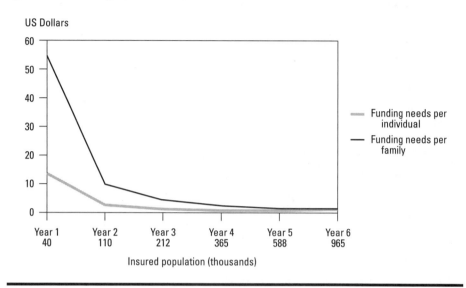

US Dollars

Year 1	Year 2	Year 3	Year 4	Year 5	Year 6
40	110	212	365	588	965

Insured population (thousands)

— Funding needs per individual
— Funding needs per family

CRITICAL UNCERTAINTIES AND RISKS

The success of *Social Re* is subject to the same uncertainties as any other business venture in a developing country. In general, good economic performance in the Philippines should improve the chances of success, because more people in the informal economy will be able to pay for membership in a microinsurance unit. Poor economic performance will likely reduce the number of people in the informal sector who could pay contributions for microinsurance, and the benefit packages could be more restrictive and less attractive, and thus narrow the *Social Re* market. Political instability could also likely make it harder to grow *Social Re*. A strong Philippine economy and stable political environment might generate larger tax revenue that could allow the government to extend PhilHealth coverage in the informal sector, mainly by lowering the premiums.

How *Social Re* is regulated may be less problematic than one might think (box 22.1). Management freedom will be greater if *Social Re* is not licensed as a registered insurance company early in its development. Because *Social Re* must be adequately capitalized and run in a business-like manner, it will meet some of the requirements imposed on registered insurance companies. The conversion to licensed status should be addressed during the pilot phase. The business plan here calls for funding that would allow the minimum capitalization requirements to be met from inception.

With many insurers, the adverse development of risks in the early years could destroy an experiment. We think this risk is muted with *Social Re*. So little is known about the dynamics of risk in microinsurance that initial loss ratios may be higher than anticipated. There is some risk of moral hazard on the part of microinsurers. *Social Re* will need to do much analytic work and refine its policy language so that it can differentiate epidemics, accidents, and random combinations of claims from poor microinsurer cost control. But this is part of the purpose of the *Social Re* pilot—to develop these techniques. As the analysis shows, the difference between a 75 percent loss ratio and 125 percent loss ratio is never more than US$72,000 per year in the baseline scenario, and is only US$144,000 if the number of insureds doubles. If *Social Re* lines up the funding called for in this business plan, it should be able to survive even if the loss ratio is higher than presumed.

The two biggest uncertainties are closely related. First, can *Social Re* sell its product to the microinsurers? The clear benefits that statistical analysis shows it offers (stabilization of financial performance and accumulation of discretionary budgets—see chapter 7) may not be enough by themselves to persuade some microinsurer decisionmakers to agree to pay a premium collected from poor members. Thus, *Social Re* will need to find donors who agree to finance a cut in the premium, or to offer incentives in terms of benefits enhancement.

That raises the second question: How large should introductory discounts be? Rate cuts and promotional benefits are standard in any business. But they can delay the point at which reinsurance becomes self-sustaining. Benefit enhancements can be continued only if a donor remains willing to cover the costs. Thus, *Social Re* has to resist the temptation of accepting business that depends only on excessive rate cuts or benefit enhancements. To the extent that it decides to make these offers, it must have a clear plan to wean client microinsurers from subsidies and move toward a relationship where premiums cover the ceded risk and most or all operating expenses. Otherwise, *Social Re*'s initial performance will not be sustainable after the pilot period. Donor funds will probably be available to cover the costs of discounts or benefit enhancements only for a short time. But *Social Re* would not be able to continue the premium subsidies on its own.

ANNEX 22A

TABLE 22A.1   Cost Factors Used on Financial Model

Cost factor	Value used	Sources
Revenues		
Premium from microinsurers	PHP 500–1,200 per family per year	ORT Health Plus (La Union) charges PHP 840–1800 per year with 85 percent compliance
		Tarlac charges PHP 2,160 per year; with 64 percent compliance collects 1,160
		Contributions to local health plans range from PHP 120–720 per year
		PHP 350 per year is average premium report
Premium subsidies		None assumed
Grants and donations		Amount necessary for operating revenue to cover expenses, plus any additional capital contribution required
Net investment income	6 percent	Return on amount invested at beginning of year
Expenses		
Reinsurance premiums		*Social Re* does not purchase reinsurance in early years of program
Incurred loss expenses		
Claims paid		15 percent of annual contribution per family to microinsurer times assumed loss ratio
Operating expenses		
Personnel		
Salaries		See attached schedule
Benefits		
Social Security	US$20	Per employee per month; reported by Manila-based consultant
Health insurance	US$100	Per employee per month; US$7 per month minimum for PhilHealth; US$142 per month reported by Manila-based consultant for private sector
Pension	10 percent	Of salary
Executive package		
Home rental, Makati	US$3,600	Per month; reported range = US$3,000–US$4,000
Househelp/guard	US$780	Per month for 3 people at PHP 12,000, 13 months per year
Utilities	US$360	Per month
Airfare for home leave	US$15,000	Estimated at US$3,750 per person, family of 4
Consultants		
Systems developer	US$50,000	Per year/years 1 and 2
Senior insurance advisor/ coach to Filipino C	US$20,000	Per quarter (10 days at US$2,000) start-up + year 1, US$10,000 per quarter (5 days at US$2,000) years 2 and 3
Research and evaluation consultant	US$5,000/US$20,000/ US$25,000	Years 1/2/3

(Table continues on the following page.)

TABLE 22A.1 (continued)

Cost factor	Value used	Sources
General office		
Occupancy	US$3,400	Per employee per year, based on monthly cost of US$17.90/sq m per month for rent, utilities and air condition, allowing 16sq m per employee
Additional start-up costs for build-out	US$12,000	Estimated at US$140/sq m,[a] 16sq m per employee less US$1,150 allowance for furniture; US$1,000 per employee
Office equipment	US$9,500	Per employee
Telephone	US$300	Per employee (current U.S. cost)
Computer	US$2,450	Per employee (current U.S. cost)
Computer for microinsurers	US$5,000	Microinsurer or new microinsurers
Software	US$600	Per employee (current U.S. cost)
Furniture	US$1,150	Per employee (50 percent of current U.S. cost)
Office supplies	US$25	Per employee per month; based on general experience
Communications		
Internet	US$400	Per month quoted by Manila-based consultant
Telephone		
Manila	US$150	Per employee per month = amount budgeted for international office in Manila
Geneva	US$8,000	
Printing and copying		
Copier purchase	US$10,000	High-end copier in United States; US$13,000
Service	US$100	Per month (half U.S. rate)
Printed program materials	US$5,000	Per year estimated
Postage and shipping	US$400	Per month; amount budgeted for office of 13 in Manila
Travel and meetings		
Fares/rates		
Airfare, round trip, Europe or United States to Manila	US$2,500	Actual cost, 2001 (US$2,243) + 10 percent
Per diem, Manila or Europe/United States	US$160	International Labour Office per diem, 2001
Airfare, domestic (round trip Manila/Davao)	US$145	Reported by Manila-based consultant
Per diem, outside Manila	US$111	Reported by Manila-based consultant
Number of trips		
Chair (Geneva-based)		Start-up: 1 8-day round trip to Manila per month for 6 months, then 6 8-day round trips to Manila per year + 4 other trips at US$2,500
CEO (Manila-based)		4 5-day round trips to Europe/United States
Technical support staff		18 3-day round trips within Philippines per staff person
Microinsurer training		3 5-day round trips to Manila per microinsurer + additional 3 5-day round trips to Manila for new microinsurers

Cost factor	Value used	Sources
Advisor to CEO (Europe/ United States–based) Evaluation consultant		5-day round trip to Manila: start-up = 2 round trips, year 1 = 6 round trips, years 2 and 3 = 4 round trips 2 2-week trips to Manila + 1 5-day trip to Geneva, years 2 and 3
Professional services and other fees		
Directors' fees		Covered by sponsor agency
Legal Manila Corporate	US$5,000 US$20,000	500 hours per year at US$10 per hour Start-up cost for incorporation, and so on
Claims processing		No variable cost if *Social Re* writes aggregate excess coverage
Audit Microinsurers Manila Corporate	US$300 US$2,000 US$2,500	Microinsurer for 3 days' review @ US$100/day 20 days @ US$100/day Per year
Actuarial/epidemiological Manila Corporate	US$40,0000/ US$40,000/ US$14,800 US$15,000	2 months junior at US$30 per hour, 1 month senior at US$65/hr, 1 month external actuary at and 2; US$125/hour, years 1 and 2; 2 months junior + 2 weeks senior in year 3 Epidemiology analysis, year 1 only
Government fees (regulatory, licensing)		None assumed
Brokerage		None assumed
Banking	US$1,000	
Other		None assumed
Insurance (liability, D & O)		None assumed
Benefit enhancements		None assumed
Interest/dividends		
Taxes		None assumed

Note: CEO, Chief Executive Officer. PHP, Philippine Pesos. CFO, Chief Financial Officer. CIO, Chief Information Officer. MUI, Microinsurer.
a. Based on 12 employees.

TABLE 22A.2 Salary Schedule for Manila Office

| | | | | | | Year 1 | | | | |
| | | | | | | | Reinsurance function | | Data | Ancillary functions | |
Staff positions	Location	Level	Start-up costs (US$)	All depts.	Management	Underwriting	Claims	technical information	Technical assistance	Notes
Total salary			50,000	249,000	144,000	30,000	10,000	35,000	30,000	
1 Chair	Central	Sr./Geneva								
2 Secretary	Central	Staff/Geneva								
3 CEO	Manila	Sr. Exec.	18,750	75,000	75,000	0	0	0	0	3 mos start-up
4 CFO/CIO	Manila	Sr.	12,500	50,000	25,000	0	0	25,000	0	3 mos start-up
5 Government relations manager	Manila	Mid+	7,500	30,000	30,000	0	0	0	0	3 mos start-up
6 Principal underwriter	Manila	Mid+	7,500	30,000	0	30,000	0	0	0	3 mos start-up
7 Underwriting staff	Manila	Mid		0	0	0	0	0	0	
8 Claims manager	Manila	Mid		10,000	0	0	10,000	0	0	1day/mo /microinsurer
9 Microinsurer support staff (3)	Man/field	Mid		30,000	0	0	0	0	30,000	
10 Systems manager	Manila	Mid		0	0	0	0	0	0	
11 Technical support	Manila	Staff	2,500	10,000	0	0	0	10,000	0	3 mos start-up
12 Administrative assistant	Manila	Staff	1,250	5,000	5,000	0	0	0	0	3 mos start-up
13 Bookkeeper	Manila	Staff		7,000	7,000	0	0	0	0	
14 Office assistant ("tea lady")	Manila	Staff		2,000	2,000	0	0	0	0	

#	Number of staff	Max # MIUs	Salary rate	6	12.0	5.5	1.0	1.0	1.0	1.5	3.0
1	Chair										
2	Secretary										
3	CEO		75,000		1.0	1.0					
4	CFO/CIO		50,000		1.0	0.5				0.5	
5	Government relations manager		30,000	1.0	1.0						
6	Principal underwriter		30,000		1.0		1				
7	Underwriting staff	40	10,000		0.0		0				
8	Claims manager	20	10,000		1.0				1		
9	Microinsurer support staff (3)	8	10,000		3.0					3	min = 3
10	Systems manager		20,000		0.0					0	starts year 3
11	Technical support	25	10,000		1.0					1	
12	Administrative assistant		5,000		1.0	1.0					1 per 5 mgt staff
13	Bookkeeper	20	7,000		1.0	1.0					
14	Office assistant ("tea lady")		2,000		1.0	1.0					

Note: CEO, Chief Executive Officer. PHP, Philippine Pesos. CFO, Chief Financial Officer. CIO, Chief Information Officer. MUI, Microinsurer.
a. One position is fixed, additional variable.

NOTES

1. Five to seven years is a more likely period to become fully self-supporting.

2. This parameter will yield the percentage of microinsurers' contribution revenue allocated to reinsurance.

REFERENCES

Dror, D.M. 2001. "Reinsurance of Health Insurance for the Informal Sector." *Bulletin of the World Health Organization* 79(7):672–78.

Preker, A.S., G. Carrin, D.M. Dror, M. Jakab, W. Hsiao, and D. Arhin-Tenkorang. 2001. "Health Care Financing for Rural Low Income Populations: The Role of Communities in Resource Mobilization and Risk Sharing: A Synthesis Report." Report submitted to Working Group 3 of the Commission on Macroeconomics and Health, Jeffrey D. Sachs (chairman). Geneva: World Health Organization. http://www.cmhealth.org/wg3.htm

Data Template: A Framework for Accounting and Statistics

David M. Dror and Rakesh Rathi

T his manual explains how to use the *Social Re Data Template* (v. 1.0) software. It explains the purpose of all the data forms and gives advice on operating the system.

THE *SOCIAL RE* PROJECT

The *Social Re* project is governed by the thought that poverty and illness are linked to exposure to many risks, which can be reduced or mitigated by insurance, microinsurance, and reinsurance.

The major activity planned is to enlarge access of the poor to health insurance and sustain services offered by community-financed health schemes (microinsurance units), by guaranteeing their solvency under a plan called *Social Re.*

Social Re would provide reinsurance to microinsurers in return for payment of a premium. In addition to this premium, participating microinsurers must agree to record, validate, analyze, and transmit information. This information serves two purposes: first, it is needed to enhance the microinsurers' chances of being managed efficiently and of remaining solvent in the interest of serving the membership; second, it is needed to cede risks to a reinsurer. The second objective hinges on the microinsurers' ability to provide the statistical information needed to calculate the reinsurance premium. Stated differently, the output of the processed information serves as the input for the reinsurance calculation module (called the *Social Re Toolkit* and described in appendix B, this volume). The purpose of the *Social Re Data Template* is to identify the information microinsurers need to provide, and to format it as a user-friendly and simple computer application that can interface electronically with the *Toolkit.*

For reviewing a draft of this appendix, the authors thank Robert Fonteneau, Senior Specialist, Caisse Nationale d'Assurance Maladie, Paris, detailed to the Social Protection Sector, International Labour Office, Geneva.

OVERVIEW OF THE *DATA TEMPLATE:* OPTIONS AND NAVIGATION

The software application contains all the cumulative data on members, the contributions they pay, and the benefits they can receive. The confidentiality of such a database must be protected and secured so that only authorized (and trained) staff can access the information. The login screen is therefore password protected (figure A.1).

Upon entry into the application, authorized users access a menu with five button-activated options (figure A.2). Each button calls up a corresponding screen that allows tracking of information about members, contributions paid, claim transactions, and details of the qualifying conditions applicable to benefits.

- *Member Details* displays a detailed form for adding/updating/deleting details about individual members.

- *Member Transaction Details* displays a form for processing individual transactions.

- *Actual Contribution Paid* displays a form to add/update contribution payments, and follow up the compliance rate for each paying member.

- *Import Data* displays a form for importing tables from other databases (notably the referential database of this application, kept separately for ease of operation).

- *Reports* displays a menu page that allows the user to view several standard reports (exportable to the *Social Re Toolkit*).

FIGURE A.1   Screen 1

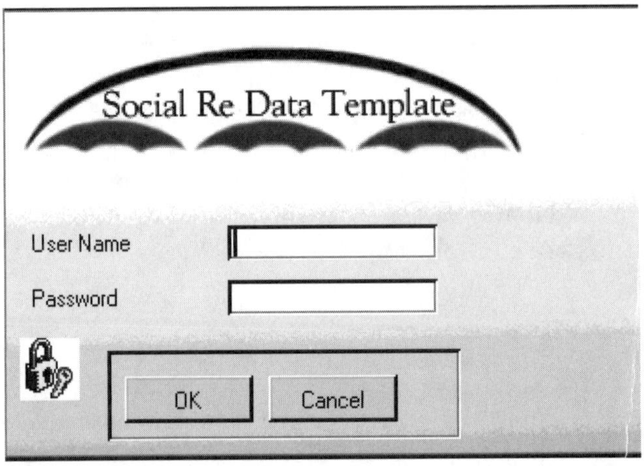

FIGURE A.2   Screen 2

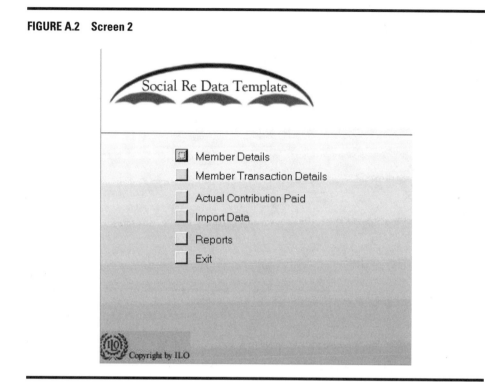

Selection 1: Member Details

When the user selects the *Member Details* option on the menu, the screen displays a form allowing the user to add/delete/update information on the member (figure A.3).

Adding a New Record

To add a new member to the system, click the *Add* button. This enables all the entry fields. All fields providing information for calculations is mandatory; other information is optional (optional fields have been included to allow microinsurers who so wish to collect the additional information).

Automatic Validation

Mandatory fields are validated automatically.

- *Member Name.* If the user leaves the "Member Name" blank, an error message is displayed.

- *Date of Birth.* The member's Date of Birth must be earlier than the current date, cannot be blank, and must be recorded in the month/day/year format;

FIGURE A.3   Screen 3

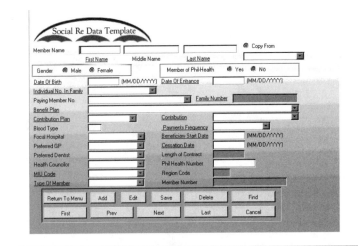

an error message is displayed in case of error, and the pointer goes to Date of Birth field.

- *Cessation Date.* The user-entered Cessation Date must be later than the Affiliation Date. If the data are invalid, an error message flashes: "Cessation Date cannot be earlier than Affiliation Date."

- *Microinsurer's Code.* If the Microinsurer's Code is not found in the database, an error message flashes: "Code Does Not Exist."

- *Duplicate Checks.* New entries are compared with existing entries by Name and Date of Birth. They are unique to each member. The unique Member Number is generated automatically.

Mandatory Fields

All of the following fields must be filled in on the Member Details Form: First Name, Last Name, Gender, Date of Birth, Microinsurance Unit (MIU) Code, Type of Member, Date of Entrance, Benefit Plan, Contribution Plan, Frequency of Payment, Waiting Period, and Cessation Date.

Optional Fields

The following fields can be filled in on the Member Details Form: Middle Name, PhilHealth number (see more details below), blood type, focal hospital, preferred medical practitioner (general practitioner, dentist), health counselor.

PhilHealth Number

This number is an identifier issued by PhilHealth for all its members. When the option "Member of PhilHealth" is selected on the form, this number must be entered. These data are optional for nonmembers of PhilHealth.

Automatic Fields

The software automatically updates the following fields: Region Code (selected from the MIU Code), Member Number (see more details below), and Beneficiary Start Date (calculated from Date of Entrance and Waiting Period).

Generation of Member Number

The Member Number is a unique identification number generated by the Data Template for every member. This number is a combination of the following multiple fields: 1. Country; 2. Region; 3. MIU Code; 4. Family Number; 5. Individual Number.

Automated Generation of Family Number

The Family Number is a 5-digit number generated on selection of Individual Number. The calculation of Family Number involves two cases:

Case a. When the Individual Number in family is 00. In this case the Family Number is a sequential number that is incremented on every save, for example, for the first record when the individual member in family is 00 the Family Number would be 00001. For the next record it would be 00002, and so on.

Case b. When the Individual Number in family is not 00. In this case the user has to select the data for Paying Member Number. Here the family number is a value picked up from the Paying Member Number. The characters 10–14 of the Paying Member Number represent its family number. This value is used as the Family Number for the dependent member. For example, for Paying Member Number INDR01P010001000 the family number would be 00010.

Multiple Choice Fields

Several fields may have more than one valid value; all valid values are accessible in the *Drop Down Boxes*. Fields with a pull-down menu include benefit plan, contribution plan, frequency of payment, and the choice of services provider(s) where applicable (for example, Focal Hospital, Preferred General Practitioner, Preferred Dentist, Health Counselor).

Confirming New Records

To save the record, click the *Save* button. To prevent a new record from being saved in the database, click the *Cancel* button.

Find Record

To find a member, select the *Find* button. A dialog box is displayed in which the user must type the member's name. Clicking the *Find First* or *Find Next* buttons takes the user from one record to the next. If the record is not found, a message will be displayed that it has not been found.

Delete Record

To delete a record from the database, first find that member's record, then click the *Delete* button.

Navigation

Arrow buttons take the user to the First, Previous, Next, or Last record. Clicking *First* displays "You are on First Record," and the *First* and *Previous* buttons are disabled. Clicking *Next* displays the next record, and enables the *Previous* and *First* buttons. To move to the previous record, click the *Previous* button. Repeated clicks on this button take the user from the current location to the first record in the database. By repeatedly clicking the *Next* button, the user can reach the last record. At that point, the *Next* and *Last* buttons are disabled. To go straight to the last record, click the *Last* button.

Wild Card Search

This option allows the user to perform a character-based search of names. The option allows the user to search members whose name begins or ends with certain characters.

Case a. To see the members whose names start with "R" type R* and click on the *Find* option. This will show a list of members whose names start with "R". Use *First*, *Next*, *Previous*, and *Last* to navigate through the records.

Case b. To see the members whose names end with "sh" type *sh and click on the *Find* option. This will show a list of members whose names end with "sh." Use *First*, *Next*, *Previous*, and *Last* to navigate through the records.

Case c. To see the members whose names have "ro" type *ro* and click on the *Find* option. Use *First*, *Next*, *Previous*, and *Last* to navigate through the records.

Selection 2: Member Transaction Details

This option displays a screen that allows the user to record claim transactions (use and cost of services) (figure A.4).

FIGURE A.4   Screen 4

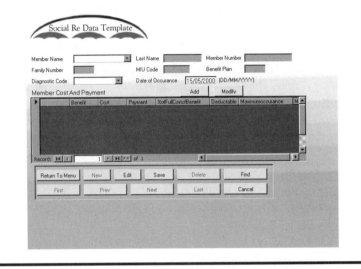

Adding a Member Transaction

The user can add a new record, or find, update, or delete an existing record.

- *Identification.* Click the *Add* button to add information about a member's use of a health service covered by the benefit package; then select the Member Number (list provided electronically). This automatically connects the transaction record with the referential details (for example, the applicable benefit package and family details essential for dependents).

- *Transaction details.* Select a Diagnostic Code from the list provided, then enter date of treatment (default Date of Occurrence is the current date). The user selects the relevant Benefit Type from those included in the Benefit Package for which the member is registered. Last, the cost data are entered, and the system automatically calculates the amount payable by the microinsurer, according to qualifying conditions that have been predefined for the specific benefit type and benefit package.

- *Saving and duplication check.* The entry is recorded by clicking the *Save* button. Once saved, the same transaction cannot be entered again.

Finding, Updating, or Deleting a Record

Any future reference to a recorded transaction requires finding it first. Transactions are always recorded for a member, and clicking the *Find* button will display a dialog box, where the user must type in the Member Number. Once the right record is found, clicking *Delete/Update* allows the user to make changes. To delete a record, find the record, and then click the *Delete* button.

Displaying Qualifying Conditions of a Benefit

When the user selects the Benefit utilized by the member, the system displays the actual payment made by the MIU, percentage of full cost of Benefit, Deductible, Maximum Occurrence, and Maximum Amount for one occurrence, which are defined in the screen designed for this purpose (figure A.5).

Selection 3: Actual Contribution Paid

This option displays a form to add/update members' contribution payments. This form automatically calculates the updated Compliance Rate (for each month and the average).

Calculation of the Compliance Rate

All payments made by a member are recorded on a screen designed for this purpose (figure A.6). Based on payments made and payments due, the Compliance Rate is automatically calculated.

FIGURE A.5   Screen 5

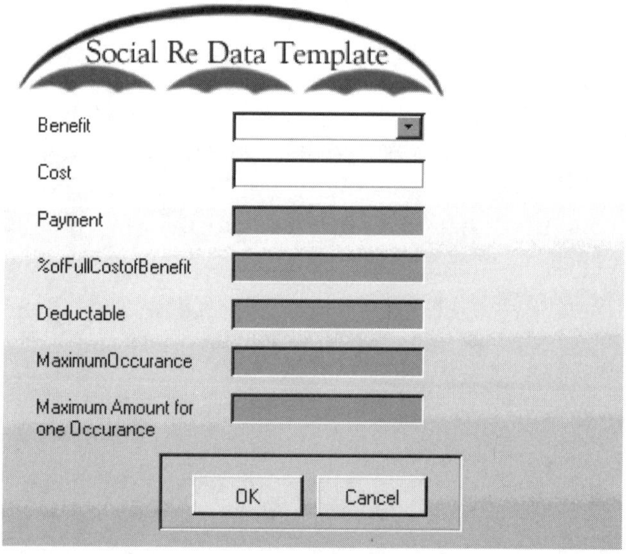

FIGURE A.6   Screen 6

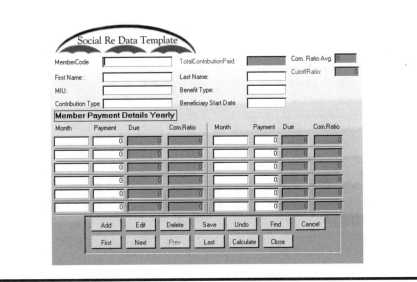

The Compliance Rate for each month is a ratio of the total contribution paid until the current month divided by the total amount due until the current month. For example, if the amount paid is 500 and the amount due is 100, then the compliance rate would be 500/100 = 5.

The Compliance Rate Average is calculated for a period of 12 months (or a calendar year) and is a ratio of the total Compliance Rate and 12. For example, if the total Compliance Rate is 100, then the Compliance Rate average would be 100/12 = 8.3333.

Selection 4: Import Data

This option displays a form for importing tables from other databases (notably the referential database of this application, kept separately for ease of operation).

To import a referential table, the user has to enter the exact name of the database, followed by a selection of the table from the pull-down menu. Failure to identify the database will cause an error message: "Database Name Not Specified." Failure to select a table will also cause an error message: "Table Name Not Specified."

Selection 5: Reports

This option takes the user to some standard reports. These reports can be viewed on screen and can be printed. The data for the reports are extracted from the previous screens.

HOW THE *DATA TEMPLATE* WORKS

The microinsurer needs to offer all members a coherent contract, under which every person knows up front what she or he must pay and what she or he can expect to get from the plan. The microinsurer also needs to furnish the reinsurer with financial information that will be necessary for the reinsurance contract. The main purpose of the *Data Template* is to facilitate the task of the microinsurer in deciding which items of information are necessary. The following sections will describe the use of the *Data Template* for the relationship with the membership and with the reinsurer.

Relations with Members

The contract between the microinsurer and each member is determined by two conditions: fixing the coverage of the member ("the benefit") and fixing the contribution the member needs to pay. The benefit package may change from one microinsurance unit to another, depending on the members' priorities and the resources available. The contributions may also vary from one place to another, not only because incomes and prices diverge but also because the priorities of different communities may drive them to select a different subscription unit (for example, individual, nuclear family, extended family). This is why the exact conditions of the contract must be written down in advance: the list of specific benefits the microinsurer agrees to pay and the contribution structure that the member agrees to pay.

In principle, total income must be large enough to cover the cost of benefits plus the cost of administering the scheme. This is why a balance sheet is needed, to reflect the financial status of the microinsurer. The relationship between the reinsurer and the microinsurer is also based on this information.

Relations with the Reinsurer

When reinsuring, the microinsurer transfers part of its risk to another agent and also agrees to transfer part of the contribution income as the reinsurance premium. The reinsurer agrees to cover the cost of claims above a certain level and must be satisfied that the microinsurer can pay all costs up to this predefined threshold. To calculate the premium, the reinsurer has to know the expected total benefit cost[1] and the total contributions due[2] and must also estimate the risk it is taking (that is, its own probability of survival with the amounts of premium it collects and the degree of risk it agrees to cover). These estimates are usually based on the mean and the standard deviation of the observed cost of care[3] and its probability. Since most microinsurers cannot provide this information, the reinsurer has to estimate these figures by using various alternative techniques, based on data that can be collected.

As stated above, the *Data Template* gives the microinsurer a structured format to record the data elements it needs for orderly management of its relations with the members. The *Social Re Data Template* will be used in the field, in poor, rural areas. Many of these locations are far from cities or large medical centers. Many microinsurers cannot afford to employ skilled technicians or medical personnel trained in statistics or accounting. The *Data Template* has been developed to reduce the cost and anxiety of collecting the data needed for reinsurance. The application is designed to be operated on an uncomplicated platform and by operators that can be trained within a few days. Once collected by the microinsurer, data can be transferred for complex statistical calculations to the reinsurer.

PLATFORM

The *Social Re Data Template* application is designed to operate from a low-cost, widely used and available platform. The operating system is Windows NT or Windows 2000 /XP versions, and the software is MS Access 97/2000, with C++ scripting and Visual Basic for Applications (VBA scripting).

The application will also have referential tables that can be maintained on a separate database, written in MS Access 97 or 2000. The two databases are seamlessly interfaced to allow electronic transfer of data ("importation") in both directions.

NOTES

1. The cumulative amount of *expected benefit costs* payable by a specific microinsurer to all members during one *financial period.*

2. The amount the microinsurer expects to collect from its members during a *financial period*, according to the applicable *contribution plans.*

3. This would include both what the microinsurer pays as benefit and the amount paid by the member as *out-of-pocket.*

Toolkit Users' Manual

Stéphane Bonnevay, Gérard Duru, and Michel Lamure

Here, we describe version 1.1 of the toolkit related to the model proposed for stabilizing microinsurance schemes from a financial point of view. The toolkit simulates the workings of a system in which several microinsurance units (MIUs) are reinsured by *Social Re*. Input data are of two kinds, depending on whether the user wants to work with benefit packages proposed by the microinsurers or with diagnostics. Input data are stored in an Excel (XLS) file with two preformatted sheets: one for benefit packages, the other for diagnostics.

All numerical results of simulations are also stored in XLS files, one file for each microinsurer and one for *Social Re*. The XLS files related to microinsurers include a sheet for each time period in the simulation. The *Social Re* file includes only one sheet containing results for the final simulation period. Graph outputs can be captured with any type of image-transformation software.

HOW TO LAUNCH A SIMULATION

To launch the toolkit, double click the program icon. The first window appears (figure B.1).

By clicking the appropriate button, the user can select a working environment for the simulation—based on diagnosis data or on benefit package data. Clicking the *Ok* button prompts display of a new window. By clicking the *Help* button, the user can get information on how to use the toolkit. To leave the application, click the *Quit* button.

Whichever white square is checked, clicking the *Ok* button displays the corresponding window (figure B.2).

The new window includes a panel and three buttons. The *Simulate* button cannot be clicked until the data are read. The panel allows the user to define the global parameters of the simulation:

- The number of time periods in the simulation. The default value is 3.

- The number of replications in the simulation. The default value is 50. For computation time reasons, the default value should not be set too high. The toolkit

FIGURE B.1   Window 1

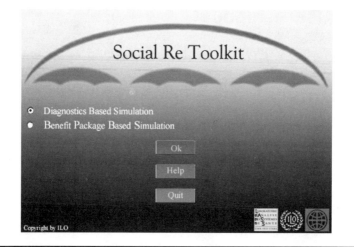

FIGURE B.2   Window 2

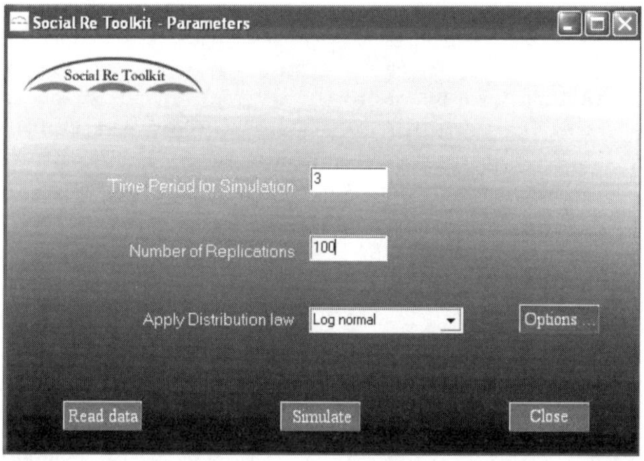

simulates the way reinsurance of microinsurers works for 21 different values of the parameter W that determines financial characteristics (for example, excess, reserve fund—see model). In the toolkit, the parameter Ω varies from 0 to 1 by step of 0.05.

- Type of probability distribution to model charges distribution. In that version, we implemented five distributions: Chi square distribution, Erlang distribution, Exponential distribution, Gamma distribution, and Lognormal distribution.

As mentioned above, before launching the simulation, the user must read the data by clicking the *Read data* button. Clicking that button displays the next dialog box (figure B.3).

FIGURE B.3   Window 3

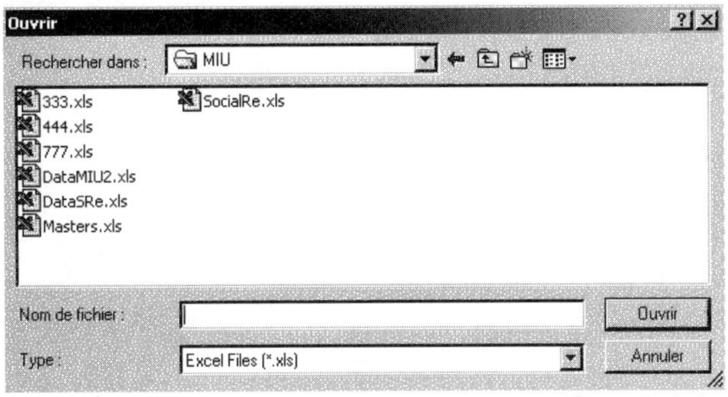

The user can select the appropriate XLS file (here, the file "DataMIU2.xls), read the data, and the *Simulate* button becomes active. By clicking it, the user launches the simulation.

By clicking the *Close* button, the user closes the window in figure B.2 and returns to the first window (figure B.1). Then, the user can select a different working environment or quit the application.

DISPLAYING THE RESULTS

There are two kinds of results:

- Numerical results, stored in XLS files

- Graph results, displayed in separate windows

For each microinsurance unit, the following numerical results are given for each time period and each value of the Ω parameter (see model):

- Microinsurer's average discretionary budget

- Microinsurer's minimum discretionary budget

- Microinsurer's maximum discretionary budget

- Standard deviation of microinsurer's discretionary budget

- Microinsurer's survival probability, if not reinsured

- Microinsurer's survival probability, when reinsured (always equal to 1)

- Premium paid to *Social Re*

- Amount of excess (a constant)

- Size of microinsurer's reserve fund

For *Social Re*, the following numerical results are given for the last time period and for each value of the W parameter (see model):

- *Social Re*'s average discretionary budget

- *Social Re*'s minimum discretionary budget

- *Social Re*'s maximum discrctionary budget

- Standard deviation of *Social Re*'s discretionary budget

- *Social Re*'s survival probability

There are three kinds of graph outputs:

- On discretionary budgets

- On excess and premium

- On survival probabilities

The graphics windows are displayed in reduced size. To enlarge the image, click on the middle rectangle at the top right of the window.

Outputs on microinsurers' discretionary budgets are given time period by time period. Each diagram shows three curves for different values of the m parameter:

- Minimum discretionary budget

- Average discretionary budget

- Maximum discretionary budget

Those diagrams must be displayed for each microinsurance unit and for each time period. To avoid filling up the screen, we display only one window by type of curve to be drawn. Each of those windows shows three parameters: maximum, average, and minimum discretionary budget size for one microinsurer in one time period (figure B.4). At the bottom of the window, there are two dialog lists, one for selecting the microinsurance unit, the other for selecting the time period. Thus, by combining those two selections, the user can display all results he or she wants.

With specialized software (for example, Paint Shop Pro™), the user can insert any diagram into a report.

Each diagram shows, according to the values of the Ω parameter, the survival probability of *Social Re* and of the microinsurer, when not reinsured. A microinsurer's survival probability can be displayed by selecting the microinsurer from the dialog list at the bottom of the window (figure B.5).

Again, those diagrams can be captured for other uses by appropriate software.

AN INTERACTIVE WINDOW

Simulations for different values of the Ω parameter give computed pairs of values (Ω_i, Pr_i), i = 1,..,21, where Pr_i denotes the survival probability of either *Social Re* or a microinsurer, when not reinsured.

FIGURE B.4   Window 4

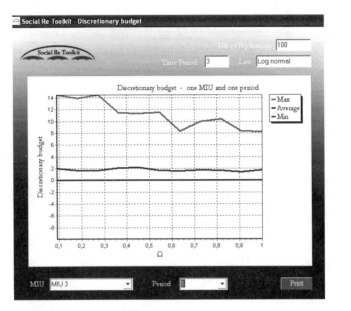

FIGURE B.5   Window 5

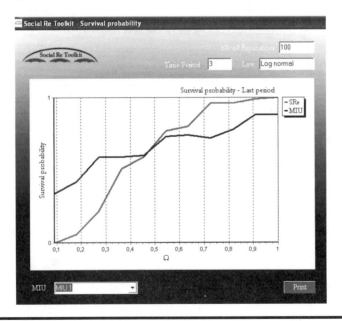

Using the curve-fitting technique of cubic splines, we can determine the survival probability of *Social Re* or any microinsurer for any value of Ω, between 0 and 1. We can compute the balance of the *Social Re* for any value of Ω between 0 and 1 the same way.

The principle of cubic splines allows the approximation of the curve by arcs of polynomial functions of degree 3 as, at each computed point of the curve in the simulation, the polynomial function is a continuous and derivable function. This yields a smooth curve with good mathematical properties. Computing that curve is quick and easy. The toolkit includes computations of that fitted curve for three items:

- *Social Re* survival probability

- Microinsurer's survival probability when not reinsured

- *Social Re* balance

Glossary of Terms

GLOSSARY OF TERMS, GENERAL

Ability/willingness to pay. Often inappropriately assumed to be equivalent. Willingness to pay (WTP) is mediated by ability to pay (ATP) and by individual and cultural aspects that determine the perceived benefit to self and to the community. There are two ways to assess WTP:

- Data on past health care utilization and expenditure

- Contingent valuation methods based on surveys

Ability to pay (ATP). Largely determined by affordability. ATP for health insurance must be considered in the context of copayments and transaction costs. The concept of fairness may be an important consideration in designing a microinsurance scheme and setting premiums.

Accountability. Result of the process that ensures that decisionmakers at all levels actually carry out their designated responsibilities and that they are held accountable for their actions.

Actual premium. The premium arrived at by estimating the average benefit payout and adding a safety margin for contingencies.

Actuary. This person compiles statistics on events and works out their probabilities (including joint probabilities) and premiums.

Adverse selection. Problem of asymmetric information that disturbs the operation of the insurance market, resulting in an inequitable transaction. The insured, knowing the likelihood of events, chooses to insure against only those that pose a strong risk. The insurer, having less information, accepts a contract that does not include premiums for low-risk events. The insured gains from the insurer's inability to distinguish "good" and "bad" risks.

Affordability. See Ability to pay.

Agent. Another term for insurer.

Ambulatory care. Outpatient medical care provided in any health care setting except hospitals.

Asymmetrical information. Parties to a transaction have uneven access to relevant information that governs an informed choice. Such asymmetry can result in an inequitable transaction in favor of the party with the most information, or it can result in the abandonment of the exchange.

Balance sheet. Statement showing the financial position at a particular point in time (for example, at the end of the financial year), listing all assets and liabilities at that time.

Bayesian method. A method (originally enunciated in 1763) for revising the probability of an event's occurrence by taking into account data as they come to hand. The usefulness of this approach depends on the relevance and power of the additional data.

Beneficiary or principal. The person designated to receive payouts from the scheme. This is typically the policyholder or a family member, but it may be an employer.

Benefit exclusion. Refusal of access to a specific benefit for an insured. Because this exclusion could be subject to abuse if it is based on arbitrary decisions made at the time of claim rather than as set out in the contract, it tends to be regulated. Reasons for exclusion that are typically allowed include a qualifying period and preexisting illness.

Benefit package or compensation. A list of specific benefits agreed upon in the health insurance contract. While private insurance typically offers modules of benefits from which to choose, microinsurers may offer a standard package for simplicity and fairness.

Beta distribution. Beta is a distribution (first used by Gini, 1911) for a real random variable whose density function is null outside the interval [0, 1] and depends on two strictly real parameters. The shape of this distribution depends on the values of the parameters: it can be U-shaped, or J-shaped, or hat-shaped. For this reason, this distribution is very often used for modeling proportions or probabilities.

Binomial distribution. A statistical method for understanding the probability of events that have only two possible outcomes—"success" or "failure." These probabilities are constant. In insurance, the binomial distribution is applied to estimate the number of persons in a community who will seek (ambulatory) care in a given period.

Bottom-up. See Top-down global strategy.

Broker. An intermediary who sells on behalf of another.

Capacity. Has two meanings:

- Insurers' ability to underwrite a large amount of risk on a single loss exposure or many contracts on one line of event. Reinsurance enables a greater capacity among primary insurers.

- Organizational and individual skills. Organizational capacity implies appropriate systems for information and management and adequate resources for handling operations.

Capacity building. Increasing organizational and individual skills and establishing frameworks for that increase to continue.

Central limit theorem. States that, as the sample size increases, the characteristics of the sample will more closely approximate those of the population from which that sample was drawn. This theorem is valuable in health insurance as it enables estimates of risk in a population to be based on sample data.

Cession and retrocession. The relationship between the primary insurer and the reinsurer is based on the clear definition of the premium to be paid by the microinsurer in return for transferring (ceding) risk to the reinsurer. The risk transferred to the reinsurer is called cession. The insurer may also transfer risk to another primary insurer, which is called retrocession.

Claim load. The amount of benefits paid to the insureds in a period. Fluctuations in claim load in the short term are covered by contingency reserves and in the long run by contribution increases.

Coefficient of variation. The ratio of the sample standard deviation to the sample mean. It measures the spread of a set of data as a proportion of its mean. It is often expressed as a percentage. This coefficient enables, for example, estimation and comparison of ranges of likely expenses for various communities.

Coinsurance. Spreads a risk too great for a single insurer over several companies that together act as coinsurers.

Collection rate or compliance rate. The proportion of possible subscriptions from members that the microinsurer collects. Lack of complete compliance can result from cultural as well as economic factors. It may be used as a measure of a microinsurer's efficiency/commercial orientation. Members are more likely to pay contributions if their perceived risk is higher.

Community. A group of people with a common interest. Often implies locality, but can be occupation-, leisure-, or religion-based.

Community financing scheme. See Community-based health insurance.

Community participation. Sharing by citizens in any kind of community in communal decisionmaking processes and definitions of problems.

Community rating. A method for determining insurance rates on the basis of the average cost of providing health services in a specific geographic area. This method ignores the individual's medical history or the likelihood of the individual's using the services.

Community-based health insurance. Community initiatives to generate health care financing through voluntary prepayment schemes.

Compensation. Benefit payout.

Compliance. Payment of contribution owed by members.

Compliance gap. Difference between contributions due and contributions collected.

Compliance rate. The ratio of actual contributions over potential contributions. See Collection rate.

Compulsory insurance. Any form of insurance the purchase of which is required by law. Governments typically require the purchase of liability insurance with respect to three types of potential loss-causing activities: those whose severity could be particularly great, with the possibility of large numbers of innocent persons being harmed because of a single event; those whose frequency is sufficiently great to affect large numbers of innocent persons independently; and those judged to be inherently dangerous.

Confidence interval. A range of values that is estimated to contain the population parameter. To be 95 percent confident that a range contains the parameter requires a larger range than to be 90 percent confident. For example, analysis of data from a community might suggest a 90 percent chance that the number of people seeking hospitalization in a year will be between 1,100 and 1,500, but the confidence interval for 95 percent confidence is 978 and 1,747.

Contingency reserves or equalization reserves. Funds held by the insurer that are in excess of expected benefit payouts in order to cover unexpected events (contingencies) that cause fluctuations in benefit payouts. They are typically regulated in order to ensure the insurer's solvency.

Contribution base. The amount that would be available to the insurer if all members contributed fully. When contributions are set as a percentage of income, this base relies on full disclosure of income (disclosure rate).

Contribution rate. The percentage of contribution base actually or expected to be collected.

Contribution. Payment of an agreed sum of money by a member to a social insurance system in return for specified benefits. The implied assumption is that other sources of income complement members' payments. See also Premium.

Cooperative. A group of people who have united voluntarily to realize a common goal, by establishing a democratically run company, providing an equitable quota of the necessary capital, and accepting a fair share of the risks and the profits of this company. Members also take an active part in its operation.

Copayment or cost sharing. The portion of medical expenses paid by a member/beneficiary. This amount is the balance remaining after the insurer has paid its portion.

Cost sharing. See Copayment.

Covariance. A measure of the relationship between two variables. Covariance does not specifically imply a cause-and-effect relationship ("causation"), although it may intuitively be inferred to exist, as can its direction. For example, if health problems vary with housing density, it may be possible to infer that density affects health, but the observed covariance of the frequency of schizophrenia with social status may not have a simple unidirectional explanation.

Covariant risk. When events are not independent, the occurrence of one may affect the occurrence of another. For example, the risk of one family member's catching influenza is covariant with that of another family member. Disasters and shocks are classic cases where proximity influences covariation. When insuring against risk of events, the actuary must consider the covariation between those risks.

Cream skimming (Preferred risk selection). An exercise whereby an insurer selects only a part of a larger heterogeneous risk group ("preferred risks"), in which all individuals pay an identical risk-adjusted premium. When the insurer reduces its loss ratio compared with the expected average cost that determined the premium, the insurer can retain a profit from cream skimming. This profit depends on the insurer's ability to distinguish several subgroups with different expected costs within the larger group, and to predict the (lower) future health care expenditure of individuals in the preferred group.

Cross-subsidies. Amounts effectively paid when the wealthy members pay more than poor, or when the healthy pay the same as the sick for lower expected benefits. The poor and the sick are said to receive cross-subsidies from the wealthy and healthy.

Crude birth rate. A summary measurement of the total number of live births in a specified population at the end of a specific time period (generally one year), divided by the midyear total population count. Expressed as the number of births per 1,000 people within that population.

Crude death rate. A summary measurement of the total number of deaths in a specified population at the end of a specific time period (generally one year), divided by the midyear total population count. Expressed as the number of deaths per 1,000 people within that population.

Data template. Social Re has developed a standard system to record, organize, analyze, audit, validate, manage, interrogate, and report data. That system is embodied in the data template.

Declaration rate. See Contribution base.

Deductible. A provision requiring the insured to pay part of the loss before the insurer makes any payment under the terms of the policy. Deductibles typically are found in property, health, and automobile insurance contracts. The purpose of establishing deductibles is to eliminate small claims and reduce the average pure premium and administrative costs associated with claims handling. Deductibles can also reduce moral hazard by encouraging persons to be more careful with respect to the protection of their property and prevention of loss. Annual deductibles and waiting periods are the most common forms of deductibles in health insurance contracts.

Defined benefit. The amount, usually formula-based, guaranteed to each person who meets defined entitlement conditions. The formula usually takes into account the individual number of contribution or insurance years and the individual amount of earnings during the same period.

Delphi method or nominal group technique. A method of business forecasting that consists of panels of experts expressing their opinions on the future and then revising them in light of their colleagues' views so that bias and extreme opinions can be eliminated.

Demand. The amount of a good or service that consumers seek to buy at a given price. *Solvent demand* implies the ability to pay as well as the willingness to pay. *Elasticity of demand* is a measure of the responsiveness of total spending on a particular good or service to a change in its price. *Elastic demand* implies that as the price goes up the total expenditure falls. *Inelastic demand* implies that as the price goes up total expenditure also goes up. Necessities typically have inelastic demand (given an adequate income base). For example, the imperative to have an aching tooth removed means that the dentist is in a position of power to charge a high price; such dental services have inelastic demand and it is unlikely that a lower price would attract people not suffering from toothache to have a tooth removed. The concept of "necessity" and therefore of what has an inelastic demand is cultural. In some cultures prenatal care may not be considered a necessity. Demand for some procedures may be truncated in poor communities. *Truncated demand* means that although the demand for surgery (for example) is inelastic and does not change with price, above a certain price it becomes zero. As half an operation is not an option, the demand is truncated because of poverty.

Dual theory of risk. The theory that describes the attitudes of individuals toward insuring themselves, by weighing on the one hand their wealth and on the other hand their aversion to risk. Two possible modifications could swing the balance in favor of insurance: decreasing the premium, or increasing aversion to risk. Even with identical feelings toward monetary loss, individuals would likely adopt different attitudes toward insurance because their feeling is different toward the probability of monetary loss; the higher that assessment, the more attractive insurance is. Consequently, two individuals sharing the same utility index for certain wealth cannot have a different degree of aversion to risk (and the converse).

Endemic disease. A sickness habitually present in an area or population.

Epidemic. The occurrence of any disease, infectious or chronic, at a frequency greater than expected, based on prior patterns of disease incidence and prevalence.

Epidemiological transition. The changing pattern of health and disease within a specified population from a predominantly infectious disease pattern of low life expectancy and high mortality, to a predominantly chronic disease pattern of high life expectancy with high morbidity. In the intermediate stage of transition, high survival rates from endemic infectious disease combined with high rates of chronic illness in survivors results in a "double burden of disease." The latter is typical of many developing countries.

Epidemiology. The study of any and all health-related issues in specified populations at specified times, including but not limited to the occurrence and frequency of medical conditions, diseases, or other health-related events; identification of the determinants of medical conditions, diseases, health-related events, and health status; the evaluation of medical procedures and diagnostic tests; the evaluation of a health care system; the evaluation of a population's demand and use of health care services; evaluation of the safety and efficacy of a pharmaceutical product; post-market surveillance of pharmaceuticals to determine product effectiveness and occurrence of side effects or adverse events; and the evaluation of quality of life, access to care, and health status in general.

Equalization reserves. See Contingency reserves.

Escrow account management. Implies the use of a special account for managing payments of various obligations. For example, a savings account may be set up to establish funds for paying insurance premiums and loan repayments.

Estimation. The process by which sample data are used to indicate the value of an unknown quantity in a population. Results of estimation can be expressed as a single value, known as a point estimate, or a range of values, known as a confidence interval. The outcome of estimation is the *estimator.*

Excluded population or excluded communities. Typically agricultural, self-employed, or poor people who have neither formal employers nor steady wages as the basis for access to government-run or commercial health insurance. They may also be excluded from housing, education, disaster relief, and other social services. They may also be unable to access financial services or to secure formal recognition of property they control or own, including property obtained under traditional (tribal) law.

Experience rating. A system where the insurance company evaluates the risk of individuals or groups by examining their health history.

Externalities. Benefits or costs with an impact beyond the parties to a transaction. That impact is not considered in the buy/sell decision and so is not reflected in the price. Pollution is an example of an external cost; safe waste disposal has external benefits.

Fairness. See Ability to pay.

Fertility rate. A measure of the total number of live births in a specified population during a specific time period (generally one year) in relation to the midyear total number of women in the specified population. Expressed as the number of live births per 1,000 women within that population.

Fiduciary. A person who holds something in trust for another.

First-line insurer. See Insurer.

Formal sector. The part of the economy/society that is registered with authorities and that is subject to regulations and standards.

Free riding. Exists in health care when persons can benefit from a health care system without contributing to the system.

Gatekeeper. A primary care physician responsible for overseeing and coordinating all of a patient's medical needs. The gatekeeper must authorize any referral of the patient to a specialist or hospital. Except in cases of emergency, the authorization must be given prior to care.

Government failure. Occurs where government does not provide goods and services or an adequate regulatory or support framework for the private sector to provide them.

Gross domestic product (GDP). The annual total value of goods and services produced in a country for use in that country.

Imperfect competition. Occurs in markets or industries that do not match the criteria for perfect competition. The key characteristics of perfect competition are a large number of small firms; identical products sold by all firms; freedom of entry into and exit out of the industry; and perfect knowledge of prices and technology. These four criteria are essentially impossible to reach in the real world.

Income effect. A price reduction that gives buyers more real income, or greater purchasing power for their income, even though money or nominal income remains the same. This price reduction can cause changes in the quantity demanded of the good.

Independence. Two events are independent if the occurrence of one of the events gives no information about whether or not the other event will occur; that is, the events have no influence on each other. For example, falling ill with measles may be independent of being injured in a cyclone.

Induced demand. Demand created by physicians who face inelastic demand and so can set both the price and the level of care. This ability to determine their own income is difficult to control, and has great repercussion on health budgets.

Informal risk-protection mechanism. See Informal sector.

Informal sector. The part of the society/economy that is not registered with authorities and, whether with legal exclusion or without it (de jure or de facto), is not subject to public regulation and does not benefit from public services or goods. For example, support given by a family, friends, and members of a community in times of loss or illness effectively forms an informal risk-protection mechanism. Despite the presumption that such care is voluntarily given, in some cases (for example, providing care to foster children), payment may in fact be given.

Inpatient. Individual admitted to a hospital for health care and allocated a bed for the duration of that admission.

Insolvency. Inability to meet current expenses from current income plus reserves, leading, in the long run, to bankruptcy.

Institution. Social constructs that contain "rules of the games" and thereby both constrain behavior and enable behavior within those rules. By enabling the individual and organization to understand and predict behavior, the social constructs facilitate economic and social interaction. Institutions include regulations and policies of organizations and governments. They also include community-based traditional patterns of behavior and those that have developed in the face of modernization.

Insurability. A risk is insurable if it is random, and there is a party willing to accept the risk for an agreed premium and another party is prepared to pay that premium (this means it is solvable). This situation implies that the probability is known, it is free of moral hazard and adverse selection problems, that it is a legal proposition, and that the premium is affordable. Practical problems associated with information availability may render otherwise insurable risks uninsurable.

Insurance. Insurance is any activity in which a company assumes risk by taking payments (premiums) from individuals or companies and contractually agreeing to pay a stipulated benefit or compensation if certain contingencies (death, accident, illness) occur during a defined period.

Insurance threshold. Insurers typically request that the insured pay the first part of any claim. This cost sharing is a form of deductible, used to simplify administration by reducing the number of small claims.

Insured. Also called Principal; the end user contracting with an insurer for insurance coverage.

Insured unit. See Subscription unit.

Insurer (first-line, primary, or ultimate). The company that contracts with the end user for insurance. The first-line insurer may be the ceding insurer if it chooses to reinsure.

Internal rate of return. The discount rate that makes the net present value of an investment project equal to zero. This is a widely used method of investment appraisal as it takes into account the timing of cash flows.

Law of large numbers. The concept that the greater the number of exposures, the more closely will actual results approach the probable results expected from an infinite number of exposures.

Load. The cost of insurance (administration, finance, and so on) as distinct from payouts (benefits). Efficient companies have a low load relative to benefits

Local government unit (LGU). The term used in the Philippines to describe public authorities at lower-than-national levels (region, province, municipality, barangay).

Macroeconomic. Refers to factors that operate at the national and global level, for example, exchange rates, inflation rates, and interest rates. The origins of any factors operating at the local level are large scale. Macroeconomic shocks are changes in the large-scale factors that affect the economy and society.

Market failure. A condition in which a market does not efficiently allocate resources to achieve the greatest possible consumer satisfaction. The four main market failures are public good, market control, externality, and imperfect information. In each case, a market acting without any government-imposed direction does not direct an efficient amount of resources into the production, distribution, or consumption of the good.

Maximum likelihood estimator (MLE). Provides the best estimate of a population value that makes the sample data most likely. For example, given that a survey of 50 households in a community indicates that 5 percent of individuals have tuberculosis, what is the proportion of tuberculosis sufferers in the community that is most likely to have given rise to this statistic? The MLE techniques enable such calculation.

Mean. Average. It is equal to the sum of the observed values divided by the total number of observations.

Members. See Subscription unit.

Microfinance institution (MFI). Provides financial services to the poor on a sustained basis. The services include saving and credit societies, agricultural insurance, property insurance schemes and, more recently, health insurance schemes.

Microinsurance. A mechanism for pooling a whole community's risks and resources to protect all its participating members against the financial consequences of mutually determined health risks.

Microinsurance unit (MIU). A very small finance institution specifically designed to offer health insurance to the poor by pooling risks across a community.

Monte Carlo simulation. A statistical technique in which an uncertain value is calculated repeatedly using randomly selected "what-if" scenarios for each calculation. The simulation calculates hundreds and often thousands of scenarios of a model. Uncertain quantities in the model are replaced with fuzzy numbers to see how that uncertainty affects results. Ideally, the simulation aids in choosing the most attractive course of action, providing information about the range of outcomes such as best- and worst-case, and the probability of reaching specific targets.

Moral hazard. An insurance-prompted change in behavior that aggravates the probability of an event in order to access benefits, for example, an insured demanding tests not required on medical grounds. Provider-induced moral hazards include overservicing.

Morbidity. Refers to illness from a specified disease or cause or from all diseases. It is a change in health status from a state of well-being to disease occurrence and thereby a state of illness.

Mortality. Refers to death from a specified disease or cause or from all diseases.

Multilateral utility. See Utility.

Nominal group technique. See Delphi method.

Nongovernmental organization (NGO). Generally refers to a not-for-profit or community organization.

Normal distribution. Statistically speaking, values of events fall in a pattern around the average value with known frequencies. For instance, if the average stay in hospital after childbirth is three days, the values of each stay would be distributed around three, some more, some less, approximately symmetrically, with greater concentration around three than around any other number. The normal distribution is a particular distribution of this kind that is rigorously defined mathematically and gives the typical bell-shaped curve when graphed. This distribution is very powerful in enabling insurers to calculate costs and utilization.

Outlier. Denotes events that fall outside the norm. For example, in a "review of utilization" a provider who uses far fewer or far more services than the average is called an "outlier."

Outpatient. Person receiving health care in a hospital without admission to the hospital or accommodation in it. The length of stay is less than 24 hours. The care may be a consultation or a technical act (diagnosis or therapeutic procedure).

Pandemic. A disease that is prevalent throughout a locality or population.

Parameter. A number that describes a characteristic of a population. For example, the life expectancy of men in a community might be 56 years. Health insurance uses statistical techniques to estimate the parameter, and the estimation of the parameter is called the statistic. One sample of 50 men taken from the community might estimate the average age statistic to be 54 years while another sample might estimate it to be 57.5 years.

Pay-as-you-go. Refers to a system of insurance financing under which total expenditure (benefit expenditure plus administrative expenditure) in a given period is met by income (contributions and other sources) from the same period. Pay-as-you-go financed insurance schemes do not accumulate reserves, except contingency reserves; surpluses and deficits translate into increases or decreases in the premium.

Per-capita premium. The practice of applying a single premium per head across the population.

Point estimation. An estimate of a parameter of a population that is given by one number.

Poisson distribution. Typically, a Poisson random variable is a count of the number of events that occur in a certain time interval or spatial area. For example, the number of people seeking critical care for malaria in a wet season month in a particular village. The Poisson distribution can sometimes be used to approximate the binomial distribution when the number of observations is large and the probability of success is small (that is, a fairly rare event). This is useful since the computations involved in calculating binomial probabilities are greatly reduced.

Population density. A measure of the size of the population in comparison to the size of a specified geographic area (region, country, province, city). Typically, it is a count of the number of residents per square kilometer.

Preferred risk selection. See Cream skimming.

Premium. Fee paid by an insured to an insurance company in return for specified benefits. Under social insurance the premium is called contribution. See also Contribution.

Prevalence. The total number of cases or people who have a specified disease, health condition, attribute, or risk factor within a specified population at a specific point in time.

Preventive health care. Medical care directed primarily toward early detection and treatment or prevention of disease or ill health (for example, immunizations, prenatal care).

Primary health care. The first level of contact by individuals, families, and communities with the health system, bringing health care as close as possible to where people work and live. The organization of primary health care depends upon the socioeconomic and political characteristics of the country, but should address prevention, curative, and rehabilitation services and include education of the population about major health problems and their prevention and control. Such care may be provided by a variety of health workers, acting together as a team, in partnership with the local community.

Primary insurer. See Insurer.

Principal. Denotes the client, in the relationship between an insurer (agent) and the insured (principal) See Insured.

Probability. A quantitative description of the likely occurrence of a particular event. Probability is conventionally expressed on a scale from 0 to 1; a rare event has a probability close to 0, a very common event has a probability close to 1.

Probability distribution. The probability distribution of a discrete random variable is a list of probabilities associated with each of its possible values. It is also sometimes called the probability function or the probability mass function. For example, the probability of a woman's delivering a single live baby might be 98 percent, twins 1.78 percent, triplets 0.218 percent, more than triplets 0.002 percent.

Providers. Doctors, nurses, hospitals, clinics, laboratories, imaging facilities, pharmacies, and other deliverers of medical services. The insurer or regulating body typically requires that a provider be qualified and/or registered in order to be included in a health insurance scheme.

Public goods. There are two aspects to public goods: it is difficult to prevent nonpayers from consuming them (nonexcludable), and their consumption by one party does not affect their consumption by others (nonrival). Vaccination is an example— those who do not pay and are not vaccinated cannot be excluded from enjoying the lower prevalence of disease; and the fact that they are healthy as a result does not affect another's ability to be healthier as a result of the program. Government usually provides public goods, because private businesses do so profitably.

Pure premium. The pure premium can be defined as the average loss per exposure unit for a specific coverage or, more specifically, the product of the average severity and the average frequency of loss. The result is the amount, which the insurance company should collect to cover all the losses to be met under the predefined types of coverage.

Qualifying conditions. Requirements for acceptance into an insurance plan; also describes the provisions that must be met before a benefit is payable.

Random variable. A function that provides a single numerical value to a particular event or outcome. The value of the random variable will vary from trial to trial as the experiment is repeated. For example, if 10 people visit a hospital as outpatients in a morning, and 7 of them have injuries rather than disease, the random variable for that event is 0.7. Another example: if the life span of a particular baby born 10 weeks premature in a community is 2 days, 4 hours, and 7 minutes, the random variable of that event is that duration.

Rating. See Risk rating

Recovery gap. An excess of benefit payouts over income, when the *compliance gap* is assumed to be zero. The recovery gap is not random and so cannot be solved by reinsurance.

Reinsurance. The transfer of liability from the primary insurer, the company that issued the contract, to another insurer, the reinsurance company. This mechanism allows a diversification of the risk and enlarges the risk-pooling base, thereby reducing the risk of insolvency. However, reinsurance extends only to risk defined in the cession contract (called Treaty). For example, a treaty to cede fluctuations in payouts will not cover the primary insurer against the financial risk of insolvency, for example, because of poorly run or unviable insurance.

Reinsurance premium. The amount charged by the reinsurer to accept an agreed amount of risk.

Reinsurance threshold. Reinsurers typically require that the insurer retains the first proportion of risk for any event. That proportion is the threshold as it is equivalent to the deductible or excess borne by the insured when making a claim against property insurance.

Reserves. Funds held either for a possible but unknown event (contingency funds) or because of regulation. A major financial management goal is to minimize reserves and thus maximize funds available for current use.

Reciprocating arrangements. Agreements existing between primary insurers to co-insure, the objective being to stabilize funds. These arrangements are sometimes considered an alternative to reinsurance, in that they enlarge the pool and reduce risk variance.

Retrocession. See Cession.

Risk. The probability or likelihood that a specified health event (for example, the occurrence of a disease or death) will occur to an individual or population group within a specific period of time.

Risk factor. An attribute (for example, a lifestyle factor or a personal characteristic) or an exposure to an environmental factor associated with an increase in the probability that a specified health event (for example, onset of disease) will occur.

Risk pooling. The process by which fluctuations in risk are reduced by averaging the risk over large numbers and heterogeneous memberships. Insurers risk pool through reinsurance.

Risk rating. Calculation of health insurance premiums based on the risk of each client. When the premium is calculated based on the risk not of a single individual but of a group, this is called *community rating* or *group rating*. When the premium is set in relation to the client's income, this is called *income rating*.

Risk segregation. Each individual faces his or her own risks without pooling.

Risk sharing. Individuals agree to split the cost of risky events. Insurers share risk through reciprocal relationships and reinsurance. Loan guarantees and insurance are among the many ways of sharing risks.

Safety coefficient. A measure of the difference between the expected annual result of an insurance scheme and the worst possible loss that can be borne. Information on the safety coefficient enables management to make better decisions about re-serve levels.

Self-insurance or self-protection. Refers to all the arrangements made by an individual or group to protect themselves from risk. It includes not only saving and establishing contingency reserves but also changing behavior to diminish or avoid risk.

Simulation. The technique of imitating behavior and events during an experimental process. Typically involves a computer.

Social capital. Refers to the multidimensional "glue" that binds community members together. While concepts of social capital vary from culture to culture, Putnam (1993) defined it as including trust, community involvement, tolerance of diversity, value of life, and extent of connectivity (socially and professionally).

Social exclusion. Inadequate or unequal participation in social life, or exclusion from a place in the consumer society, often linked to the social role of employment or work.

Social insurance. An insurance program that is shaped by broader social objectives than just by self-interest of each individual principal or agent, while retaining insurance principles that persons are insured against a definite risk.

Social protection. Policies and programs designed to reduce poverty and financial vulnerability. Social protection policies typically focus on labor market policies, social insurance, social assistance, community-based schemes, and child protection.

Social Re *data template.* See Data template.

Social reinsurance, Reinsurance undertaken in pursuit of social goals rather than profit.

Social utility. The gain to society from, in this case, insurance. Where insurance has zero or negative social utility it may be banned; where it has high social utility but low private utility it may be mandated. The choice of rendering a public utility mandatory or not depends on political will or the power of authorities, including community leaders.

Soft budget. A budget with a flexible limit.

Solidarity principle. Applying rules that spread risks and resources across members of a group in a way that provides both insurance coverage and egalitarian distribution. *Risk solidarity* would imply that high-risk individuals receive a subsidy from low-risk individuals, allowing all risk levels an equal access to health care coverage. Solidarity between high- and low-income individuals, or "*income solidarity,*" implies income redistribution through organized transfers. In insurance, the solidarity principle is juxtaposed to the *equivalence principle*, which implies that the insurer has to break even on each insurance contract, by applying *risk rating*.

Solvable. An insurance transaction is said to be solvable if the risk is observable; there is no antiselection (adverse selection), and the premium is acceptable to both parties.

Solvent demand. See Demand.

Spot market transaction. The "spot market" implies transactions for immediate delivery of services as distinct from the insurance requirement of prepayment against (possible) future delivery of services. Populations that are excluded from health insurance rely on spot payments to access health care.

Standard deviation. A statistical term for a measure of the variability in a population or sample.

Subscription unit. Refers to the people covered by a single membership. This may be the individual (usually in developed economies) or the household (usually in developing economies).

Target group. Refers to both current and future beneficiaries of the insurance system. The target group can comprise several subgroups of people with similar characteristics (for example, income, economic sector). *Social Re's* target population is the microinsurers that serve communities excluded from other health insurance programs (not just current members, but all members of the community).

Toolkit. The Toolkit simulates the workings of a system in which several microinsurers are reinsured by *Social Re.* Varying key elements in this system allow comparison of outcomes.

Top-down global strategy. Implies that a public policy, for instance the approach to improving access to health care or health insurance, was directed by a powerful global body to national governments and down through the rank and file to the community. This contrasts with the "bottom-up" approach based on the empowerment of communities.

Transaction costs. The costs additional to the price of a good or service, arising, for example, from search costs, travel costs, marketing and distribution, or transfer of ownership costs.

Ultimate insurer. See insurer.

Underwriter. A company that receives the premiums and accepts responsibility for the fulfillment of the policy contract; the company employee who decides whether or not the company should assume a particular risk; the agent who sells the policy.

Underwriting. The process by which the insurer decides what risks to cover. The profit objectives may conflict with social obligation. For the reinsurer, underwriting considerations determine the risks of the primary insurer that can be accepted for reinsurance, and which the insurer will retain.

Underwriting assistance. Reinsurance companies gather extensive data on the insured and events. They can share this information with insurers to improve the performance of insurers.

Unilateral utility. See Utility.

Uninsurable. See Insurability.

Unit cost. The average cost of particular health care treatments. These costs are negotiated between a microinsurance unit and providers. Insurance enables a move away from fee-for-service toward averaging out-of-unit costs.

Universal coverage. Implies that all members of a country (or a community) have health insurance.

User fees. Charges payable by users, usually at the point of service. See Spot market transaction.

Utility. The satisfaction gained from having the desire for goods and services met. Multilateral utility means that several parties benefit from outcomes. These parties can be a group of insureds or the insurer and the insured. Unilateral utility means that only one party gains. The balance between group and individual utility is a delicate component of relations within a community, between insurer/insured, or between insurer/reinsurer.

Utilization. Refers to utilization patterns of medical services in a location over a period. Data on recent utilization, collected at the national and community levels, is a valuable asset in predicting future patterns.

Variation coefficient. See Coefficient of variation.

Vector-borne infectious disease. Infections caused by human contact with an infectious agent, transmitted from an infected individual by an insect or other live carrier. For example, malaria is biologically transmitted from an infected individual to a noninfected person by the same mosquito (the vector) biting both people.

Working capital. Current assets minus current liabilities. It is the capital available for an organization's short-term financing.

Willingness to pay (WTP). See Ability to pay.

GLOSSARY OF TERMS, *DATA TEMPLATE*

Member Details

Dependent(s). Every person who is covered by virtue of payments made by one *paying member.* The record of every dependent must identify the paying member she or he depends on.

ID number. The unique identification number of every member (both paying member and dependent). The ID number is composed of ISO country code (3 position, alphanumeric) + region code (3 digits) + MIU code (3 digits) + family code (5 digits) + individual code (2 digits).

Paying member. A person paying the *contribution due*. According to the *contribution plan*, a paying member may also cover other members of the family as his/her *dependents*. The record of every paying member must identify all his/her dependents.

Contributions

Compliance rate. The *actual contribution paid* divided by the *contribution due*. Compliance rate can be calculated on a monthly basis, or for the current financial period, or on a rolling 12-month period. It can also be calculated for a single individual, a single microinsurer, or for the entire pool of reinsured microinsurers.

Contribution plan. A set of contribution rates that determines the price of being insured.

Contribution due. The price an individual must pay the microinsurer for a *benefit package* during a *financial period*, according to the applicable *contribution plan*.

Contributions due, total. The amount the microinsurer expects to collect from its members during a *financial period*, according to the applicable *contribution plans*.

Contribution paid, actual. Actual contributions are estimated as the product of potential contributions multiplied by the compliance rate. The amount an individual in fact pays the microinsurer during a defined *financial period*.

Contribution paid, total actual. The amount all members in fact pay the microinsurer during a defined *financial period*.

Prorated affiliation. Membership for part of the *financial period*, expressed as a percentage of the full period. Prorated affiliation could entail eligibility to a prorated portion of certain *benefits paid by the microinsurer*.

Benefits

Benefit cost, expected. The estimated amount payable by a specific MIU to one member for one claim.

Benefit cost, total expected. The cumulative amount of *expected benefit costs* payable by a specific MIU to all members during one *financial period*.

Benefit cost, observed. The amount paid by a specific microinsurer to a specific individual for a specific *claim*.

Benefit cost, total observed. The cumulative amount of *observed benefit cost* for all *claims* of all members during the current *financial period*.

Benefit package. A set of *benefit types*.

Benefit type. A definition of the microinsurer's responsibility for each cost-generating event. The characteristics of this responsibility include the maximum number of occurrences, maximum amount per occurrence, a *deductible*, the rate (or amount) of *copay*.

Claim. The bill presented to the microinsurer (by the member) for one *cost-generating event*.

Copay. The part of the cost of a *claim* payable by the member, as defined in the *benefit package*.

Cost-generating event (CGE). An event requiring medical attention for which the provider presents a bill.

Deductible. An amount payable by the member before the microinsurer pays *benefits*, defined in the *benefit package*.

Cost of care, observed. The sum of the *observed benefit cost* plus the amount paid by the member as *out-of-pocket*, for a specific *claim*.

Cost of care, total observed. The cumulative sum of the *observed cost of care* for all *claims* in the *financial period*.

Out-of-pocket. The part of a *claim* paid by a member, composed of *deductible* amounts, plus *copay*, plus the services that are not covered under the *benefit package*, plus the *contribution due* for insurance.

Reinsurance

Administrative costs. Costs of operating the microinsurance or the reinsurance that are neither the *total cost of care* nor the total amount paid by the reinsurer.

Amount paid by reinsurer. The amount paid by the reinsurer to a specific microinsurer.

Amount, total paid by reinsurer. The cumulative *amount paid by the reinsurer* to all client microinsurers during the current *financial period*.

Claims. The costs presented by the microinsurer for payment by the reinsurer, as defined in the reinsurance treaty.

Discretionary budget. A saving constituted when *the observed total benefit cost* is lower than the *reinsurance threshold*. The microinsurer can use this amount at the end of the *financial period*.

Financial period. The period used for the accounting, usually the calendar year.

Income, microinsurer's. The sum of the t*otal actual contribution paid* plus *subsidies* and any *other income* recorded by the microinsurer.

Income, microinsurer's other. Income recorded by the microinsurer that is neither contribution income nor subsidies (for example, interest on surplus).

Loss ratio. The ratio of incurred claims to collected premium.

Premium. The price of reinsurance, paid by the microinsurer to the reinsurer.

Reinsurance threshold. An amount that the microinsurer is responsible for paying out of its own means, before the reinsurer agrees to pay.

Reserves. The sum of the *reinsurance threshold* plus the *premium.* The microinsurer must have this amount at the beginning of each *financial period* to ensure its solvency.

Subsidies. Payments made to the microinsurer intended as compensation for specific financial commitments (for example, to compensate it for setting *contributions due* below break-even level), or to fund a specific enhancement of benefits (for example, micronutrient supplementation), or to support certain noncore activities (for example, training).

SOURCES

This glossary was compiled from the works in this book and the following sources.

Amos Web-Economic Gloss Arama. 2001. http://www.amosweb.com/ (cited May 2002).

Canadian Institute of Actuaries. n.d. "Lexicon, English-French, French-English." http://www.actuaries.ca/publications/other_lexicon_e.html (cited May 2002).

Cichon, M., W. Newbrander, H. Yamabana, A. Weber, C. Normand, D. Dror, and A. Preker. 1999. *Modelling in Health Care Finance: A Compendium of Quantitative Techniques for Health Care Financing.* Geneva: International Labour Organisation and International Social Security Association.

Cyert, R.M. 1987. *Bayesian Analysis and Uncertainty in Economic Theory.* Totowa, N.J.: Rowman and Littlefield.

Dror, D.M., and G. Duru. 2000. "Financing Micro-insurance: Perspective and Prospective." Proceedings (vol. I) of the 7th International Conference on System Science in Health Care. Organized by International Systems Sciences Congress in Health Care & Semmelweis University, Budapest, May 29–June 2, 2000.

Easton, V., and J. McColl. 2001. "Statistics Glossary." http://www.stats.gla.ac.uk/steps/glossary/index.html (cited May 2002).

European Commission. 1996. *Glossary of Public Health Technical Terms.* EU Commission, Brussels.

ILO Recommendation 127 on Cooperatives of the International Labour Organisation.

ILO-STEP (International Labour Organisation/Strategies and Tools against Social Exclusion and Poverty). 2000. *Methodological Guide for Undertaking Case Studies/Health Microinsurance Schemes.* Geneva, ISBN 92-2-112317-0, 89 pp.

Nielson, N. 2001. "Glossary of Insurance and Financial Planning Terms." http://www.ucalgary.ca/MG/inrm/glossary/gloss-c.htm (cited May 2002).

North, D.C. 1991. *Institutions, Institutional Change and Economic Performance.* Cambridge, Mass.: Cambridge University Press.

OECD (Organisation for Economic Co-operation and Development). 1999. *Glossary of Insurance Policy Terms*. Paris: OECD.

Outreville, J.F. 1998. *Theory and Practice of Insurance*. Boston: Kluwer Academic Publishers.

Putnam, R., R. Leonadi, and R. Nanetti. 1993. *Making Democracy Work: Civil Traditions in Modern Italy*. Princeton, N.J.: Princeton University Press.

Rochaix, L. 1995. "La fonction de demande de soins ou l'Arlésienne du marché." *Risques* 21:69–85.

Ron, A., and A. Kupferman. 1996. "A Community Health Insurance Scheme in the Philippines: Extension of a Community Based Integrated Project." Macroeconomics, Health and Development Series. Geneva: World Health Organization.

Rutherford, D. 1992. *Dictionary of Economics*. London: Routledge.

Scholz, W., M. Cichon, and K. Hagemejer. 2000. *Social Budgeting*. Quantitative Methods in Social Protection Series. Geneva: International Labour Organization and International Social Security Association.

Statistics Glossary. http://www.stats.gla.ac.uk/steps/glossary/probability.html#indepevents (cited May 2002).

Tonglet, R. 1994–95. *Syllabus d'épidémiologie*. Ecole de Santé Publique UCL.

Trojan, A. 1998. Bürgerbeteiligung - Die 12 stufige Leiter der Beteiligung von Bürgern an lokalen Entscheidungsprozessen; BZgA 1996, Leitbegriffe der Gesundheitsförderung - Glossar zu Konzepten, Strategien und Methoden der Gesundheitsförderung.

World Health Organization. 1978. *Primary Health Care*. Report of the International Conference on Primary Health Care, Alma-Ata, September 6–12, 1978. Geneva: WHO ("The Alma Ata Declaration").

_____. 1994. *Terminology for the European Health Policy Conference*. Copenhagen.

About the Coeditors and Contributors

THE COEDITORS

David M. Dror is a senior health insurance specialist, International Labour Office, Geneva. Since the mid-1970s, he has been involved in social security issues, first at the national level, then internationally, in various roles in the ILO. He has specialized in health insurance since 1988, both as a practitioner, responsible for managing a health insurance plan, and as a consultant and expert. Since 2000, he has served as the leader/manager of the *Social Re* project. He is the author of numerous reports, studies, and journal articles. Mr. Dror studied in Israel, the United States, Switzerland, the United Kingdom, and France. He holds a Ph.D. from University of Lyon 1 Claude Bernard, France, in economics, and D.B.A., M.B.A., and B.A. degrees in international health services, business administration, and liberal arts, (plus an academic teaching diploma).

Alexander S. Preker is chief economist for Health, Nutrition, and Population and editor of the HNP Publication Series, the World Bank, Washington, D.C. In this capacity, he oversees the World Bank's analytical work on health financing and delivery. He coordinated the team that prepared the World Bank's 1997 Sector Strategy on health care in developing countries, was one of the authors of the *World Health Report 2000* on Health Systems, and is currently a member of the Commission on Macroeconomics and Health. He has published and taught extensively on topics related to health systems development, is on the editorial committee of several journals, and is a frequent speaker at major international conferences. He has an appointment as Adjunct Associate Professor at The George Washington University. His training includes a Ph.D. in economics from the London School of Economics and Political Science, a fellowship in medicine from University College London, a diploma in medical law and ethics from King's College London, and an M.D. from the University of British Columbia/McGill.

THE CONTRIBUTORS

Erwin Alampay is an associate, Institute of Public Health Management, and a professor at the National College of Public Administration and Governance of the

University of the Philippines. Prior to joining the government, he was involved in operations management in a number of Philippine companies. He has written many papers on volunteer management, identification of indigents for social health insurance, and e-governance. He obtained his bachelor's degree in industrial engineering and master's in public administration at the University of the Philippines at Diliman, and his master's in the politics of alternative development strategies at the Institute of Social Studies, The Hague, Netherlands.

J.P. Auray is director of research, Centre National de la Recherche Scientifique, and director of the Laboratoire d'Analyse des Systèmes de Santé, UMR-5823 of CNRS, a laboratory on decisionmaking in health systems. He holds a doctorate in applied mathematics from the University of Lyon 1 Claude Bernard, France.

Bernd Balkenhol heads the Social Finance Programme, International Labour Office, Geneva, which explores the use of financial instruments and institutions for social objectives. From 1986 to 1990, Mr. Balkenhol served as expert to the Central Bank of West African States in Dakar, advising this institution on policies to promote small and medium enterprise finance by banks and other financial institutions. For two years he also worked in an ILO program on employment policies, based in Ethiopia. His publications deal with credit unions, informal finance, and financial-sector policies. Mr. Balkenhol is an economist with a Ph.D. from Freiburg University and an M.A. from the Fletcher School of Law and Diplomacy.

Yolanda Bayugo, M.D., is an associate, Institute of Public Health Management, and a consultant on provincial health systems in Cambodia. She has served as a municipal health officer and has worked with indigenous people for a nongovernmental organization in the Philippines. During that period, she started up a social health insurance program for women health workers. She studied anthropology at the University of the Philippines and obtained a master's degree in public health at Heidelberg University, Germany.

Sara Bennett is senior research adviser, Partners for Health Reform Plus project, and a lecturer on the Health Economics and Financing Programme, London School of Hygiene and Tropical Medicine. She has worked on health insurance issues, including microinsurance, in Georgia, Thailand, and Zambia and has published widely on health care financing and health policy in developing countries.

Stéphane Bonnevay is a research fellow, University of Lyon 1 Claude Bernard, MA2D Group, Laboratoire d'Analyse des Systèmes de Santé. He holds a doctorate in computer science from the University of Lyon 1 Claude Bernard, France. His thesis deals with texture analysis in images. Actually, he works on processes of decisionmaking, knowledge extraction, knowledge representation, knowledge structure, and data fusion. (Web site: http://lass.univ-lyon1.fr/membres/bonnevay/)

Logan Brenzel is senior program associate/health economist, MSH. She has nearly 15 years of experience in designing and implementing health financing and health reform research and activities in developing countries. She is currently responsible for the Latin American and Caribbean Health Sector Reform Initiative as senior health economist, Health and Child Survival Fellows Program, U.S. Agency for International Development. Ms. Brenzel has a doctoral degree in health economics from the Johns Hopkins University School of Public Health and a master's degree in health policy and management from the Harvard School of Public Health.

Reinhard Busse, M.D., M.P.H., is professor and department head for health care management at Technische Universität Berlin. He pursues research in three areas: analysis of European health systems, health technology assessment, and hospital management with particular emphasis on health outcomes. Until April 2002, he was head of the Madrid hub of the European Observatory on Health Care Systems, for which he is now an associate research director, supervising the "Health Care Systems in Transition" profiles of the central European countries and co-directing the study on "Social Health Insurance Countries in Western Europe."

Craig Churchill is with the Social Finance Programme, International Labour Office, Geneva. Before joining the ILO, Mr. Churchill served as director of research and policy at Calmeadow, a Canadian microfinance nongovernmental organization. His decade of microfinance experience also includes stints with ACCION International, the MicroFinance Network, and the Get Ahead Foundation in South Africa. In addition to serving as the editor of the *MicroBanking Bulletin* and on the editorial board of the *Journal of Microfinance*, he has published more than 20 articles, working papers, and technical guides on the subject.

Gérard Duru is professor of mathematics and econometrics at Claude Bernard Lyon I University. He also is president of the scientific committee of the Groupement Scientifique Santé, GDR 875 (CNRS, Hospice Civils de Lyon, Université Lyon 1, Lyon 3, Aix Marseille 2, Toulouse 3, Rennes 1), and the group's director of doctoral studies in analytical methods of health systems (Méthode d'Analyse des Systèmes de Santé) at Lyon 1, Lyon 3, Aix Marseille 2, Toulouse 3, and Rennes 1 universities. Professor Duru is the president of the International Society For System Sciences in Health Care, past president of the Société Internationale de Démographie d'Economie et de Sociologie Médicale, vice president of the French Collège des Economistes de la Santé, and head of the health section of the Applied Econometrics Association. He has many years' experience as consultant, notably to the Council of Europe and several government agencies in France. He is chief editor of *Health and System Science* (Editions Hermes - Paris - London) and a member of the editorial board of *Journal d'Economie Médicale*. Professor Duru holds a degree of Docteur en Mathématiques (3ème cycle) and of Docteur ès Sciences (Mathématiques) and has been awarded the Chevalier des Palmes Académiques distinction.

Frank G. Feeley is a clinical associate professor, University of Boston School of Pubic Health, and teaches classes in health regulation and financing and comparative health systems. He worked for five years in the Commonwealth of Massachusetts in the Medicaid program and as assistant commissioner for regulation in the Department of Public Health. In the past decade, he has served as an adviser to the American Psychiatric Association on its sponsored insurance programs and has worked in many countries, most recently as director of a project, funded by the U.S. Agency for International Development, to provide technical assistance in the reform of health law and regulation in the Russian Federation.

Jonathan Flavier, M.D., has been a specialist in community-based health for the last 13 years. Over this time, he has been learning with and from people in mostly rural communities as a rural health physician of the Department of Health, as an employee of the Philippine Rural Reconstruction Movement; and from work with international development agencies like the GTZ-SHINE, the John Snow Inc. Research and Training Institute, and EngenderHealth. He is an expert not only because of his education but also because of his broad experience from his associations with people in his health and development work.

Robert Fonteneau is a senior specialist, Caisse Nationale d'Assurance Maladie, Paris, detailed to the Social Protection Sector, International Labour Office. He was co-founder of the French College of Health Economists (CES).

Donato J. Gasparro is president of NiiS/APEX Consulting Group, N.J. He is a recognized leader in the health care arena, with more than 21 years of experience in the health care actuarial and underwriting business. Mr. Gasparro leads his company's effort in strategic planning, underwriting, audit, and actuarial consulting to the senior management of the firm's clients. His clients include domestic and foreign entities that assume financial and/or actuarial risk such as insurance and reinsurance companies, provider-sponsored health plans, MGUs, employers, and government agencies.

George Gotsadze, M.D., is director, Curatio International Foundation, Tbilisi, Georgia. He has worked in various countries in the Caucasus, Asia, and Africa. Since 1996, he has been actively involved with health-sector reforms in the Caucasus region. He has acted as consultant to various municipalities, NGOs, and multilateral agencies, and has published a number of papers on health care financing and community health insurance.

Jeannie Haggerty, is a public health researcher and professor in the Départements de Médecine familiale and Médecine sociale et préventive at the Université de Montréal in Canada. Her domain of research relates to accessibility and quality of primary care both in Canada and in developing countries, particularly assessing the impact of clinical and health system policies and reforms. She has extensive experience using administrative billing data for profiling the practice of health care providers and for surveillance of quality of care. She holds a Ph.D. in epidemiology and biostatistics.

Melitta Jakab was a researcher, Human Development Network, the World Bank, Washington, D.C., while working on the *Social Re* project. Currently she is completing a Ph.D. degree in health economics at Harvard University. Prior to her assignment to the Human Development Network, she had worked in the Bank's Resident Mission in Hungary as a research and operations assistant. She has an M.A. in health policy and management from the Harvard School of Public Health and a bachelor's degree in economics and political science from McGill University.

Avi Kupferman, has more than 35 years of managerial and consulting experience in establishing and operating companies in developing countries. From 1993 on, he drew on this experience first as country director, then as regional director, of ORT–Asia, a branch of the World ORT Union, an international nongovernmental organization based in London. His work entailed development of community-based health insurance schemes in various locations in the Philippines, including rural communities and urban squatter populations. Mr. Kupferman holds bachelor degrees in business administration and electronics from New York University, New York.

Michel Lamure is a professor of computer sciences (informatics) and applied mathematics, University of Lyon 1 Claude Bernard, France. He is the head of the Methods and Algorithms for Aided Decision Making group, Laboratory for the Analysis of Health Systems (LASS), National Scientific Research Council (UMR 5823, CNRS), France. From 1992 to 1995, he was vice chairman of the Computer Sciences section of the National Council of French Universities. From 1996 to 1998, he was chairman of the Computer Sciences section of the National Council of French Universities; pedagogical councilor for Mathematics and Computer Sciences at the French Ministry for Education and Research; general secretary of the International Society for Systems Science in Health Care, and chief editor of *Revue Santé et Systémique* (Hermès, Paris). He is a specialist in computer-aided decision methods. His work entails analysis of the whole process of decisionmaking, from data collection to decision, including knowledge extraction and representation and preferences aggregation.

Jack Langenbrunner is a senior economist, the World Bank, Washington, D.C. His focus at the Bank is on national health accounts and health financing and, in operations, on Eastern Europe and former Soviet Union Republics. He served on the Clinton White House Task Force on Health Reform. He holds a master's degree and a doctorate in economics and public health from the University of Michigan, Ann Arbor.

William Newbrander is director, MSH's Center for Health Reform and Financing. A health economist and hospital administrator, Mr. Newbrander joined MSH in

1992 after having served with the World Health Organization for eight years in Papua New Guinea, Thailand, and Switzerland. He had previously managed hospitals in the United States and Saudi Arabia. Today, in addition to managing the Center for Health Reform and Financing, he provides technical assistance for MSH in health reform and health policy, social health insurance, issues on equity and the poor, hospital management, and decentralization. His numerous publications reflect his work in health reform and issues of equity. He holds master's degrees in hospital administration and in economics as well as a Ph.D. in health economics from the University of Michigan.

Anne Nicolay is the adviser of the GTZ-supported "Social Health Insurance" component (formerly the SHINE Project, Social Health Insurance—Networking and Empowerment) of the German Support to the Philippine Health Sector. As a health economist, she has worked over the past 12 years in African, Caribbean, and Asian countries on health care financing issues, from the district to the national level, notably in projects funded by the European Union, the Inter-American Development Bank, and German Technical Cooperation.

J. François Outreville is executive secretary, United Nations Staff Mutual Insurance Society, Geneva. He was previously economic affairs officer with the United Nations Conference on Trade and Development (UNCTAD) and Associate Professor of Finance and Insurance at Laval University, Quebec. He has also been visiting professor at McGill University, the University of Texas at Austin, the National University of Singapore, and Nijenrode University in the Netherlands. He is a member of the American Risk and Insurance Association and the Academy of International Business and an Associate Editor of the *Geneva Papers on Risk and Insurance* and the *Journal of Actuarial Practice*. He has published numerous articles in economics and insurance journals.

M. Kent Ranson, M.D., Ph.D., currently works as a research consultant at SEWA Social Security in Ahmedabad, Gujarat. He received his M.D. from McMaster University, a master's in public health from Harvard University, and a Ph.D. from the Health Policy Unit, London School of Hygiene and Tropical Medicine. His current research aims to assess the impact of SEWA's social security scheme and to identify ways in which it can be improved. Dr. Ranson's previous research looked into the cost-effectiveness of interventions for trachomatous visual impairment (Harvard Center for Population and Development Studies), and for tobacco use and malaria in India (the World Bank).

Rakesh Rathi is IT Systems Manager, World Health Organization, Geneva. Mr. Rathi has worked extensively on strategy, planning, and management, IT coordination and analysis, web and Internet services, application development, end user computing, and server administration with international organizations in Geneva, including United Nations Volunteers and the International Labour Office, in addition to the WHO. He holds a bachelor of engineering in computer science.

Tracey Reid has 11 years of epidemiological research experience, primarily in the areas of health services utilization, quality of care and physician prescribing and practice behavior. Ms. Reid has focused on data management and analysis as well as writing and editing study reports, manuals, and journal manuscripts. She holds an MSc from the Department of Epidemiology and Biostatistics, McGill University and a B.A. in history from Concordia University.

Aviva Ron is director, Health Sector Development, World Health Organization, Western Pacific Regional Office, Manila, and previously worked with the WHO International Cooperation Office, Geneva, mainly providing technical support to developing countries in health care financing. As a consultant to the International Labour Organisation, her major project was the development of the social security system for Thailand. Later, as a social security specialist, Ms. Ron was a member of ILO's South-East Asia and Pacific Multidisciplinary Advisory Team (SEAPAT), based in Manila. She is the author and editor of several books, chapters in books, and numerous other publications in health services systems development and social health insurance. Ms. Ron obtained master's and doctor of science degrees from the School of Hygiene and Public Health, the Johns Hopkins University, Baltimore, Maryland, where she served on the faculty of the Department of Medical Care and Hospitals.

Elmer S. Soriano, M.D., is executive director, Institute of Public Health Management. Dr. Soriano has served as senior research associate at the Asian Institute of Management, lecturer at the Ateneo de Manila, and manager of a cooperative health financing program in the Philippines. He has acted as consultant to various municipalities, nongovernmental organizations, and cooperatives and has published a number of papers on health care financing, social health insurance, and health and governance. He obtained his master's degree in development management from the Asian Institute of Management.

Katherine Snowden is senior consultant, Third Sector New England. She has been a consultant to nonprofit and public sector organizations for more than 20 years, including 10 years as an economist and senior consultant with Arthur D. Little, Cambridge, Mass. Her areas of special knowledge include financial analysis, budget projections, business plan development, institutional strategic planning, market assessment, and strategy formulation. She has worked for nonprofit organizations, private schools, and government agencies.

Michel Vaté is professor of economics, IEP Lyon, Université Lumière Lyon 2, France. He holds a doctorate in economics, and postgraduate degrees in business administration and political science. He has taught and written on risk analysis, forecasting, and decisionmaking. He has been the dean of the faculty of economics at University of Lyon 2, France.

Axel Weber holds a Ph.D. in social economy and has been an independent consultant in health insurance and social protection in Africa, Latin America, Asia, Eastern Europe, and Central Asia. He did feasibility studies on community-based health insurance in Africa and Asia. He has worked for International Labour Office as a consultant in the fields of actuarial studies, health insurance feasibility studies, social protection strategies, and social budgeting. He recently joined the Asian Development Bank as a social protection specialist. He has worked in the German Ministry of Labor, in the Federation of German Regional Health Insurance Funds (AOK) in the planning department, and in the European Commission, Brussels, in the section dealing with social economy (mutuals, associations, cooperatives, foundations). He is author of articles and books about social protection and health insurance, including the guidelines for planning social health insurance published by ILO and WHO in 1994.

Hiroshi Yamabana is an actuary in the Financial, Actuarial and Statistical Services Branch, International Labour Office, Geneva. He is currently working on actuarial valuations of the ILO member countries and the development and training of actuarial methodologies and techniques in social security. Before joining the ILO, he worked as an actuary for the Japanese Ministry of Health and Welfare. His experience at the ministry included actuarial planning in Japan's pension and health insurance schemes. He holds a master's degree in mathematics from Kyoto University, Japan.

Index